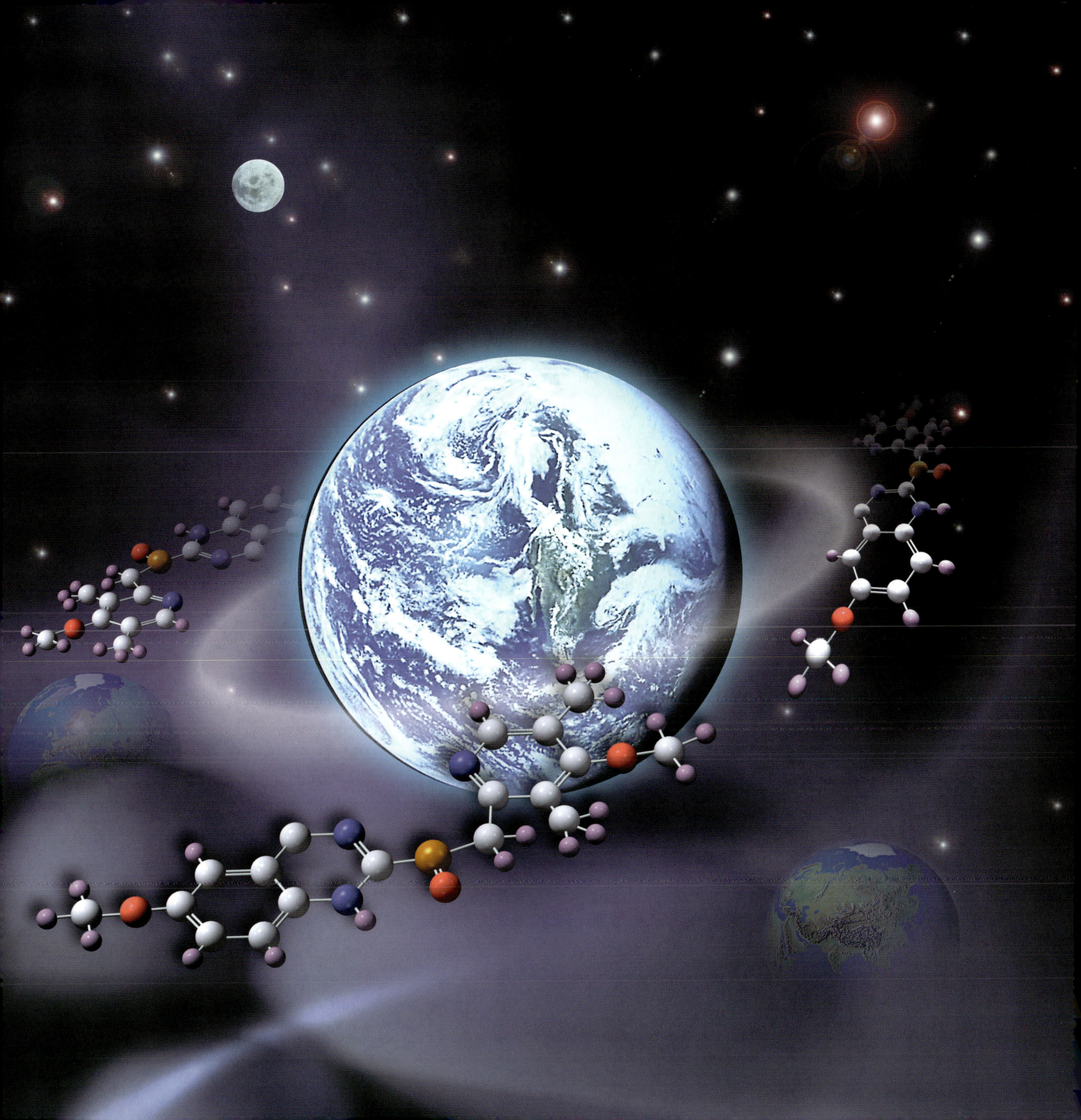

Irvin M. Modlin, MB ChB, MD (Hon Causa),
MA (Hon Causa), PhD, FRCS (Ed),
FRCS (Eng), FCS (SA), FACS
Professor of Surgery and Director, Gastric Surgical
Pathobiology Research Group
Yale University School of Medicine
Department of Surgery
New Haven, Connecticut

George Sachs, MB, ChB, DSc
Professor of Physiology and Medicine
Wilshire Chair in Medicine
University of California, Los Angeles
Senior Medical Investigator
Veterans Administration Medical Center
Los Angeles, California

Editorial Directors:
Prof. Irvin M. Modlin and Prof. George Sachs

Senior Editor: Brenda D. Frank

Illustrations:
Steven M. Lustig
BioDesign Communications Inc.
Huntington Beach, California

Michaela Battaglin, Milan, Italy
Irvin Modlin, New Haven, Connecticut

Art Direction and Typesetting:
Henny Schultz
Schultz Squared, Inc.
Boothwyn, Pennsylvania

Published by CoMed Communications, Inc., Philadelphia, Pennsylvania

ISBN 0-943035-00-7

Prescribing information and registration status for the different products mentioned herein differ among countries. Please consult prescribing information for these products in your country.

THE LOGIC OF OMEPRAZOLE:
Treatment by Design

The funding for this book was provided by AstraZeneca.

AstraZeneca

From the very earliest days, digestion has been recognized as a matter of critical relevance to well being. Quality of life has over many centuries been closely related to the stomach and its sensations. Seated on the marble terraces of Kos, Hippocrates opined lucidly on the nature of digestion *(pepsis)* and expounded on *coction* or cooking as the basis of *pepsis*. Although he was aware that malfunction of digestion or dyspepsia was a serious and common problem, he could do little more than speculate as to its causation and counsel his patients to moderate their dietary habits. His cognate Grecian and Roman successors had little more to offer either as *medici* or philosophers. Celsus was prescient in suggesting avoidance of acrid or acid food while Dioscorides and Scipio proposed a diverse variety of herbal remedies and even charcoal to counter the irritant effects of the evil humors that could grip the stomach in their painful clutches. For almost two millennia, spirits, irritants, and nervous disorders were variously held to be the causation of apepsia, dyspepsia, and even polypepsia, as physicians and patients struggled with a problem that was intractable and for which they possessed neither explanation nor remedy.

In 1823, Prout determined that gastric acid was hydrochloric, and that dyspepsia was related to acid secretion by the stomach. As a result of this seminal observation, peptic ulcer disease was recognized as a consequence of acid secretion and a rational basis established for a consideration of its management. In the early twentieth century Schwarz published his famous dictum, "*No acid, no ulcer,*" and the disease and its etiology became firmly embedded in the dogma of the times. Over the subsequent fifty years, the treatment of peptic ulcer disease vacillated between bland diets (eg, Sippy, Doll) and heroic pharmacologic approaches including effective doses of atropine and immense amounts of "white medicine." Ablative gastric surgery (total gastrectomy, partial gastrectomy) was augmented by visceral neural surgery (vagotomy and its endless permutations of truncal, selective, and highly selective), and large components of normal structures were sacrificed with substantial morbidity and mortality in an effort to decrease acid secretion. Although gastrin, discovered by Edkins at the turn of the century, had initially been declared humbug, its unequivocal existence and effectiveness as an acid secretagogue was established by Komarov and, thereafter, by Gregory. The recognition by Popielski in 1918 — that histamine stimulated gastric acid secretion — fell by the wayside as gastrin became regarded by most gastric physiologists as the dominant secretagogue.

Fortunately, the pharmacologist James Black, who had pioneered the synthesis of selective β-adrenergic antagonists at ICI, believed not only that histamine was the dominant secretagogue, but that histamine acted in the stomach at a different receptor from those attacked by the histamine antagonists that had been synthesized by Boivet. In the reorganization of Smith, Kline and French that occurred in 1967, the team led by Black at the Welwyn Garden City branch of SK&F continued research on the synthesis of H2 receptor antagonists that had started in 1963, while a team at the SK&F headquarters in Philadelphia, led by Virgil Wiebelhaus and under the guidance of Peter Ridley, undertook the task of discovering pump-based rather than receptor-based inhibitors of acid secretion. By 1970, a screen had been developed measuring the effects of compounds on a potassium-stimulated p-nitrophenyl phosphatase (a partial reaction of the pump), and some lead structures had been discovered. However, Black and his colleagues succeeded in synthesizing the first H2 receptor antagonist — burimamide in 1970 — and metiamide, the first such antagonist to be tested in man. In November 1973, they introduced Cimetidine (Tagamet®) at a symposium in London. The characteristics of this compound and its anticipated success resulted in discontinuation of the search for other acid inhibitors in Philadelphia.

Meanwhile, across the North Sea from Great Britain, a Swedish company, Hassle AB, had discovered compounds that inhibited gastric acid secretion in their rat ulcer model. They pursued this avenue of research, picking up from the "antigastrins" projects of Searle and, later, Servier in France. Servier synthesized pyridine-2-thioacetamide; then, in 1974, Hassle AB produced pyridine 2-methyl thio-benzimidazole, an effective inhibitor of rat gastric acid secretion. The benzimidazole was supposed to mimic 2-ethylamino-imidazole, or histamine. This compound was followed, in 1976, by the synthesis of pyridyl 2-methyl sulfinyl-benzimidazole, now called timoprazole. The chemists involved in this project, Ulf Lunggren, Arne Brandstrom, and, later, Per Lindberg, were part of a team headed by Sven-Erik Sjostrand. This compound was 10 times more potent in inhibition of acid secretion.

In 1975, an in vitro model of acid secretion, the rabbit gastric gland, had been developed by a graduate student, Thomas Berglindh, who was working with Karl Johan Obrink, a pioneer in the field of acid secretion. Hassle AB requested that timoprazole be tested using the rabbit gastric gland model. Testing revealed that timoprazole, like the H2-receptor antagonist cimedine, inhibited histamine- and gastrin-stimulated secretion. However, unlike cimetadine, timoprazole also produced inhibition of carbachol-stimulated acid secretion. Studies of timoprazole in rats resulted in side effects on the thyroid and the thymus, and this prevented further development of this compound. Timoprazole was unstable in solution, so, in 1977, a new compound, picoprazole, was made. Its mechanism and site of action were unknown, but it had a lesser effect on iodine uptake by the thyroid.

In 1977, a symposium on acid secretion was held (in conjunction with the International Congress of Physiology) on proton transport. Gaetano Saccomani, a member of an acid-transport research group in Birmingham, Alabama that had shown that gastric H^+,K^+ ATPase was the proton pump of the stomach, presented a talk on a polyclonal antibody against H^+,K^+ ATPase, showing that it reacted strongly with the stomach and weakly with thyroid on radial immunodiffusion. After the talk, Erik Fellenius, a member of a research team at Hassle AB asked George Sachs, the leader of the Alabama group, whether this antibody had been tested against the thymus. It had, but Sachs told Fellenius that he would have to explain the reason for the question before providing an answer. Fellenius then recounted the effect of timoprazole on acid secretion, gastric glands, thyroid, and thymus. Sachs then revealed that the polyclonal antibody did indeed show reactivity with thymus extracts. These data had not been presented, as he had no plausible hypothesis as to why any thymic reaction occurred and had perhaps an implausible hypothesis for the thyroid reactivity with the antibody. Given his involvement with SK&F in the discovery of inhibitors of the gastric acid pump 10 years earlier, he was eager to test the Hassle AB compounds on the acid pump. Fellenius then visited the laboratory in Birmingham where Berglindh was working as a postdoctoral fellow and decided to send timoprazole and picoprazole for testing as inhibitors of the gastric proton pump.

In those days, two general assays were being run on ATPase: one in which no acid gradient was developed, and another where acid transport was measured. It turned out that the compounds, especially picoprazole, did little to inhibit ATPase when no acid gradient was developed (at first a great disappointment), but (a revelation!) they were effective when the enzyme was transporting acid. This type of drug was therefore an acid-activated inhibitor of the gastric acid pump. These data were presented to Hassle AB in October 1978 by Sachs and Berglindh, who had demonstrated that these drugs were therefore prodrugs converted to the active form after accumulation in the acidic secretory canaliculus of the parietal cell.

A young student in the group at Hassle AB, Bjorn Wallmark, joined the group in Birmingham to carry out research on the kinetics of gastric ATPase for his PhD thesis. A new compound, omeprazole, was synthesized in 1979, and was chosen as the candidate compound for development as an antiulcer agent. Oddly, that same year in Perth, Western Australia, a pathologist named Robin Warren first observed the presence of spiral organisms in biopsies of gastric ulcers.

Upon the departure of Sven-Erik Sjostrand and Erik Fellenius, Enar Carlsson became the leader of the Hassle AB group in Gothenburg. The group included numerous chemists and biologists, including Bjorn Wallmark, and Lars Olbe, a professor of surgery at the University of Gothenburg, who was also working on the physiology of acid secretion.

This figure includes some of the people who were involved in defining the road to omeprazole and its success. Clockwise from top: George Sachs, Ian Talmage, Thomas Berglindh, Arne Brandstrom, Enar Carlsson, Per Lindberg, Bjorn Wallmark.

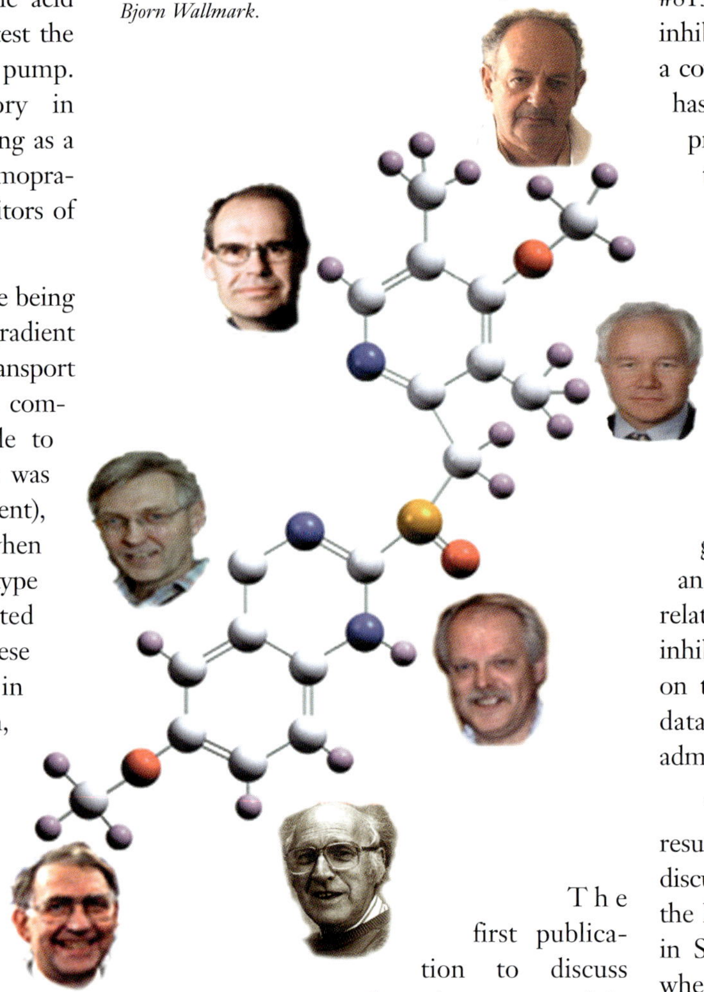

The first publication to discuss these drugs appeared in *Nature* in 1981 and was followed by presentation of the first human studies in 1982—1983, pioneered by Anders Walan, Christer Cederberg, and Lars Olbe. With this attention, other companies rapidly became interested in similar compounds: Upjohn in the USA; Takeda, Eisai, and Nippon-Chemifar in Japan; Byk Gulden in Germany; and Fisons in the UK, to name just a few.

The chemistry of inhibition was resolved by Brandstrom and Lindberg, as well as by Senn-Bilfinger in Germany and Schussitzki in the UK. The hypothesis was that, after acid-space accumulation, a sulfenamide was formed in an acid-catalyzed reaction that then reacted with one or more cysteines on the outside surface of the pump to form a disulfide derivative. Later work by the Sachs group demonstrated that the omeprazole became bound to cysteine at position #813 in the catalytic subunit of H^+,K^+ ATPase inhibiting enzyme activity and acid transport in a covalent manner. However, more recent work has raised the possibility that sulfenic acid, a precursor of sulfenamide, might actually be the active form of omeprazole.

Development of the compound as an acid inhibitory agent continued in spite of the concerns of management at Astra Hassle AB that it could not compete with either cimetidine or ranitidine. However, in 1984, clinical development was halted because of the appearance of ECL cell carcinoids in rats on high-dose, lifelong treatment. Rapidly thereafter, the group in Gothenburg led by Enar Carlsson and Hillevi Mattson showed that this effect was related to the hypergastrinemia resulting from inhibition of acid secretion and had no bearing on the safety of omeprazole itself. Indeed the data could be mimicked by ranitidine administration.

This finding allowed the clinical studies to resume. The first large public symposium to discuss omeprazole was held in association with the International Congress of Gastroenterology in Sao Paolo, Brazil, in the summer of 1986, where the lighting system failed during the presentations. At the 1988 International Congress in Rome, the first set of presentations dealing with clinical findings about this drug, now called a proton pump inhibitor, were aired in an audience-participation session. The launch symposium followed rapidly thereafter in Monaco, chaired by Andre Blum and George Sachs, and under the direction of Ian Talmage and Anders Vedin of Astra Hassle AB.

France first, then Sweden, approved omeprazole; thereafter, other European countries soon followed suit. The drug obtained

Food and Drug Administration (FDA) approval in the USA in 1989 by Merck & Co., Inc., the company that had acquired rights to the drug in North America. Further indications for the clinical use of omeprazole were added following the presentation of Roger Berlin of Merck & Co., Inc. to an additional FDA advisory committee meeting.

The advent of this proton pump inhibitor on the worldwide market heralded a new era in effective treatment of acid-related diseases, especially heartburn associated with gastroesophageal reflux disease. In spite of the presence of several different H2 receptor antagonists on the market, omeprazole, aided by a bevy of clinical investigators, has become the world's largest selling proton pump inhibitor.* Not coincidentally, combination therapy with proton pump inhibitors is now also the mainstay of treatment for eradication of *Helicobacter pylori*, the organism initially identified by Robin Warren in 1979, the year of synthesis of omeprazole. As H. L. Mencken so shrewdly noted in 1919:

> "*Life is a struggle, not against sin, not against Money Power, not against malicious animal power, but against hydrogen ions.*"

This book relates the story of the struggle against *gastric* hydrogen ions and details how far we have progressed in winning this battle with the development of the proton pump inhibitor omeprazole

*Data on file, DA-PR134, since June 1998, IMS Health.

THIS BOOK IS DEDICATED

By George

To Joyce, Paula, Pauland, Lara, David, Stevie, Margot,
Natalie, Nicholas, Oscar, Lucas, Stevie and Winston

And

By Irvin

To Alex, Jonnie, Julie, Monte, Maria and Newton.

Home is where one starts from.
As we grow older
The world becomes stranger,
the pattern more complicated
Of dead living.
Not the intense moment
Isolated, with no before and after,
But a lifetime burning in every moment
And not the lifetime of one man only
But of old stones that cannot be deciphered.

To arrive where you are, to get from where you are not,
You must go by a way of wherein there is no ecstasy.
In order to arrive at what you do not know
You must go by the way which is the way of ignorance.

Thomas Stearns Eliot
Four Quartets. East Coker. (1940).

ACKNOWLEDGEMENTS

We are deeply indebted to a number of people including M. Kidd and Jian Fahardi (New Haven), David Scott, David Weeks, Jai Moo Shin, Keith Munson and Klaus Melchers, and Eva Lacayo-Barquero (Los Angeles) for their contributions to the way we think. We are also beholden to Douglas Levine and Tom McCourt, without whose overview and ongoing support this work would never have seen the light of day. Lois Brothers, Mark Mallon, and Mary Carpenter maintained a fine perspective on the subject during the course of our enterprise. The combination of their wise contributions and the generous support provided by AstraZeneca facilitated the culmination of this endeavor.

Steve Lustig and Michela Battaglin provided artistic input of rare quality, and the legacy of their pictorial skills, as displayed in this book, attests to their talents.

GS believes prolonged exposure to Chateau Y and a glass of milk fertilized the seeds of this endeavor, and IMM, that the serenity induced by La Tâche broadened our scientific horizons and honed thought processes in a fashion that may only be achieved by short carbon fragment-induced mild inebriation. Neither of us has succumbed to the perils of the Tynanian dictum, and we have resisted the temptation to "write heresy, pure heresy — rouse tempers, goad, lacerate and raise whirlwinds." Consequently, this book is lacking in rebarbative comment of which we are both so fond, believing it to be the one truly definable cause of non-ulcer dyspepsia.

A great debt is due to Yale University School of Medicine and, in particular, the History of Medicine Library that provided IMM with the ideal milieu to pursue these studies. In particular, Irvin wishes to gratefully acknowledge the sagacity of Solly Marks *(amolikke tzeiten)*, who has, over the years, claimed to perceive some faint merit in his endeavors and whose maieutic skills facilitated pursuit of the elusive proton and its history.

Numerous institutions and persons generously provided us with access to material and allowed its use, including the Yale University History of Medicine Library, the Hunterian Museum and Library of the Royal College of Surgeons of England, the Royal Society of Medicine, the Royal College of Physicians of England, and the Wellcome Institute for the History of Medicine. Innumerable colleagues, scientific collaborators, and friends have generously allowed us to use information emanating from their labors: *Ars Gratia Artis.* We are both entirely responsible for any errors, oversights, and misinterpretations of either history or scientific data expressed in this text.

Finally, we wish to acknowledge William Prout, William Beaumont, Robin Warren, and Barry Marshall for exciting in us a curiosity regarding muriatic acid and neutralophiles. Their speculations, although centuries and continents apart, altered the entire thinking of the world of gastroenterology and the treatment of countless millions of patients. Indeed each labored *Per Ardua ad Astra* to convince an unbelieving world of new knowledge. The most profound debt is due to the intrepid pioneers of the proton pump and its inhibition, who, in the basements of Hassle, Gothenburg, and the laboratories of Birmingham, Alabama, successfully overcame intellectual obstacles and vaulted the boundaries of contemporary therapeutic limitation. They, like the intrepid maritime explorers of the past, voyaged on the Sea of Acid and healed the dyspeptic masses. *"Qui genus medici ingenio superavit."* In one decade, the entire world of physicians and patients alike can acknowledge the evolutionary and remarkable contributions of omeprazole to acid peptic disease therapy.

NOTE TO PRESCRIBER

PRILOSEC® (omeprazole) is indicated first line for heartburn and other symptoms associated with gastroesophageal reflux disease (GERD), erosive esophagitis, maintenance of healed erosive esophagitis, active duodenal ulcer, active benign gastric ulcer, pathological hypersecretory conditions, and in combination with clarithromycin and amoxicillin or with clarithromycin for *Helicobacter pylori*-associated duodenal ulcer disease.

The most frequently reported adverse events with PRILOSEC are headache, diarrhea, and abdominal pain. Symptomatic response to therapy does not preclude the presence of gastric malignancy. Atrophic gastritis has been noted occasionally in gastric corpus biopsies from patients treated long term with omeprazole.

CONTENTS

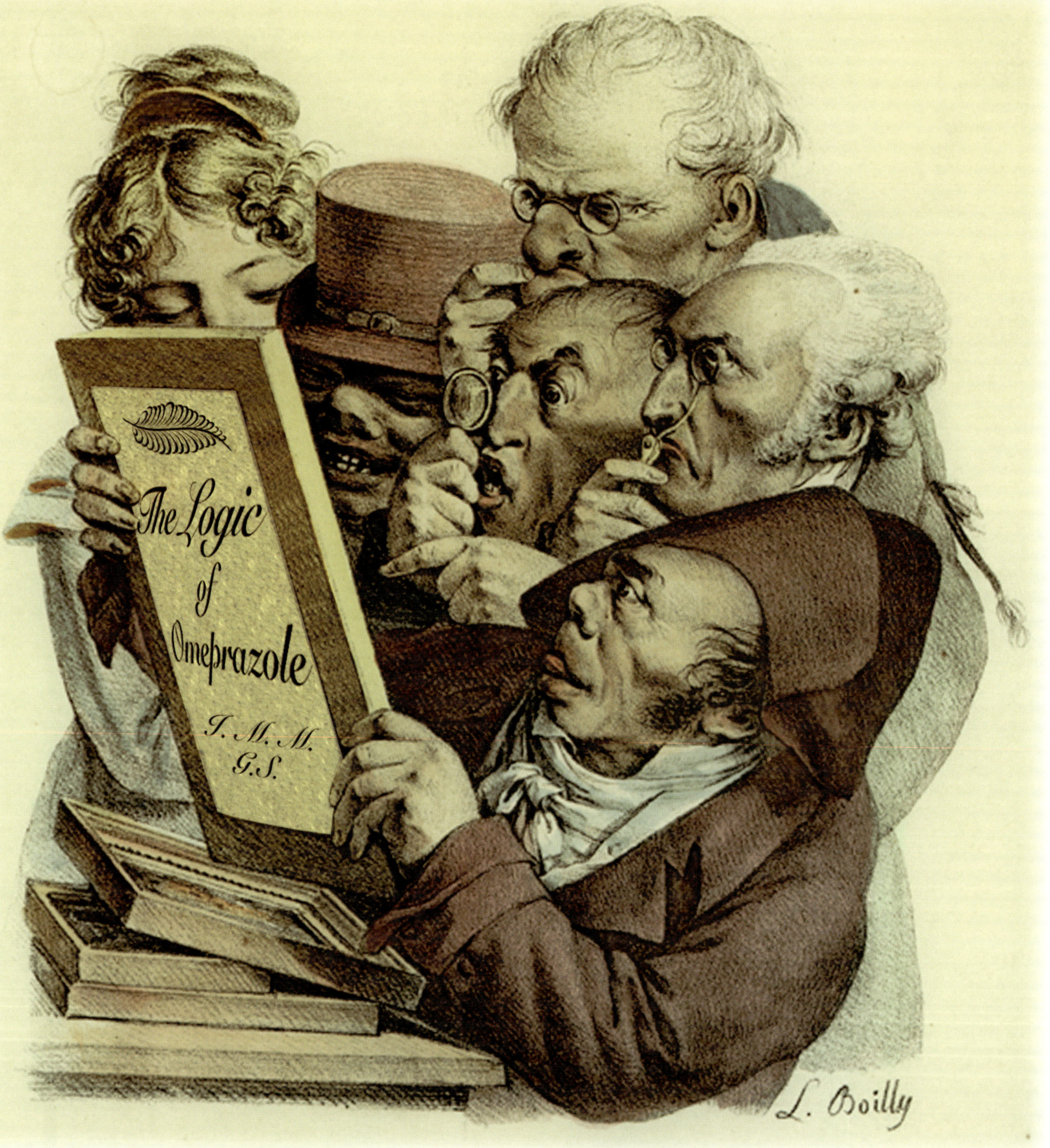
The Logic
of
Omeprazole
T. M. M.
G.S.
L. Boilly

Chapter I

Dyspepsia, Dogma, and Acid

Epidemiology

Origins

Understanding Dyspepsia

Anatomy

The Stomach

Regulation of Secretion

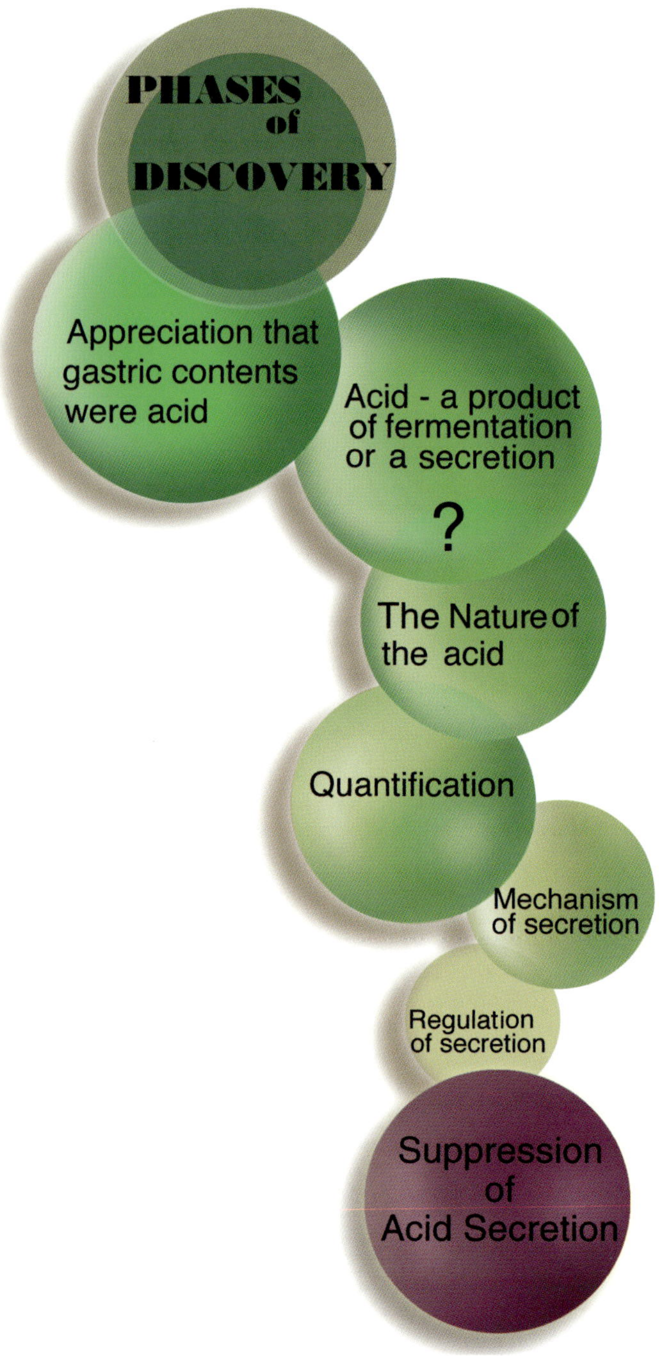
PHASES of DISCOVERY
Appreciation that gastric contents were acid
Acid - a product of fermentation or a secretion ?
The Nature of the acid
Quantification
Mechanism of secretion
Regulation of secretion
Suppression of Acid Secretion

DYSPEPSIA, DOGMA, AND ACID

Figure 1. *— A Man Suffering From Indigestion. Colored etching by G. Cruikshank, 1835, after A. Crowquill (Courtesy of the Wellcome Institute Library, London). This dramatic early 19th-century depiction of a man suffering from abdominal discomfort indicates the widespread public awareness of the chronic symptomatology and misery generated by dyspepsia and indigestion. The position of the patient's hand, the blue devil's crow bar, and the attempt to cool down the shoulder tip pain or relieve rigors suggests that the "indigestion" depicted may have been of a biliary nature.*

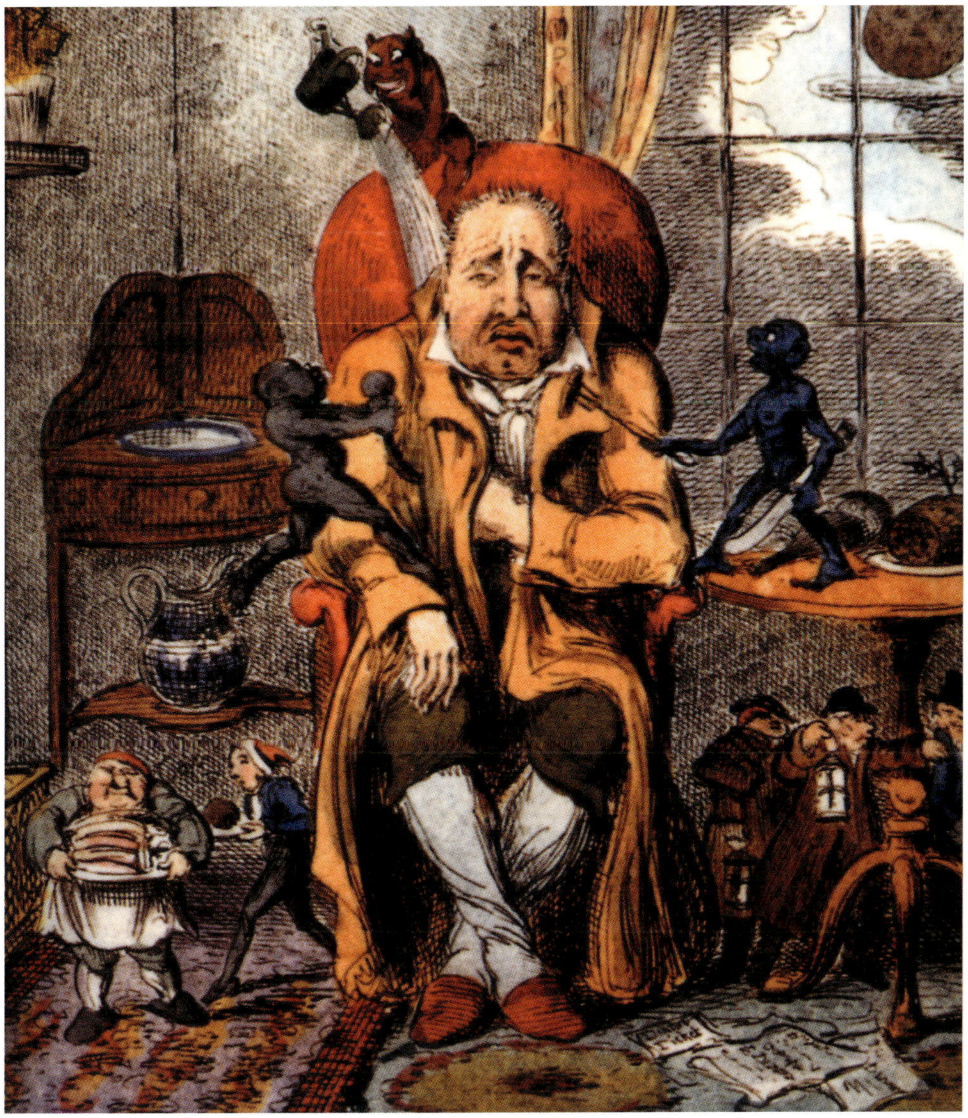

People have always been preoccupied with pleasure, comfort, and a sensation of well being. Although philosophical discourse has been an important part of the evolution of the species, the pursuit of food and sex has dominated. Failure to satisfactorily achieve the latter has resulted in frustration, depression, and aggression. Similarly, difficulties with food—its acquisition, quality, desire for, and digestion of—has manifested in dyspepsia.

In 1888, Dr. Adolphus Bridger, a London physician, wrote in the preface to his book, *The Demon of Dyspepsia*, "ten years of medical practice devoted very largely to this branch, has convinced me that the subject is not only one of the greatest individual, but also of the highest national importance..." Scores of similar books were published to meet the Victorian appetite for works on the physiology of digestion and the preoccupation with digestive disorders, then referred to as *dyspepsia*. In the second half of the 19th century, such books became a distinct genre, with titles such as *Digestion: The Passport to Health* and *Common Sense Management of the Stomach*. One text was titled *Anatomy of Dyspepsia, Being a Practical Enquiry into the Derangements of the Organs of Digestion, Shewing Their Connexion with Cutaneous Disease, Renal Disorders and Nervous Affections; Embracing Hints to Tropical Invalids, with Remarks on Exercise.*

A tract published in the last year of Queen Victoria's reign, *Dyspepsia*, was the second volume in *Heywood's Penny Medical Library*, a series of popular handbooks, and carried the advertising slogan "price a penny; will save a pound":

> Dyspepsia has been called the national disease, and it is not only the national disease of this country, but for most, if not all, civilized countries. It is not surprising that more has probably been written about this ailment than about any other. The literature regarding it would, if collected, form quite a big library...

Epidemiology

Approximately 25% of the general population in any western country may have recurrent dyspepsia over a 12-month period. There appears to be neither a significant difference between Europe and the United States nor between men and women, although prevalence declines significantly as age increases. Whether this is due to an adaptation to the stresses of life or is more organically based is unknown.

The long-term outcome of patients with dyspepsia of unidentified etiology is uncertain. Between 10% and 15% of persons will become asymptomatic, and overall symptoms tend to decrease with age. However, in control population groups, approximately 12% to 15% of subjects develop symptoms of dyspepsia and heartburn annually for which no cause can be identified.

Although a specific disease process in the upper gastrointestinal tract may not be definable, even after serious investigation of symptoms, the disease entity per se represents a considerable socioeconomic problem. As dyspepsia accounts for between 20% and 70% of all gastrointestinal consultations with general practitioners, a significant amount of physician time is spent evaluating the problem. Up to a third of patients are referred to gastroenterologists for further evaluation. The majority of these patients are treated, even if no objective evidence of mucosal ulceration is detectable. No studies are available to determine whether the use of medication improves the long-term outcome of the disease process.

In Sweden, in 1996, it was calculated that the costs of functional dyspepsia were greater than $55,000 per 1000 persons. Such costs are significantly higher in the United States and will continue to increase as the cost of health care grows. Patients with the diagnosis of functional dyspepsia have been reported to have a twofold to threefold increase in the number of days of reported sickness from their work. When studied with quality-of-life scales, they attain scores significantly lower than those of their cohorts. Thus, functional dyspepsia, whether subdivided into functional heartburn or dyspepsia with motility-related disturbances, remains a difficult therapeutic and diagnostic area. Clearly, some of these patients have centrally mediated problems that may be outside the care of the gastroenterologist, but others likely have organic pathology that has as yet not been identified.

Epidemiologic studies have reported that 15% of the population suffers heartburn at least once a week, and 7% have heartburn daily. This number is greater in pregnant women and persons who are either overweight or whose occupation involves frequent stooping or bending. In persons whose heartburn and reflux symptoms are significant enough to seek medical advice and endoscopy, 30% to 60% may exhibit evidence of esophagitis. Although the overall prevalence of erosive esophagitis in the general population is approximately 2%, which is 15 times less than the prevalence of reflux symptoms, on endoscopic evaluation, reflux esophagitis can be documented in up to 15%. It is evident that most patients whose symptoms may be classified as dyspepsia or heartburn never seek medical advice and, instead, self-medicate. The reasons for this are complex and include the fear of the detection of serious disease. Also, there is often anxiety that the physician will initiate investigations that prompt further conflict or prescribe medication and suggest alterations in life style that will cause further conflict and discomfort.

Origins

In the earliest times, physicians believed that the various organs were seats of separate spiritual agencies that, in a divine manner, controlled bodily function. The ancient Greeks proposed that digestion was a process of concoction or heating and, in this evolution, food was converted initially to chyle and then to the four humours (blood, phlegm, yellow bile, and black bile) before use by the mortal body. Hippocrates called the process of digestion *pepsis* and proposed that it was not dissimilar to the preparation of food by cooking. Galenic physiology proposed that successive cooking processes occurred sequentially in the stomach, intestine, and liver until food was finally converted into blood.

Over the succeeding two millennia, opinion continued to vacillate widely among what exact course the disease might follow, how it should be described, and what its cause might be. Thus, as late as the 17th century, Robert Lovell, a physician from Coventry, still depicted the disease *dyspepsy* (or dyspepsia) within the framework of Galen of Pergamum. He stated that "imbecility of the stomach is a vice of the concocting faculty, by reason of which, it concocteth not at all slowly or depravedly; it's called apepsy, bradypepsy or dypepsy." By the 18th century, the words *apepsy* and *bradypepsy* had fallen into disuse. The word *dyspepsia* itself was thereafter considered more in the context of altered nervous function, and the ancient concepts of *humours* had fallen into disuse after nearly two millennia. The old connotations of coction and pepsis promulgated by Hippocrates of Kos and amplified by Erasistratus and Herophilus of Alexandria were subsumed as a neural or nervous basis.

This alteration in perception of the origin of dyspepsia is evident in the changes made in John Quincy's *Lexicon Physico-Medicum*, first published in 1719, and that given in the 13th edition, nearly a century later in 1811. The semantic transformation of

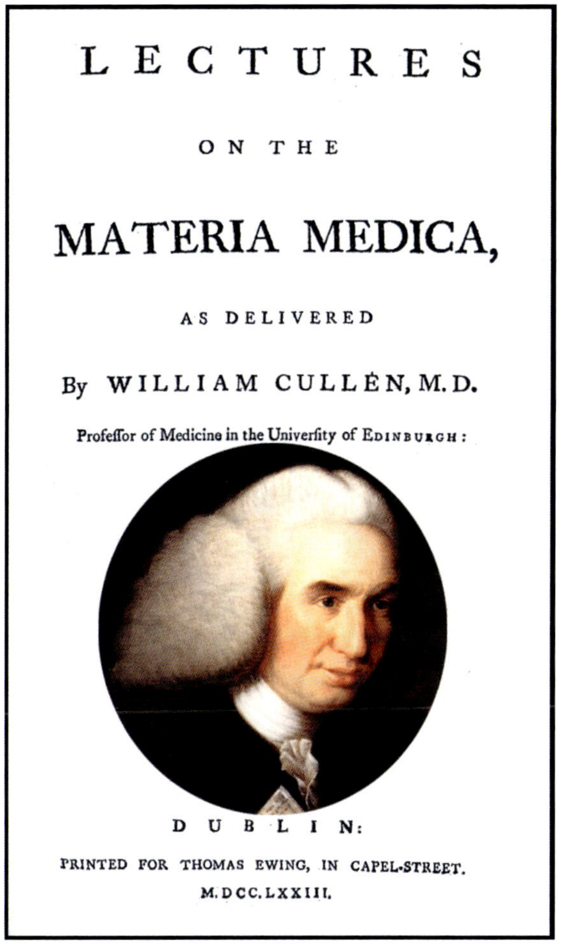

LECTURES

ON THE

MATERIA MEDICA,

AS DELIVERED

By WILLIAM CULLEN, M.D.

Profeſſor of Medicine in the Univerſity of EDINBURGH:

DUBLIN:

PRINTED FOR THOMAS EWING, IN CAPEL-STREET.

M.DCC.LXXIII.

Figure 2. *— William Cullen (1712-1790) was instrumental in founding the Medical School of Glasgow in 1744. He held the Chairs of Medicine and Chemistry at both Glasgow and Edinburgh and was the first to give clinical lectures in Great Britain. These lectures were also the first (1757) to be delivered in the vernacular instead of Latin. Cullen was an inspiring teacher and particularly noted for his kindness in assisting needy students. Although it is accepted that he introduced a number of new remedies into practice, critics of his skills, such as Sir William Hamilton, stated that "Cullen did not add a single new fact to medical science." It is said that his finest innovation was the use of hydrotherapy with rapid changes in temperature for the treatment of abdominal discomfort. This form of treatment was called by Despine of Aix les Bains, "The Scotch Douche." Cullen based his teaching of medicine on the rationale that life was a function of nervous energy and that disease of any sort was a reflection of a nervous disorder. Having studied with Hermann Boerhaave in Leiden and having been exposed to the taxonomic skills of Carl Linnaeus, he had learned the skills of detailed classification. Cullen thus divided diseases into fevers, neuroses, cachexias, and local disorders differentiating more than 30 forms of rheumatism and even considering gout as a neurosis. He believed that all forms of dyspepsia represented local abdominal manifestations of a nervous disorder. This concept has persisted in a variety of different forms well into the 20th century.*

"dyspepsia" from "bad" and "to concoct" ("bad digestion") but "generally confined to the office of the stomach" had altered by 1811 to reflect symptoms that now were categorized in their many and different forms as of "nervous origin." Thus, the etiology was initially stated as "great grief and uneasiness of mind, intense study, profuse evacuations, excess in venery, hard drinking particularly of spiritous liquors, and of tea, tobacco, opium, and other narcotics, immoderate repletion, and overdistension of the stomach, a deficiency in the secretion of the bile or gastric juice, and the being much exposed to moist or cold air..."

A century later, the causes associated with dyspepsia are noted as "a long train of nervous symptoms which generally attend on this disease, such as loss of appetite, nausea, heartburn, flatulency, acid eructations, a gnawing in the stomach when empty, a sense of constriction and uneasiness in the throat...great costiveness, habitual chilliness, paleness of the countenance, languor, unwillingness to move about, lowness of spirits, palpitations and disturbed sleep." Thus, dyspepsia remained a disease, but the symptoms, in their many and varied forms, were categorized as nervous.

So concerned were the physicians of Victorian England about the depradations of dyspepsia and the havoc that it might wreak on the populace that they wrote of it in the most overblown prose. Dyspepsia was depicted as universal malady with an infinity of forms and the direst of consequences. Bradshaw, in 1864, stated with exaggerated alarm and no little concern:

> Dyspepsia is a complaint from which no race, sex, age, class or condition is exempt — it accompanies man from the cradle to the grave...From the gorgeously berobed potentate on his gilded throne attended by his parasites, to the most squalid mendicant clad in rags and surrounded by destitution, this wonderful and curious malady discovers itself under an infinity of forms, pervading every ramification of society, remorselessly, unheedingly — now sinking the body to the abysm of physical degradation — now prostrating the mind from the loftiest pinnacles of man's ennobling attributes and lowering him to a level with the very meanest animalities — now showing itself with the most marked manifestations upon the body — now apparently quitting the real seat of its tenure and developing itself upon the mind, carrying before it like some sweeping avalanche, every obstacle in its path — paralysing intellects, the most brilliant with irresistible severity — on its velvet couch, as he piteously bewails the violence inflicted on his constitution...while another dyspeptic martyr infinitely more deserving of our sympathy, bemoans over some distressing symptom not of his own creation, but one which has been bequeathed to him as an hereditament.... This universal malady needs no artistic flourish to heighten the effect of the picture, requires no elaboration to impress us with a due sense of its importance from whatever point of sight it is beheld.

Despite such concerns regarding the outcome of the disease, by the beginning of the 19th century, dyspepsia had acquired a much greater breadth and complexity of meaning. In this respect, William Cullen's influence on perceptions of dyspepsia was crucial, for he insisted, in his much-quoted comment, "that in a certain view almost the whole of diseases of the human body might be called nervous." In 1769, Cullen presented his remarkable and elaborate classification of diseases, whose concepts he had extrapolated from the taxonomies developed by 18th century botanists. As Cullen had studied with Boerhaave in Leiden and was a colleague of Linnaeus, his familiarity with clinical disease and plant taxonomy was substantial. He thus developed lists of diseases that were composed of categories and compilations of symptoms and proposed that as all life was a manifestation of nervous energy, all diseases were a form of nervous disorder. Cullen coined the word *neuroses* to represent the second of his four classes and emphasized the importance of this group in his schema of illness. The *neuroses* were in turn subdivided into four orders, each of which he divided into genera; one of the orders included "syncope, dypepsia, hypochondriasisis, and chlorosis." As a result of Cullen's influence, considerable attention was thereafter focused on the brain and the nervous system as opposed to the heart and vascular system. By 1814, George Owens Rees, physician to the London Dispensary, wrote the following on the new role of the stomach in his book *Disorder of the Stomach:*

> The stomach has hitherto been generally regarded as a receptacle for a certain fluid which promotes digestion; but besides this it performs another very important function somewhat analogous to the heart: for as the heart transmits blood and throws it forward through the arteries to every part of the system so there is great reason to believe that the stomach diffuses in a like manner a degree of nervous energy to every part of the body...

Understanding Dyspepsia

The comprehension of the origins of dyspepsia and its relationship of food to illness is shrouded in the mists of time. The interdictions placed upon unsuitable, unclean, or poisonous foods in the Mosaic code (Exodus, Leviticus) return to the initial experiments of prehistoric man with regard to things edible or inedible. As such, dietetics became the basic element in ancient therapy.

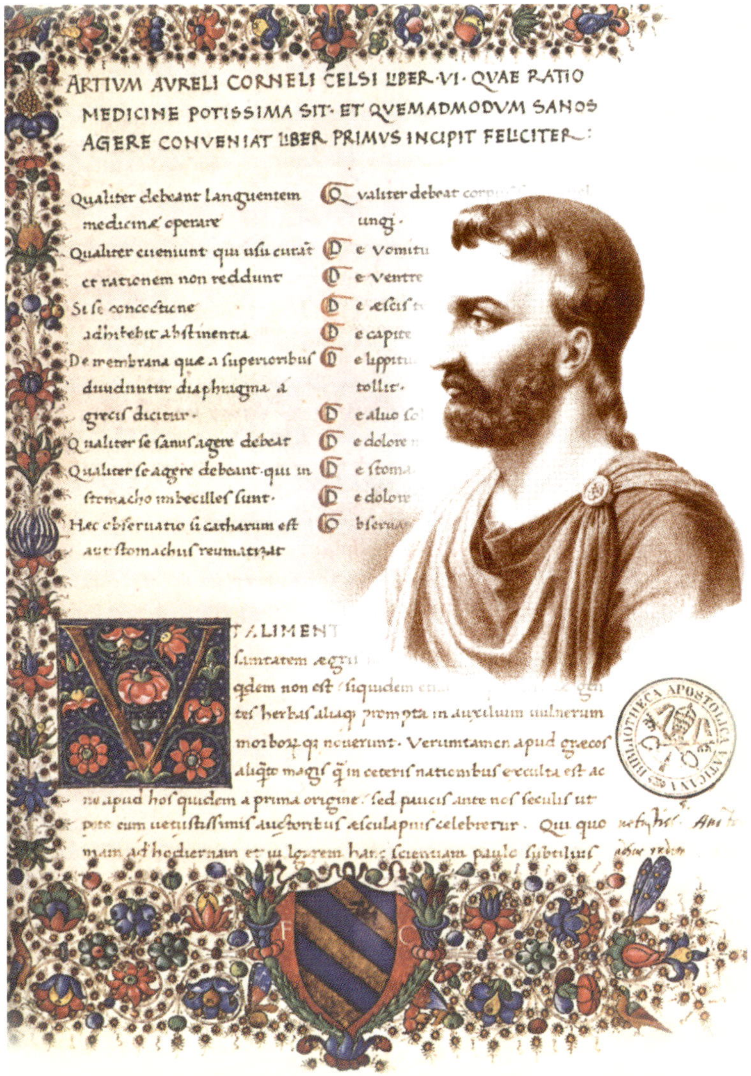

Figure 3. — Aurelius Cornelius Celsus of Rome was not a physician but an aristocrat of the noble family of Cornelii and lived during the reign of Tiberius Caesar. His classical work, De re Medicina, *was one of the first medical books to be printed and, although ignored by the Roman practitioners of his day and slighted as "mediocre" by Quintilian, he remains one of the authorities of his time. He wrote on medicine in much the same spirit in which Virgil considered veterinary matters in the* Third Book of the Georgics. *Celsus provided medical assistance free to the members of his country estate as would be expected of a wealthy Roman aristocrat. So highly rated was his writing that he was considered the Cicero of Medicine, and the eight books that constitute* De re Medicina *are masterpieces of precise literary style. The first of the four texts deals with diseases, that may be treated by diet and alteration of life style, whereas the last four describe those amenable to drugs and surgery. Celsus believed that nutritive enemata were important in treating abdominal problems and provided a diffuse and exotic list of herbal remedies that might be used to remove stomach discomfort and other digestive ailments.*

"... if the stomach is infected with an ulcer..., light and gelatinous food must be used ... and everything acrid and acid is to be avoided..."

Wheat, barley, fruit, wine, and olive oil were the main vegetable staples. Meat was more extensively consumed in the Homeric period than later; fish was hardly eaten at all. The Greek rustic learned, by long experience of trial and error, to prefer cooked food to raw and to restrict diet during acute illness. It was well understood that a slop diet eased the sick stomach and that eating should be deferred until a fever subsided. In early Greek pathology, the very efforts of the body to bring the humours from a raw, fermented status (apepsis) to normal (pepsis) were associated with cookery or coction, a view of digestive processes that survived until the 17th century.

In the archaeologic remains of ancient Egypt, concern about food is already that of an advanced civilization. Hieroglyphics and papyri depict the harvesting and marketing of fruit and grain, grape arbors and fish ponds, the kneading of dough, the brewing of beer, dining at table, and the symbolic suckling of an infant at the udders of the cow Hathor. The Ebers Papyrus features intestinal parasites and the liver complaints common to all tropical and subtropical areas. The practical knowledge of digestive disorders, scattered through the literary remains of Greek medicine, was considerable however obfuscated by Greek physicians who speculated about the etiology and by their ignorance of human postmortem appearances. Nevertheless, some of the clinical pictures of digestive disorders from Hippocrates, Celsus, Aretaeus, Galen, and the Byzantine compilers are not far from the remedies that were available at the end of the 19th century.

There were two chief problems encountered in coming to an understanding of the background of digestive disorders: the establishment of the anatomic basis of digestion and the elucidation of the physiologic background of gastric function.

Anatomy

The esophagus was envisaged as "the mouth of the stomach" and for hundreds of years became confused with the *cardia* of the pre-Galenic writers. In Galen's time and thereafter, it was known as the *stomachus*. Precordial distress *(morbus cardiacus)*, although allocated to the heart by Erasistratus, Asclepiades, and Aretaeus *(syncope)*, was thought to be of gastric (and eventually esophageal) origin by Galen, Aetius, and Alexander of Tralles. Caelius Aurelianus proposed that both a cardiac and a gastric variety could be defined but he lacked adequate criteria to be certain. Anorexia, excessive appetite *(bulimia)*, excessive thirst *(polydipsia)*, nausea and vomiting, seasickness, and hiccough were all classified primarily as esophageal disorders, yet recognized as symptomatic of gastritis and other digestive ailments. Diseases of the spleen and of the portal vein were long associated with the digestive system, and gastritis and hepatitis were recognized as separate diseases by Aretaeus, Celsus, and Alexander.

The Stomach

Functions and Junctions

Although it had been recognized since antiquity that the stomach was involved in digestion, little was known about its anatomic structure or its physiologic function. As human dissection was forbidden because of the ancients' disapproval of desecration of the body, there was conjecture as to the anatomic relationship between the stomach, esophagus, duodenum, and small bowel. Most of the information was obtained by studying war dead, execution victims, or injured gladiators. At vivisection it was apparent that the stomach was warm, as were the intestines. This led to the belief that digestion was a form of coction, much like cooking. The observations of the stomach in fish, Barbary-apes, pigs, and ungulates led to the conclusion that, in principle, the stomach was a reservoir and functioned much like a pot in which food would be stewed. As late as the 18th century, the great surgeon and scientist John Hunter would refer to the stomach as a "vat" or "stewing pot."

The issue that perplexed the ancient Greeks was how food became converted into nourishment. In Alexandria, Erasistratus recognized the concept of diffusion of substances into the tissue and even named the matrix "parenchyma." Unfortunately, he still thought that food was converted to chyle and then to the four humours that would be used to sustain life. The process by which this occurred was known in general as "pepsis" and was conceived as a form of cooking, albeit conducted in the body itself. What intrigued the ancients was the actual process by which this pepsis took place. The concept of the stomach as an organ actively secreting acid and pepsin and being responsible for digestion was not appreciated until the early 19th century. Hippocrates of Cos, Galen of Pergamum, and Erasistratus of Alexandria all reflected on the various possibilities. Unfortunately, like much of Greek medicine, theories did not culminate in solid facts.

Although early Greek practitioners of medicine were unaware of the concept of acid in the modern biochemical sense, they identified acid as bitter-sour liquid. The relationship of acids to abdominal discomfort and dyspepsia was recognized as early as 350 BC by Diocles of Carystos. He specified that sour eruptions, watery spitting gas, heartburn, and epigastric hungry pains radiating to the back with occasional splashing noises and vomiting were symptoms of a melancholy gassy illness originating in the stomach.

The Romans rejected the medical profession as charlatans and decried men who would profit from the sickness of others. In the beginning of the Christian Era, Celsus, who was not a physician, advised that "if the stomach is infested with an ulcer... light and gelatinous food must be used and everything acrid and acid is to be avoided."

The concept that secretions within the stomach were involved in digestion was evolved from the observation of stewing food in a pot of boiling water. In a world in which the laws of thermodynamics were as unknown as the principles of one-way valves, the bubbling of steaming water and gases evoked concepts of spirits and supernatural agencies in cooking.

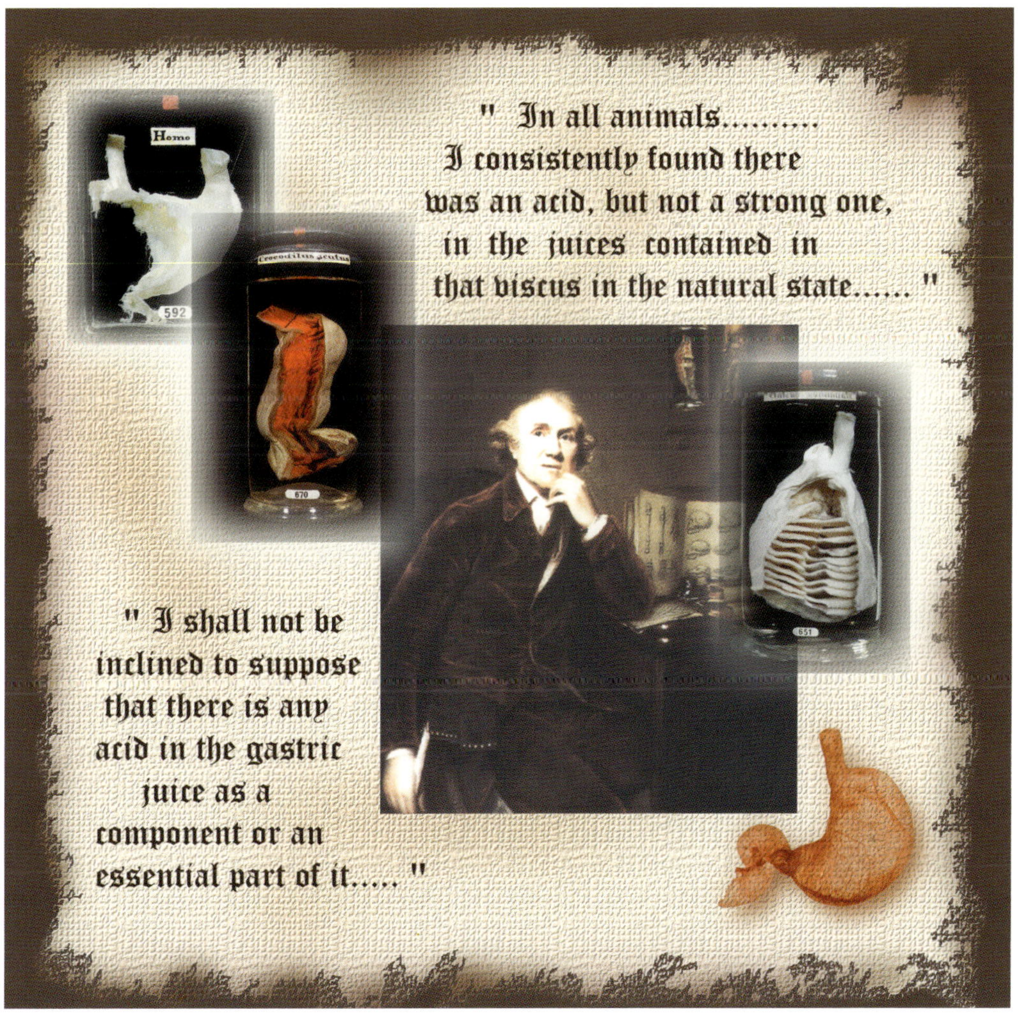

Figure 4. — *John Hunter (1728-1793) was the founder of surgical science and a rigorous investigator of physiology. In this picture, he is surrounded by a number of the stomachs contained in his magnificent collection of more than 30,000 dissected anatomic specimens. (Individual images Courtesy of the Royal College of Surgeons of England.) Hunter's observations on the stomach were far ranging and perspicacious. In 1772, he stated that he was convinced of the presence of an acid in the stomach. By 1786, he had reassessed the situation and thought that gastric acid originated from a sugar that was secreted by the stomach. His varying viewpoints reflected the confusion about gastric acid that reigned even among the most eminent physicians of his time. Of particular relevance, however, were Hunter's observations made after experiments undertaken in several species of animals including fish "which all die of violent death." Hunter confirmed that digestion neither depended on the action of the stomach nor on heat but on the gastric juice and the possession by the body of "a living principle" that departed after life was extinguished. His puzzlement that the stomach was not digested itself during digestion continues to confound physiologists and clinicians to this day. Hunter wrote, "these appearances throw considerable light on the principles of digestion. They show that it is not mechanical power, nor contractions of the stomach, nor heat but something secreted in the coat of the stomach, which is thrown into the cavity and, therefore, animalifies the food or assimilates it to the nature of blood. The power of this juice is confined or limited to certain substances, especially of the vegetable and animal kingdoms; and although this menstruum is capable of acting independently of the stomach, yet it is obliged to that viscus for its continuance."*

In the top left is the stomach of a boy, Master Stevens, with the whole cardiac extremity destroyed after death by the action of the gastric juice. The stomach at the bottom right is a human fetal stomach dried and preserved in oil of turpentine to show its general form and particularly the manner of ramification of the arteries within the wall (1782). The other two stomachs (crocodile and tope fish) are examples of the anatomic variation evident in the stomachs of different species to facilitate trituritation and digestion of food.

The portrait of Hunter is by Sir Joshua Reynolds, who considered Hunter to be a bad "sitter." Whether the look of anguish on Hunter's face reflects his feeling on sitting or is an accurate portrayal of the angina that would later kill him is uncertain. The large skeletal feet at the top right are those of the Irish giant O'Byrne, and the books at his side on the Natural History of Animals and the Natural History of Fossils indicate Hunter's diverse interest in all forms of physiology, osteology, pathology, and paleontology.

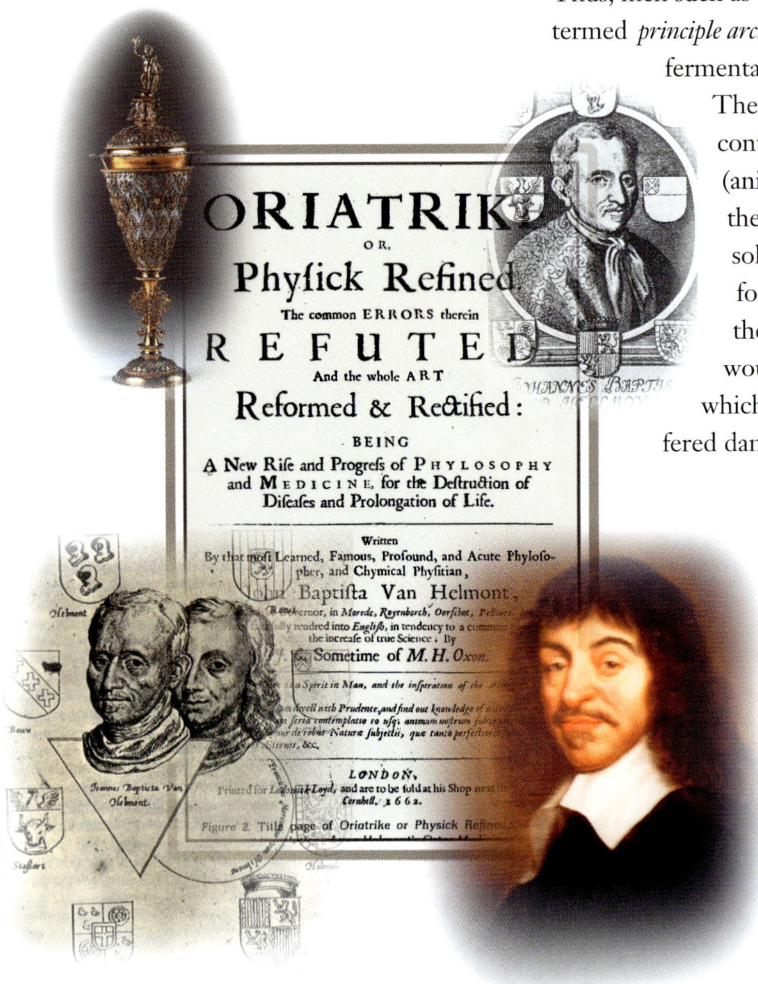

Figure 5. — Jean Baptiste von Helmont (1577–1644) (top right) *with his son* (bottom left). *Von Helmont was the founder of the Iatrochemical School and proposed that gastric acid might be a mineral acid such as nitric or hydrochloric acid. By distilling salt and clay, he actually produced "spirits of sea salt (hydrochloric acid) —* spiritus salis marina *— and demonstrated that it could be used to dissolve human kidney stones. His son posthumously published his major medical literary contribution,* Ortus Medicinae, *in 1648.*

The interest of the philosopher Rene Descartes (bottom right) *in the stomach reflected his intellectual quest for the physical site of the soul. As a supporter of the Iatromathematical school, Descartes regarded the body as a material machine directed by a rational soul, which he believed to be located in the pineal gland. The consideration of the stomach as the source of the soul or the "solar plexus" was part of the widespread desire to identify the site of the human soul and the elucidatie of its "secretion": the Holy Grail of philosophic physiology.*

Thus, men such as Van Helmont concluded that a spirit, termed *principle archeus* or *Blas* governed the intermittent fermentation that took place in the stomach. These agents were thought by him to control the sensitive and motive soul (anima sensitiva motivaque) in the "pit of the stomach," which was known as the solar plexus. Indeed, the stomach was for years thought to be the source of the soul, as a sharp blow in that area would cause a person to collapse, from which it was inferred that the soul had suffered damage and temporarily fled the body.

The quest for the soul was almost as important as the search for the Holy Grail as anatomists, physiologists, and philosophers sought it desperately within the body. Descartes concluded after years that "the pineal gland was the very source of the soul itself." He claimed that its unique position in relationship to the aqueduct of the brain was the center of the human body, and he compared it to a "small penis."

Although Van Helmont believed in spirits, he was a superb chemist and noted that in sparrows that he fed there was "a great sharpness in the throat"; he presumed that this was part of the digestive process of the bird. He also recognized that juice from the stomach of birds dissolved the leather of his glove as did the liquid distilled from sulfur alone, which was an acid, although the latter alone would not decompose food *in vitro*. He thus proposed the existence of another agent in the stomach that was responsible for digestion and termed it a *ferment*. This agent, pepsin, would be identified two centuries later by Theodor Schwann in the laboratories of Johannes Müller in Berlin. During a frenzied 2 months of investigation Schwann isolated a separate compound in the gastric juice that was capable of digesting egg and meat.

Although Van Helmont proposed that there was an acid of some kind in the stomach and called it *ensurinum*, he was unclear as to its nature and believed that the alkaline gall in the duodenum was in some way related to its function. Previous ruminations on the nature of the digestive material in the stomach had emanated from Paracelsus, who was a peripatetic alchemist physician and a proponent of chemical pharmacology and therapeutics. He believed that the acid in the stomach of humans came from the drinking of acidic spare waters (*acetosum ensurinum*, "hungry acid") and that its action was part of a catalytic process necessary to prevent the formation of precipitations and concretions within the body. This assertion was not unreasonable, given that bladder and kidney stones were extremely common medical disorders in the medieval world. Paracelsus was an unusual man who moved from city to city daily deriding his colleagues for their practice of mysticism and burning their books in the public squares; in the evening he caroused with the locals. As a brilliant maverick, he made many enemies and was stabbed to death in a tavern at Salzburg in 1541. Nevertheless, his rejection of the old notions of the four elements of earth, air, fire, and water was correct. However, his concept of forces of energy (archei) that governed the universe and maintained such physiologic processes as digestion proved erroneous.

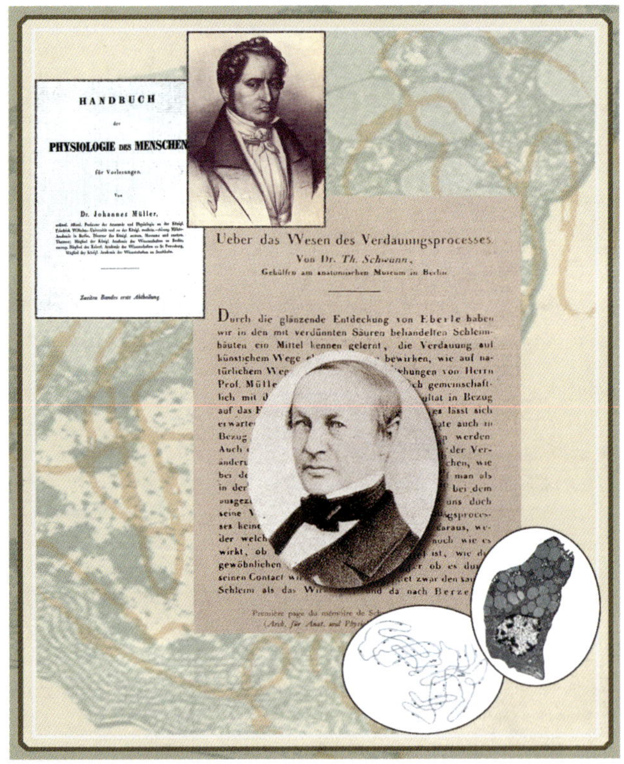

Figure 6. — Theodore Schwann (1810–1882) was a brilliant student who displayed an early aptitude for mathematics and physics. Educated as a Jesuit, Schwann (center) *studied medicine in Bonn and Wurzberg before joining the laboratory of Johannes Muller (1801–1858)* (top left) *in Berlin in 1834. In 1836, he identified a novel agent in gastric juice and named it "pepsin" after characterizing its digestive properties. Although Rudolph Heidenhain of Breslau had identified the cellular origin of secretory granules, it was John Newport Langley* (bottom right) *of Trinity College, Cambridge, who identified the cellular source and mechanism of pepsin secretion using salamanders. In 1930, Northrop was the first to crystallize pepsin and to determine its prolate ellipsoid structure* (bottom right).

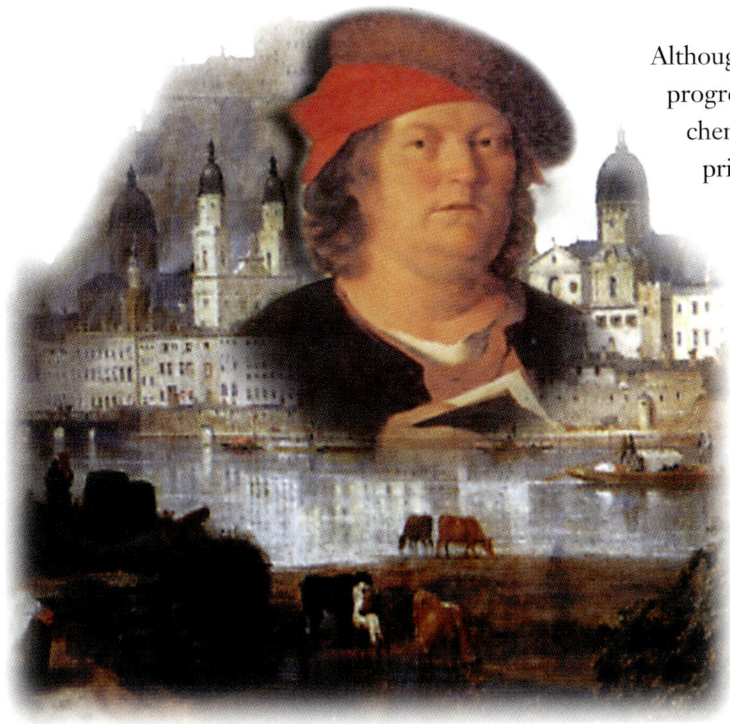

Figure 7. — Philippus Aureolus Theophrastus Bombastus von Hohenheim (Paracelsus) was born in Ensiedeln near Zurich in 1493. Assuming the role of a peripatetic alchemist-physician, he became a vociferous proponent of chemical pharmacology and therapeutics. To the discomfort of his colleagues, he insisted that the majority of medical doctrine was nonsense and demanded that extensive reform of medical thought be undertaken. Paracelsus believed that the stomach of humans contained an acid that was derived from the drinking of acidic spa waters (hungry acid) and that its action was necessary both for digestion and as part of a catalytic process to prevent the formation of precipitation and concretions within the body. The outspoken style and unpopular views expressed by Paracelsus resulted in his premature demise during a bar brawl at a tavern in Salzburg (background vista).

Although alchemists and chemiatrists had made progress in the identification of numerous chemical substances, the nature of the active principle of gastric juice and digestion was unresolved. Johann Tholle, who wrote under the pseudonym of a mythical 15th century monk, Basil Valentine, published extensively on ammonia, sulfuric acid, and sugar of lead. He is rumored to have identified hydrochloric acid by mixing oil of vitriol (sulfuric acid) with common salt.

In Leiden in the mid 17th century, Sylvius made considerable contributions to chemistry having learned from Glauber about the interaction of acids and alkalis. Ignoring Van Helmont's suggestions of a specific gastric ferment, he maintained that digestion took place in the stomach by saliva and that further digestion was due to intestinal juice. Leuret in Paris perpetuated this notion well into the early 19th century, as did such physiologists as Claude Bernard and François Magendie. Regnier de Graaf, an extraordinarily gifted pupil of Sylvius, generated pancreatic fistulae in dogs to study secretion and digestion at the behest of his mentor. Unfortunately, confusion with the pyloric caeca of the stomach of fish confused the anatomic assessment, and it was concluded that pancreatic juice was acidic. Nevertheless, de Graaf and Sylvius believed that bile and pancreatic acid in combination fermented and digested food.

Frustrated by their inability to resolve the digestive process on a purely chemical basis by iatrochemistry, physicians adopted a more mechanical form of thinking. As a result, a school of thought known as *Iatromathematics* arose, which proposed that digestion occurred as a result of the fixed consequences of the laws of physics. This group of physicians perceived that the entire body and its various functions could be explained on the basis of mechanical events and produced numerous examples and illustrations to support their view. Although such notions may be considered bizarre given the contemporary understanding of chemical doctrine, such formidable intellectuals as Descartes, Pitcairn, Borelli, Sanctorius, and Boerhaave firmly believed in these concepts. Boerhaave, however, was shrewd enough to hedge his bets and proposed that chemical activity comprised the initial phase followed by mechanical trituration to complete the process of digestion.

Giovanni Borelli, a Neapolitan mathematician, regarded all physiologic processes as mechanical and considered that a contracting muscle increased in bulk because of fermentation within its substance, which was initiated by liquid discharged into the muscle by nerves. His colleague, Giorgio Baglivi, who would later in his practice undertake the autopsy of Marcello Malpighi, was the first to determine the differences between smooth and striated muscle but somewhat lost his perspective of physiologic process. He pushed the mechanical allegory to the division of the human machine into innumerable smaller machines and thus likened the teeth to scissors, the chest to bellows, the stomach to a flask, the visceral glands to sieves, and the heart and vessels to a pump and aqueduct system.

Figure 8. — Regnier de Graaf (1641-1673) of Holland (bottom left) was one of the brilliant young men who flocked to study medicine with François de la Boe-Dubois (Sylvius) at Leiden. Sylvius considered that pancreatic juice was the main factor in the digestive process and so intrigued de Graaf with his theories of "concoction" that he undertook to resolve the issue. Using novel techniques to develop experimental pancreatic fistulas (top right), *de Graaf concluded that pancreatic juice was acid in character, and both he and Sylvius hypothesized that bile and pancreatic juice in combination fermented and digested food. Unfortunately, contamination of the duodenopancreatic fistulae with gastric contents produced an erroneous result. This was further compounded by de Graaf's dissection of the stomachs of fishes* (bottom right) *that contained numerous pyloric caeca whose conglomerate mass was mistaken as part of the pancreatic ductular system. Despite his misunderstanding of the nature of pancreatic secretion as acid, de Graaf's contributions to experimental pancreatic physiology were prodigious and only exceeded by his subsequent unique contributions to the study of ovarian structure and function. His premature death from an intestinal infection deprived science of a perceptive and prescient intellect.*

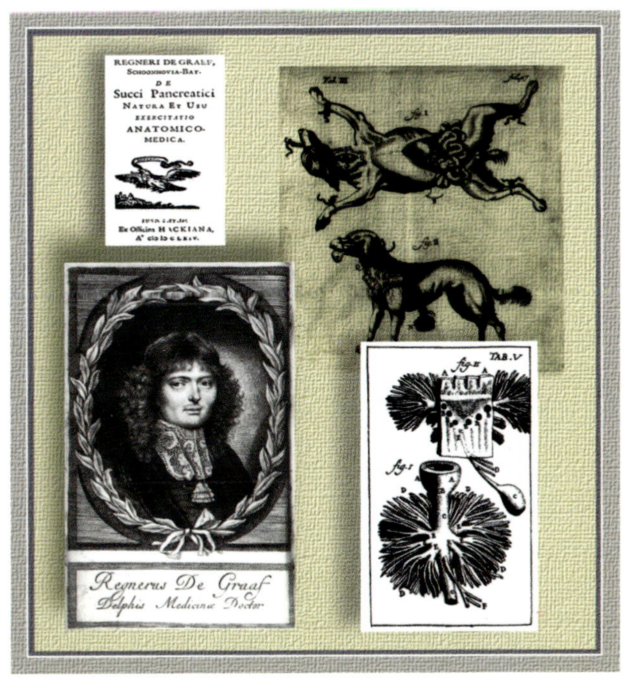

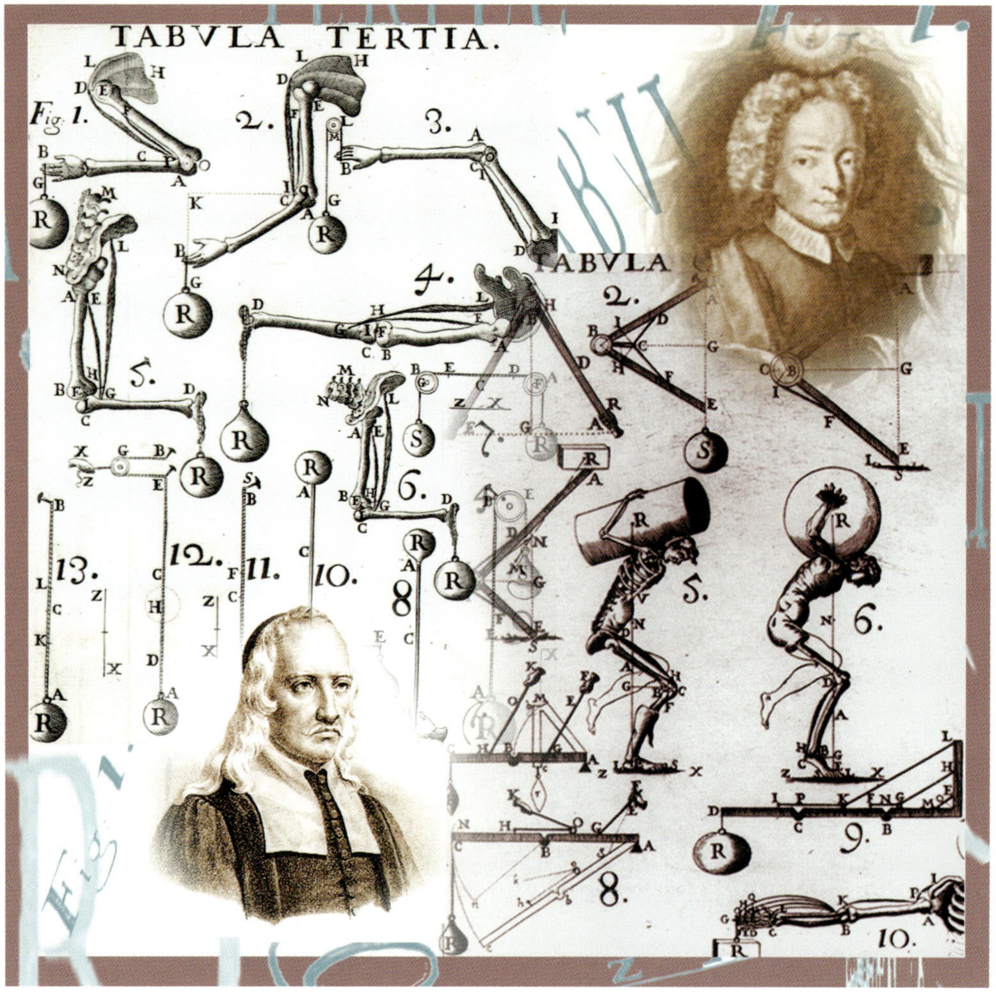

Figure 9. — The Iatromathematical School maintained that all physiologic events should be regarded as fixed consequences of the laws of physics. Thus, the stomach was regarded as a mechanical mill responsible for grinding up its contents into chyme. Giorgio Baglivi (1668-1706) (top right) was a pupil of Malpighi and the Chairman of Medical Theory at the Collegio Della Sapienza in Rome. In 1700, he was the first to distinguish between smooth and striated muscle. Baglivi referred to the stomach as a flask that possessed the muscular power of grinding food to facilitate digestion. His views were closely supported by G. A. Borelli (1608-1679) (bottom left) who, despite being a pupil of the enlightened Galileo, applied an extreme mechanistic view of human function to the process of digestion. The Iatromechanists considered that all human function could be interpreted within physical principles as an allegory of pistons, pulleys, weights, and joints. Garrison considered that "they pushed the mechanical allegory to the extent that divided the human machine into innumerable smaller machines: likened the teeth to scissors, the chest to a bellows, the stomach to a flask, the viscera and glands to sieves, and the heart and vessels to a waterworks." Archibald Pitcairn, although a staunch proponent of the iatromathematical point of view, was concerned as to why the stomach when it digested food failed to digest itself. Did he perhaps dream of an acid and a barrier?

Archibald Pitcairn, an iatromathematist who trained with Boerhaave before returning to Edinburgh, asked the most perceptive questions relating to the stomach. His question is still to a large part unanswered. First posed in 1727, we still question "why upon the digestion of food upon the stomach, which is easily as digestible as the food itself, yet the stomach itself should not be dissolved?"

By the end of the 17th century, there were two main schools of thought regarding the nature of digestion. The first believed that digestion was an act of trituration, and the second group believed that it reflected fermentation that was either due to an internal property of the food itself or agents secreted by the lining of the stomach. Early experiments with vegetable dyes allowed for the primitive understanding of acids or alkalis. In 1692, Viridet noted that a tincture of heliotrope, which turned red in the presence of acid, produced a remarkable coloration of the stomach but remained blue in the esophagus. His work was amplified by Réaumur, the French naturalist, who noted, in studies of his pet buzzard, that gastric juice also turned blue heliotrope red.

In a subsequent series of imaginative studies, Réaumur trained his buzzard to swallow small metal tubes containing sponges and used these to recover the gastric juice. He determined that this fluid prevented meat from corruption and that extracorporeal digestion of food was to some extent dependent on the temperature of the recovered gastric juice. Almost a decade later, Henry Gosse, unexcited by the studies of buzzards and sparrows turned a childhood habit of aerophagy and self-emesis into a tool of physiologic investigation. By inducing emesis at specific times after eating, he was able to demonstrate a time curve for digestion. Although his studies failed to reveal the presence of acid or alkaline gastric juice, he did, however, propose that secretion might occur by a mechanical process by which food stretched the internal lining of the stomach. Gosse may thus be regarded as the first to indirectly suggest the role of antral distension in activating gastric secretion.

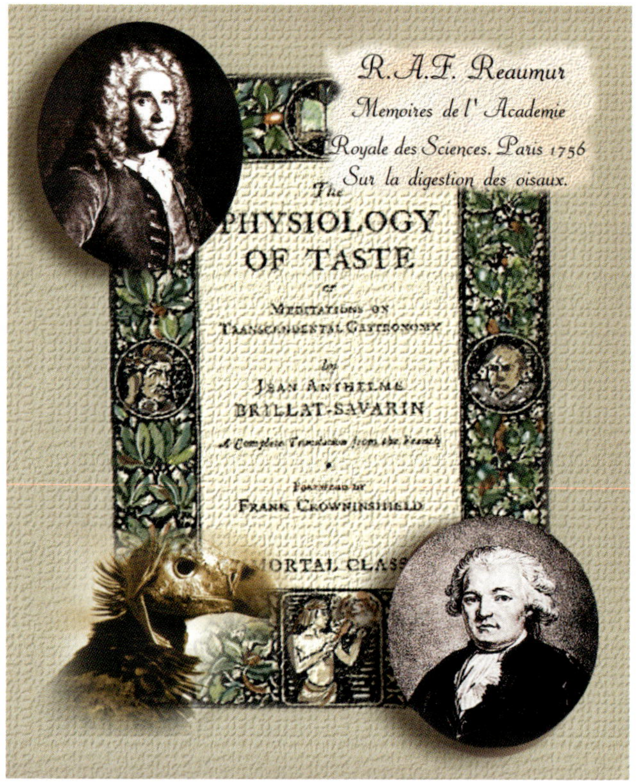

Figure 10. — The French were considerably interested in digestion both at a scientific and epicurean level. R.A.F. Réaumur (1683–1757) (top left) studied the digestion of birds, particularly his own pet buzzard, (bottom left), in detail and concluded that their stomachs secreted acid that was necessary for digestion. The premature demise of his experimental model resulted in Réaumur's loss of interest in the subject of digestion, and he thereafter turned his skills to the development of a novel technique for strengthening steel. Anthelme Brillat-Savarin (1755–1826) (bottom right) studied digestion and its effect on the higher senses by compiling an exotic compendium of culinary information and dining etiquette. His reflections on the physiology of taste background and the relationship of food to human behavior are still regarded as definitive among those who believe that the gut–brain axis is modulated and amplified by a malolactic acid transduction system.

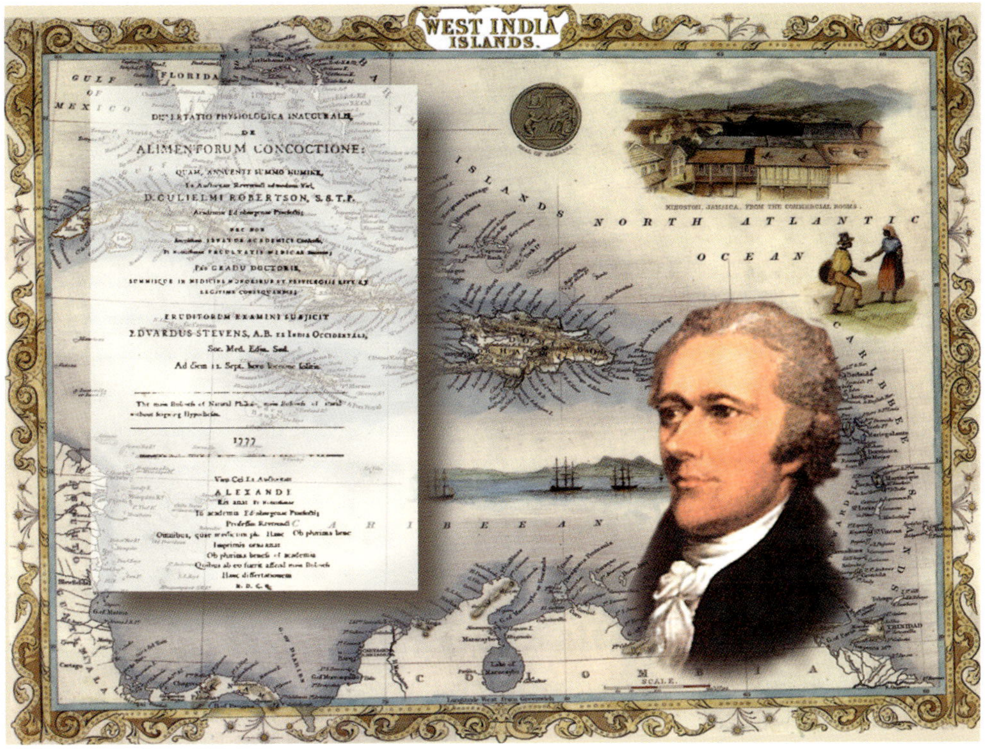

Figure 11. — Edward Stevens (1755–1804) was the presumed illegitimate half brother of Alexander Hamilton, the Secretary of the Treasury (bottom right). *Both had been born and raised on the island of St. Croix in the Caribbean Leeward Islands before seeking their fortunes elsewhere. Stevens graduated from King's College in New York (now Columbia University) in 1774 and thereafter pursued his further medical studies in Edinburgh from 1775. During this time, he became President of the Edinburgh Medical Student Society and wrote one of the first theses* (De Alimentorum Concoctione), *which accurately described the process of digestion. It was dedicated to Alexander Tertius Monro, who was the last member of a family that had held the Chair of Anatomy at Edinburgh for 126 consecutive years (1720–1846). After returning to the United States, Stevens became Professor of Medicine at Columbia University but soon thereafter lost interest in academia and accepted the position of Consul General to the island of Santo Domingo. After his early contributions to the science of digestion, Stevens failed to further pursue an investigative career, choosing rather to follow in the political footsteps of his brother. His description of the course of digestion in the peripatetic hussar remained a classic until William Beaumont's studies of Alexis St. Martin.*

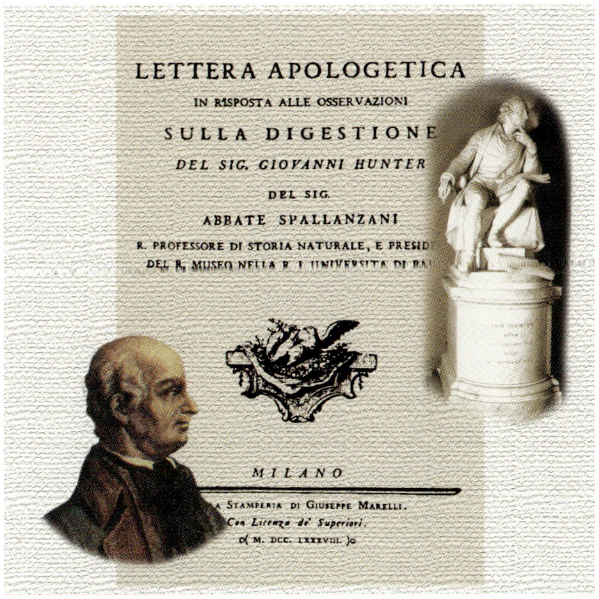

Figure 12. — The Jesuit abbot, Lazzaro Spallanzani (1729-1799) (bottom left) *was Professor of Physics and Mathematics at the College of San Carlo in Modena. Over the course of his life, he undertook important studies on the gastric secretion of a wide variety of animals and concluded that digestion was a chemical process dependent on both the digestive power of saliva as well as the solvent properties of gastric juice. His recognition that the process of gastric digestion was not due to putrefaction but represented an active process was an important contribution. In collaboration with Professor Carminati of Pavia, and the chemist Scopoli, Spallanzani was able to conclude that gastric juice from crows contained "pure water, some soapy and gelatinous animal substances ...and that the gastric juice distinctly turned tincture of heliotrope red." John Hunter* (right), *whose comments on digestion in Observations on Certain Parts of the Animal Oeconomy (London, 1786) were translated into Italian by Antonio Scarpa, evoked a sharp response from the abbot who assumed divine support for his digestive position. Their disagreement as to the presence or absence of acid in the gastric juice and whether the process of digestion required heat was finally resolved amicably in the form of a polemic letter* (background) *addressed to Leopoldo Caldani, was published in Milan in 1788. Presumably, the limited nature of the chemical techniques available to both resulted in a misunderstanding that was subsequently resolved by mutual agreement.*

A notable contribution of this era derived from the work of Edward Stevens of the West Indies, who had been sent to Edinburgh to further his medical studies. Stevens was the illegitimate half brother of Alexander Hamilton, the Secretary of the Treasury, and was possessed of the same high intellectual faculties. He became the President of the Edinburgh Medical Student Society, and his dissertation on digestion in 1777 *(De Alimentorum Concoction)* was a masterpiece of logical deduction and creative experimental work. In Edinburgh, Stevens acquired the services of a visiting Hungarian hussar whose livelihood was generated by swallowing stones and then regurgitating for the entertainment of the populace. Using perforated silver spheres constructed to hold meats, vegetables, worms, and leeches, Stevens observed that all were digested when passed through the rectum. Although he did not use a sponge and thus did not attempt to extract gastric juice and evaluate the presence of acid, he was the first to develop an orderly understanding of the nature of digestion.

In 1780, in Pavia, Italy, Lazaro Spallanzani, a professor of natural history, performed similar experiments on himself and many different kinds of animals to identify the nature of digestion. He could find no evidence of fermentation and proposed that digestion involved either an acid or a putrefactive principle. His personal observations that the ingestion of large quantities of strawberries and wine interfered with sleep by producing severe irritation from the stomach accompanied by a sharp and acidic taste may be regarded as the first definitive description of nocturnal reflux. A subsequent collaboration with Scopoli, professor of chemistry at Pavia, led to the conclusion that there was not only acid in the stomach but that it was probably hydrochloric. Unfortunately, the fact that the subjects studied in these experiments included ruminants and regurgitors produced confusing results. Therefore, Spallanzani and, Scopoli's peers did not accept a definitive conclusion. Nevertheless, a contemporary evaluation of their data leaves little doubt that they had not only identified an acidic agent but that it almost certainly was hydrochloric acid. Disagreements in this area of physiology were significant, and there were tense exchanges among individual scientists.

Thus, John Hunter and Spallanzani engaged in an acrimonious correspondence regarding Hunter's vacillation as to whether there was acid or not present in the stomach of humans. Indeed, one of the greatest intellectuals of the 18th century, Albrecht von Haller (1708-1777), from his lofty ivory tower in Göttingen, proclaimed that gastric juice was neither acid, alkaline, nor a ferment and that any acid found in the gastric juice arose from the degeneration of food. He proposed that the chief digestive agent was bile and that its function was to digest fat. Given that Haller had produced a Chaldean grammar at the age of 10 and a Latin poetry book at age 6, followed by 13,000 scientific papers and the definitive text on the physiology of the human body, his thoughts were considered authoritative at that time.

Figure 13. — William Prout (1785-1850) (right) *was born on in Horton, a remote village of Gloucestershire, England. Having studied at Guy's Hospital in London, he became a member of the Royal College of Physicians as well as a fellow of the Royal Medical Chirurgical Society. On December 11, 1823, at the Royal Society of Medicine, he presented his landmark paper "On the Nature of Acid and Saline Matters Usually Existing in the Stomach of Animals"* (left)*. Prout identified hydrochloric acid in the gastric juice of numerous species, including humans, and quantified free and total hydrochloric (muriatic) acid* (bottom)*. In addition, he related the amount of acid to the degree of dyspepsia and also proposed that chloride was secreted from the blood to the lumen by electrical means. In this hypothesis, Prout proposed (more than a century before it could be confirmed) that when gastric acid was secreted, the blood would become alkaline (postprandial alkaline tide). Apart from his definitive resolution of the nature of gastric acid, Prout was the first to propose that the atomic weights of all elements would be multiples of that of hydrogen (Prout's Hypothesis). A further major contribution to the science of gastroenterology was his classification, in 1827, of foods into the subgroups of carbohydrates (saccharinous), fats (oleaginous), and proteins (albuminous) for which he was awarded the Copley Medal.*

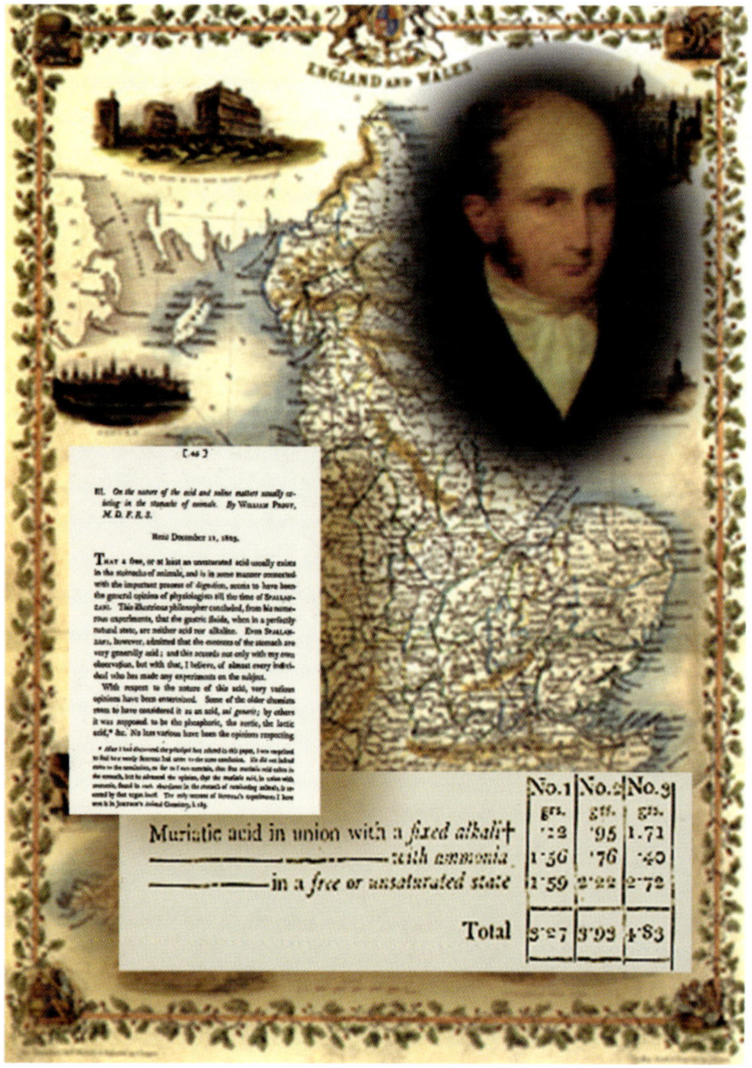

The resolution of the identification of the acid contained in gastric juice would fall to William Prout in 1823. Having made contributions in the fields of meteorology, physiology, clinical medicine, and chemistry, Prout finally turned his attention to the investigation of the nature of the acid in the stomach. No doubt, the endless pontification of quacks and homeopaths induced this impeccable scientist to address the question. On December 11, 1823, at the Royal Society of London, Prout delivered his landmark paper, "On the Nature of Acid and Saline Matters, Usually Existing in the Stomach of Animals." The presentation was unique in two ways: Prout had specifically identified hydrochloric acid in the gastric juice of numerous species, including man, dog, rabbit, horse, cat, and hare, and he was able to quantify the free and total hydrochloric acid and chloride.

The acid was measured by neutralization with a potash solution of known strength and the chloride by titration with silver nitrate. So advanced were his ideas, that he proposed that chloride may be secreted from the blood to the lumen by electrical means and that when gastric acid was secreted the blood would become alkaline (now recognized as the postprandial alkaline tide). More than 100 years were to elapse before this elegant electrochemical theory was confirmed. Prout had obtained his human specimens from the most eminent of British surgeons, Astley Poston Cooper (1768-1841) of Guy's Hospital. In his records, Prout noted that the amount of acid measured in the gastric juice obtained from these patients

Figure 14. — Astley Poston Cooper (1768-1841) was a distant relative of Sir Isaac Newton, and his uncle, William Cooper, was the senior surgeon at Guy's Hospital. After a period of study with John Hunter, Cooper soon became regarded as the greatest surgeon and teacher of his time. Although quick tempered and imperious, his sartorial elegance, keen intellect, and remarkable surgical skills earned him widespread respect and admiration. Cooper became a luminary of the Royal College of Surgeons of England (top left)*, and his lectures formed the basis for much surgical education of the time. He was particularly forceful in applying the dictum that "operating is not all a surgeon ought to know "and insisted that "without knowledge it is impossible to adopt a proper remedy." It was Cooper who provided the gastric juice from his patients at Guy's Hospital* (bottom) *for Prout to analyze. In so doing he thus facilitated the initial identification of hydrochloric acid in humans.*

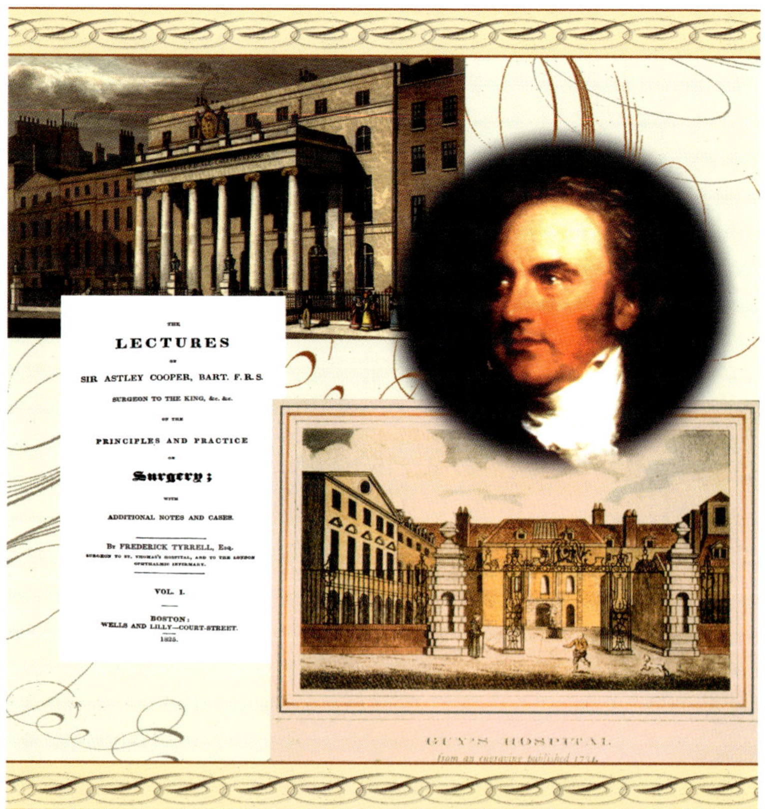

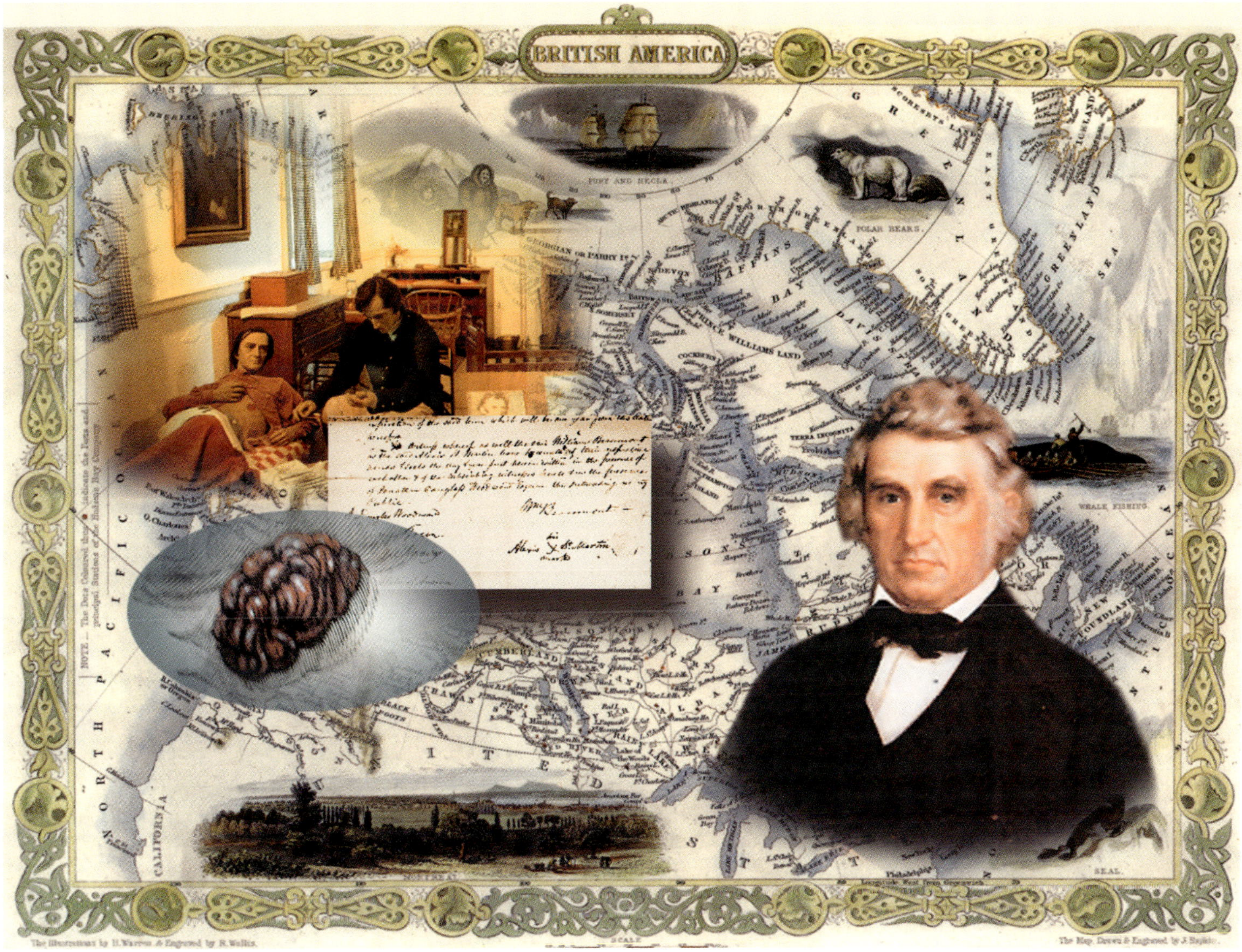

Figure 15. *— William Beaumont* (right) *was born on November 25, 1785, in Lebanon, Connecticut, and at the age of 22 began his study of medicine. During the War of 1812, he accepted a position in the army as an acting surgeon's mate and thereafter returned to civilian life. In 1819, after a brief spell in practice, his former colleague, Joseph Lovell, who had now become Surgeon General, offered Beaumont a commission, and he was assigned to Fort Mackinac on the Island of Michel Mackinac at the junction of Lake Huron and Lake Michigan. It was here at Jacob Astor's fur trading store on June 6, 1822, that Beaumont first encountered the 19-year-old voyager, Alexis St. Martin, who had been accidentally shot in the left upper abdomen and chest. On being summoned to see the critically injured patient, Beaumont remarked "the man can not live 36 hours; I will come and see him by and by." Fortunately for gastric science, Beaumont was able to save St. Martin's life, and after 10 months his wounds were all healed except for a gastric fistula* (left). *Curious as to the nature of gastric function, Beaumont thereafter undertook a series of studies on the gastric fistula of St. Martin* (left). *This work would subsequently become the scientific foundation of gastric physiology and secure for Beaumont recognition as the pioneer physiologist of the United States. Because St. Martin was a difficult patient and a relatively uncooperative experimental subject, Beaumont secured a contract* (center) *to ensure St. Martin's continuous participation. Despite his lack of training as a physiologist and his relatively unsophisticated medical background, by 1833, Beaumont produced a classic text on the gastric function:* Gastric Juice and the Physiology of Digestion. *As Beaumont had no expertise in chemistry, he collaborated with Robley Dunglison (Professor of Medicine in Virginia) and Benjamin Silliman (Professor of Chemistry at Yale College) in establishing the presence of free hydrochloric acid in the gastric juice of St. Martin. Dr. Born, in 1913, elegantly framed the contributions of William Beaumont: "Every physician who prescribes for digestive disorders, and every patient who has benefited by such as prescription, owes gratitude to the memory of William Beaumont who in 1825 on the Island of Mackinaw began his studies on digestion, which he pursued with labor and skill for the benefit of mankind."*

was greater in those patients with more severe degrees of dyspepsia. Thus, Prout is owed the credit not only for the identification of hydrochloric acid in the stomach and its quantification, but the recognition that the clinical symptom of dyspepsia bears a relation to the level of acid.

William Beaumont of Lebanon, Connecticut, was far removed from the London and Edinburgh medical societies. Trained in a modest medical apprenticeship without benefit of a medical school, he was a member of the United States military at Fort Mackinac on the Canadian frontier. Fort Mackinac was a territorial outpost of the army and also functioned as a trading post where trappers brought furs to Jacob Astor's first business venture. It was at Fort Mackinac that Beaumont met Alexis St. Martin, a French-Canadian boatman responsible for transporting fur cargoes along the Great Lakes of Huron and Michigan to the depôts for sale.

The accidental discharge of a musket resulted in a penetrating injury through St. Martin's stomach and left chest, and Beaumont was called to save the French–Canadian's life. Despite all initial pronouncements of a probable early death, St. Martin's life was saved; his wounds healed, leaving a gastric fistula. This provided Beaumont with the opportunity to become the first practitioner to scientifically study the physiology of human digestion. Beaumont, although devoid of formal scientific and chemical training, used this situation to define gastric secretion. Dunglison of Virginia and Silliman of Yale University, who helped him both with the design of experiments and the measurement of the gastric acid, ably assisted in this endeavor. The extraordinary contributions of Beaumont, published in 1829 as *The Physiology of Digestion*, are to this day regarded as representative of the highest level of physiologic experimentation. Indeed, the doyen of 20th century medicine, William Osler, was to write the following of Beaumont:

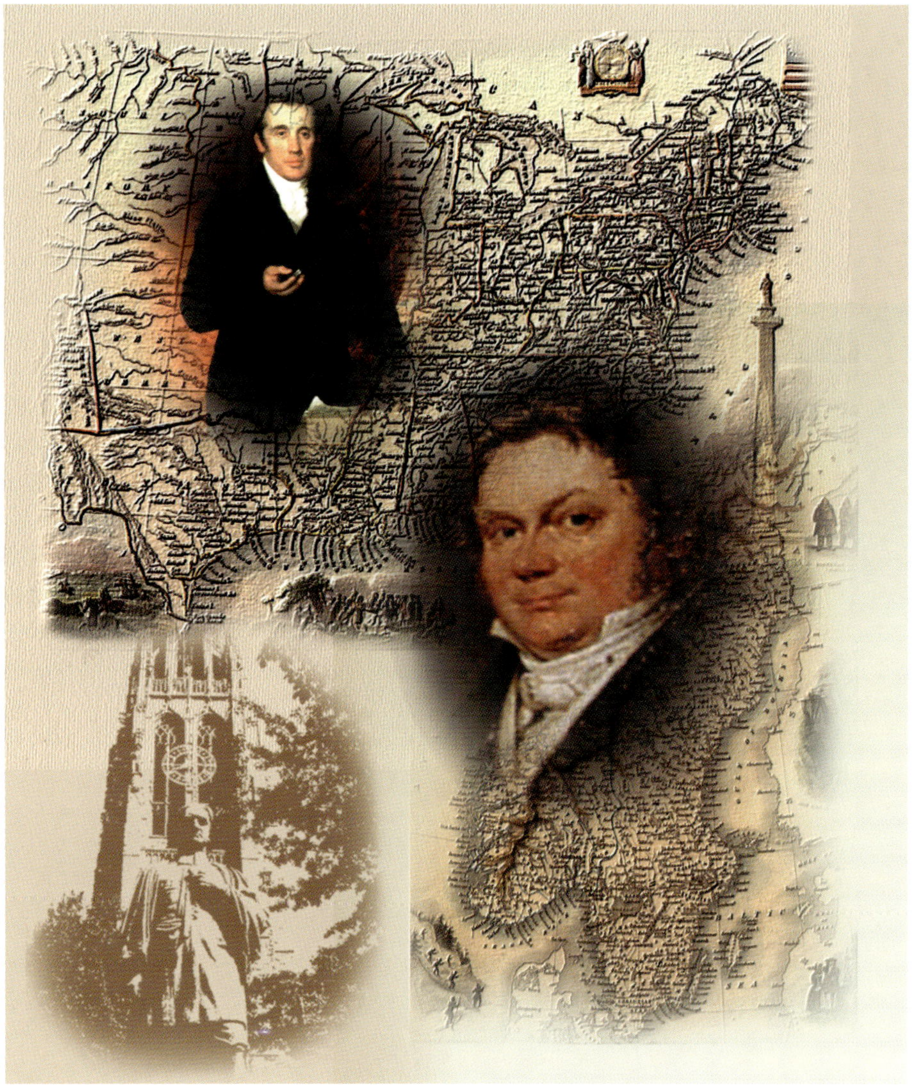

Figure 16. — Although William Beaumont possessed the intellectual curiosity and perspicacity to use the gastric fistula of St. Martin to study digestion, he possessed few scientific skills with which to address the task. To support his endeavors, he secured the support of Robley Dunglison (1798-1869), Professor of Medicine in Virginia, who had initially come to the United States from Edinburgh University at the invitation of President Jefferson. Dunglison was trained in chemistry and thus successfully identified the presence of hydrochloric acid in the gastric juice of St. Martin. In addition, he suggested a number of useful experiments and proposed that Beaumont collaborate with Benjamin Silliman (top left), *Professor of Chemistry at Yale College. Silliman duly confirmed the presence of free hydrochloric acid in the gastric juice but thought that a definitive opinion should be sought from the most eminent chemist of the day, J. Berzelius of Stockholm* (bottom right). *Silliman thus arranged for Beaumont to send a sample of gastric juice to Berzelius via the diplomatic courier of the Swedish ambassador in New York. Unfortunately, Berzelius never adequately analyzed the sample, pleading problems initially with work overload, then summer heat, and finally inadequate support personnel. As he had already adjudged that gastric juice contained lactic acid, it is likely that he was not keen to confirm his own error. Silliman's diaries clearly indicate that he suffered from a duodenal ulcer, and the statue of Abraham Pierson, the first rector of Yale* (bottom left) *suggests evidence of retrosternal burning discomfort.*

> The man was greater than his work...the pioneer physiologist of the United States and the first to make a contribution of enduring value, his work remains a model of patient, persevering research. The highest praise that we can give is to say that his life fulfilled the idea with which he set out, and which he so well expressed in the sentence: "truth, like beauty is when unadorned adorn the most and in prosecuting these experiments and inquiries, I believe I have been guided by its light."

The first serious physiologic experimentation thus undertaken in the United States was by William Beaumont in the field of gastric physiology.

The studies performed by Beaumont were particularly noteworthy. Although patients with gastric fistulas had been previously identified and studied in Europe, there was little serious advance in the understanding of gastric digestion. In 1797, Jacob Helm of Vienna studied Theresa Petz of Breitenwaida, generating a meticulous review of her digestion, intragastric temperature, and salivary function. Little novel information had been acquired; however, Helm astutely used himself and his brother, as well as a hired person, Zyriak Sieddeler, as controls for the studies. Similarly, in 1801, Rouilly in France had transferred his patient, Madeline Gore — who had sustained a traumatic gastric fistula — to the care of Dupuytren and Bichat in Paris. After studying her gastric juice, Clarion, professor of chemistry, concluded that French gastric juice was identical to saliva.

By the middle of the 19th century, Beaumont had confirmed Prout's work on hydrochloric acid in the United States as well as Friedrich Tiedemann and Leopold Gmelin's work in Germany. Nevertheless, some great scientists, including Bernard, Magendie, and Berzelius, considered lactic acid to be the active principle of gastric juice. John Richard Young, in Philadelphia, marred some fine work on digestive physiology by concluding that gastric acid was phosphoric acid. After the work of Tiedemann and Gmelin, even Berzelius of Sweden, recognized as the greatest organic chemist of the time, accepted the work of the unlettered American frontier physician and concurred that hydrochloric acid was the correct answer.

Regulation of Secretion

Having concluded that the stomach produced acid, considerable debate now ensued as to the regulation of its secretion. The late 19th century was consumed with the belief that the brain and nerves controlled both health and disease and Ivan Pavlov of Russia became a proponent of "nervism." Over a period of more than three decades, Pavlov and his colleagues, including Dolinsky and Klemensiewicz, undertook a series of complex and elegant canine studies using nerve resection, gastric pouches, and antral transpositions. These culminated in Pavlov's confirmation of a pivotal role of the central nervous system and the vagus nerve in the regulation of gastric secretion. Such observations agreed with the clinical doctrine of the time that held dyspepsia to be an abdominal problem of "nervous" or cerebral origin.

The vagus or "wandering nerve" had first been described by the Roman anatomist Marinus and thereafter accorded validity by Galen, who identified its relationship to "the nerve of the voice" and regarded it as an important structure, although he failed to recognize its gastric relevance. Further elegant delineation of its complex course by Vesalius had done little to elucidate its function, although some inklings of its action must have derived from the acquisition of an alternative name: the pneumogastric nerve. The award of a Nobel Prize validated the conclusions of Pavlov and his colleagues, and the doctrine of the neural regulation of acid secretion became widely accepted. Scientists as diverse as Rokitansky of Vienna and McCrea in Manchester claimed that gastroduodenal ulceration was due to neural dysfunction. McCrea even proposed that "local spasm with resultant anemia is a probable cause of the chronicity of ulcer aided by factors such as retention and infection set up by reflex spasm." Raymond Latarjet of Lyons, France adopted a different approach and empirically severed the abdominal vagal nerves, believing that the reduction in secretion of acid would result in healing of ulcers of the stomach and duodenum. Although he was correct in this supposition, he was unaware of the consequent deleterious effects on pyloric and antral function that engendered delayed gastric emptying and necessitated a drainage procedure or gastrojejunostomy. Out of the subsequent widespread adoption of vagotomy (the gastric surgical equivalent of prefrontal lobotomy) arose an entire corpus of surgical literature attesting to the innumerable permutations and commutations of pyloroplasties available for management of this adverse effect of gastric denervation.

Dissatisfied with the concept of neural regulation as the sole source of functional control of the digestive system, William Maddock Bayliss and his brother-in-law, Ernest Starling, addressed the issue of secretory control from a different direction. On January 16, 1901, in an epic experiment conducted at University College, London, they demonstrated the existence of a chemical messenger in the mucosa of the duodenum that would activate pancreatic secretion. This first identification of a non-neural mechanism of secretory regulation led to the formulation of the concept of a hormone and the subsequent development of the discipline of endocrinology.

By extrapolation of the work of Bayliss and Starling, John Edkins of London proposed that a similar agent was present in the gastric antrum and was responsible for the regulation of gastric acid secretion. His early work, conducted under the supervision of the neurophysiologist Sherrington, led to compelling evidence of the existence of an antral chemical messenger capable of stimulating fundic acid secretion. Following Starling's lead in naming the duodenal secretagogue as "secretin," Edkins proposed that the gastric agent be named *gastrin*. Unfortunately, the intellectual doyens of the time, including Sir Henry Hallett Dale, were obsessed with the notion of histamine and acetylcholine as the principal regulators and dismissed his theory as humbug, with the result that both Edkins and his novel proposal fell into scientific disfavor.

Apart from his fundamental observations regarding gastrin, Edkins had also worked with Langley on pepsin and had also described the presence of spiral bacteria in the gastric mucosa. Despite the frustration of the rejection of his gastrin hypothesis, Edkins persevered and established the first training program for women physiologists in England, became a notable oarsman for Cambridge, and was elected president of the British Croquet Association. It is rumored that some 40 years later, at a lecture at which Simon Komarov presented the definitive chemical evidence that gastrin existed, Edkins'

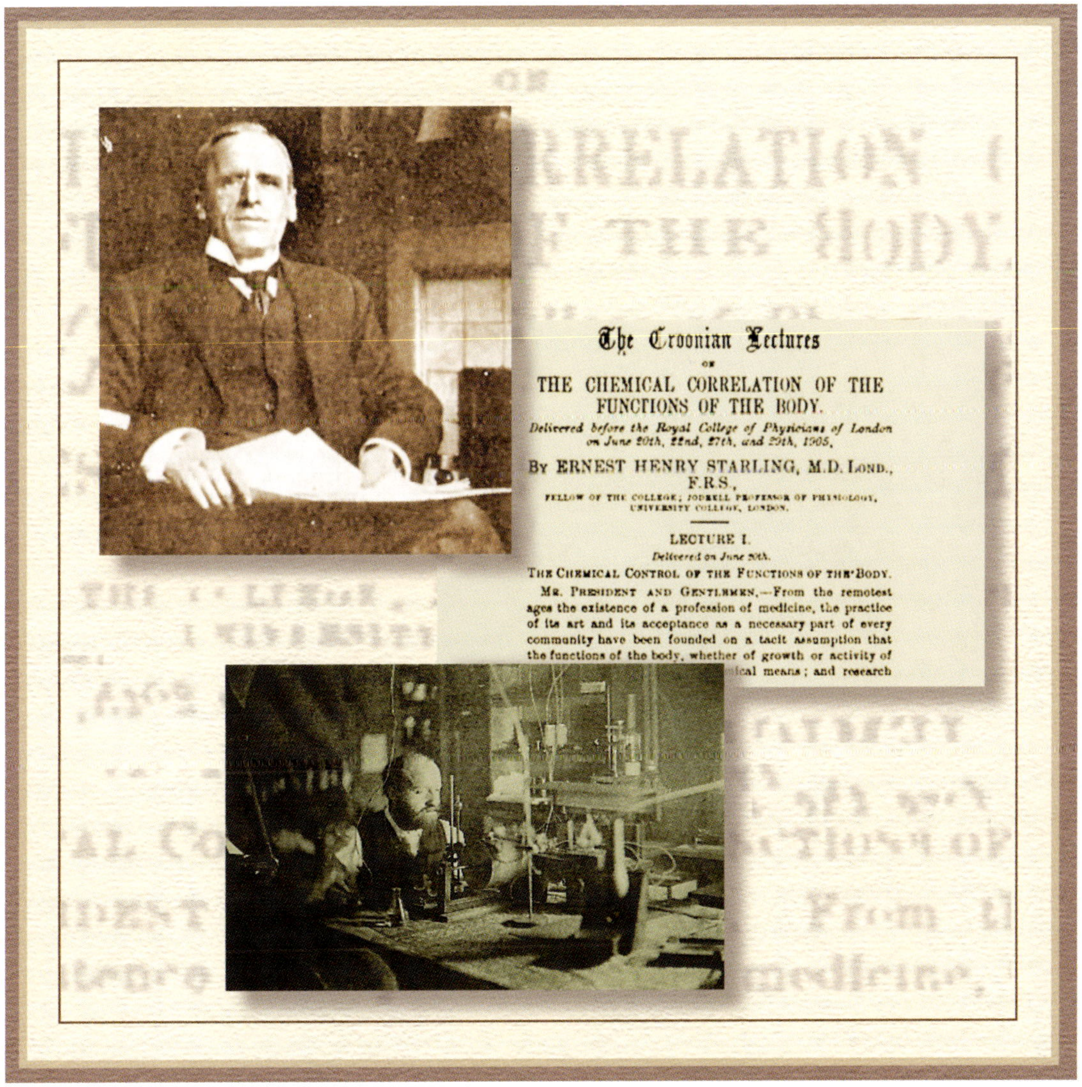

Figure 17. *— Ernest Henry Starling (1866-1927)* (top) *was a scientific pluralist of extraordinary intellectual vigor. His studies helped resolve the regulation of pancreatic function, lymph formation, peristalsis, and led to the enunciation of "the law of the heart." On January 16, 1901, at University College London, with Starling and William Bayliss (his brother in law)* (bottom), *he demonstrated that acid liberated a chemical messenger from cells of the duodenum and jejunal mucosa that stimulated pancreatic secretion. In 1905, Starling presented this epic observation as a Croonian lecture before the Royal College of Physicians of London. The title "The Chemical Correlation of the Functions of the Body" documented the first report of the existence of a chemical messenger system and thus laid the foundation of the modern discipline of endocrinology. Starling subsequently used William Hardy's original proposal of the word hormone to characterize such a messenger. In propounding the chemical messenger system, Starling conceived of an alternative to Pavlov's concept of nervism and fundamentally altered the physiologic dogma of the time. Starling also stated in his lecture that "chemical means" could control not only "activity" but also "growth." Thus, the concept of a chemical messenger responsible for not only secretion but also trophic activity, and even healing was first enunciated almost a century ago.*

tion of Popielski's work, which was not presented until 1920, when Ernst Rothlin of Zurich also concluded that although a stimulant of acid secretion, histamine was not a powerful stimulant of pepsin. Dale was subsequently awarded the Nobel Prize for his research in the area of acetylcholine and his general contributions toward the understanding of histamine function. On April 26, 1962, at a meeting in New York, chaired by Simon Komorov,

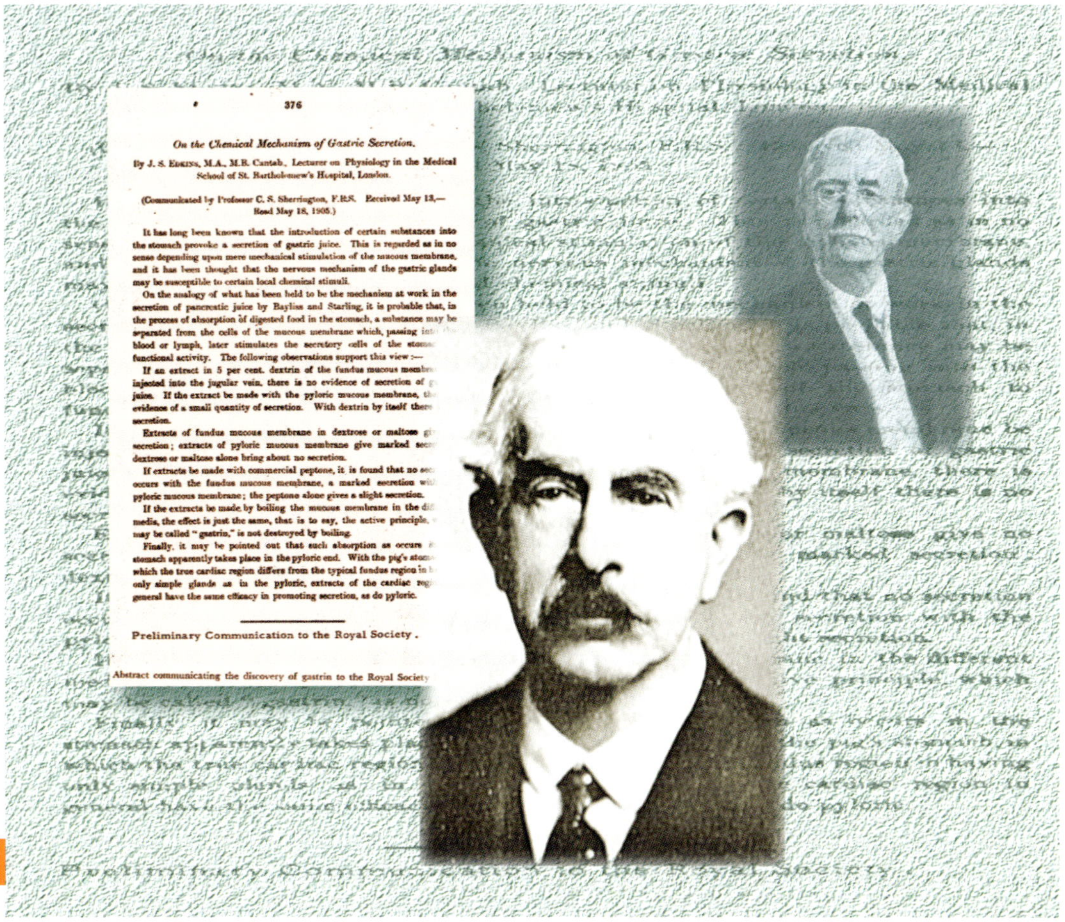

17

Figure 18. — On May 18, 1905, John Sydney Edkins (1863-1910) (center) *provided a preliminary communication to the Royal Society of Medicine in London that was read by his mentor, Professor C. S. Sherrington* (top right). *The modest paper* (left), *entitled "On the Chemical Mechanisms of Gastric Secretion," proposed the regulation of gastric acid by a substance ("a gastric secretin") that Edkins proposed be known as gastrin. The subsequent adverse reaction of the scientific cognoscenti of the day to the novel proposal of Edkins led Sherrington to disassociate himself from this work and pursue studies in neurophysiology, for which he subsequently received a Nobel Prize.*

wife, Nora Tweedy, was present. In thanking Komarov for the posthumous vindication of her husband's discovery, she told him "John (Edkins) never doubted that gastrin was a true hormone!"

Three decades later in 1938, Simon Komorov successfully documented that gastrin existed as a chemical entity separate from histamine and vindicated the work of John Edkins. Although Dale had worked extensively in the area of pharmacologic and physiologic actions of histamine between 1910 and 1927, he had utterly failed to detect its role in promoting gastric acid secretion. This honor would fall to Leon Popielski, a student of Pavlov's, who, on October 28, 1916, in Lemberg, demonstrated that beta-imidazolylethylamine acted directly on gastric glands to stimulate acid secretion, as neither vagal nerve section nor atropine abolished its effect. The First World War interfered with the publica-

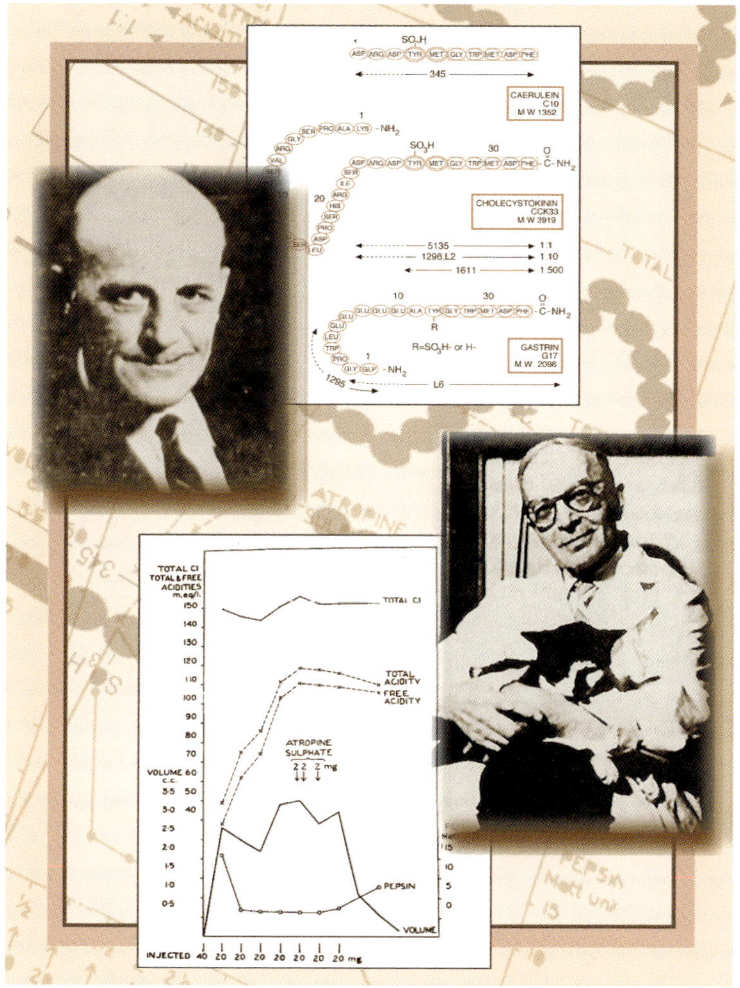

Figure 19. — Simon Komarov (bottom) *spent 3 years (1910-1913) in the laboratory of Pavlov at St. Petersburg, Russia, before moving to North America. His initial studies in conjunction with Babkin at McGill University finally led to the isolation and identification of the nonhistamine acid stimulatory extract of the antrum as gastrin* (bottom center). *"In all cases, without exception, the pyloric preparation injected in quantities equal to 5 gm of mucosa elicited a copious secretion of gastric juice, which was characterized by high acidity, low peptic power, and which was not effected by atropine even in large doses." In 1962, Rod Gregory* (top left) *and Hilda Tracey, working in conjunction with G. W. Kenner, identified the chemical structure of gastrin* (top center). *To obtain adequate material for the purification, they studied 600 hog antrums weekly for 6 months from a local manufacturer of pork pies. In the course of their elucidation of the structure of gastrin, they noted that it existed in multiple forms and proposed that such structural variations might have biologic implications.*

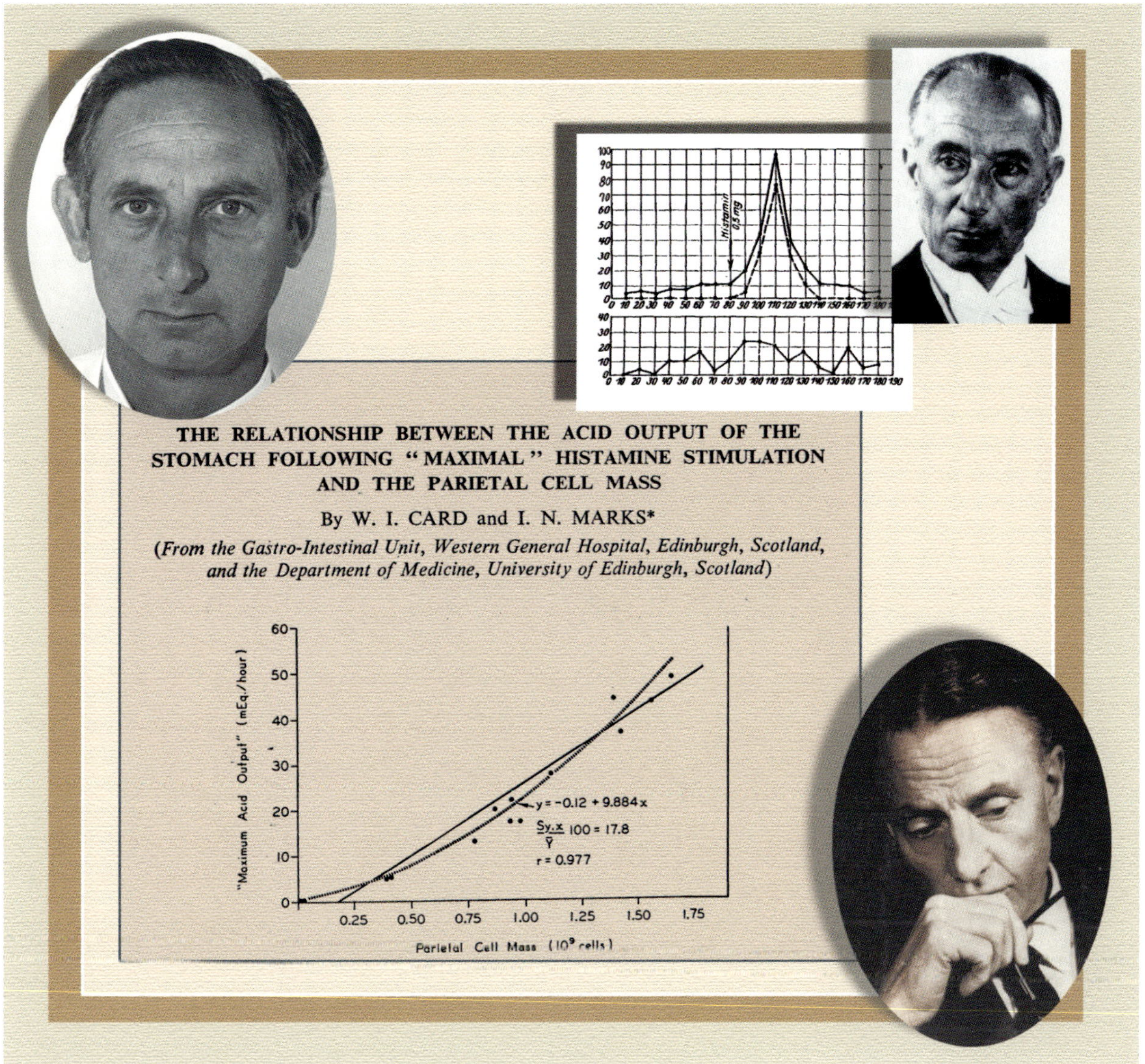

Figure 20. — *The establishment of the role of acid in the genesis of peptic ulceration was supported by studies undertaken jointly by I. N. Marks* (top left) *and W. Card* (bottom right) *of Capetown and Edinburgh, respectively, who concluded that acid secretion was a function of parietal cell mass. They established that histamine stimulation that had been introduced by Gerhardt Katsch (1887-1961) of Marburg* (top right) *could be used to assess the function of the parietal cell mass. This work facilitated the recognition that acid output, parietal cell mass, and peptic ulceration were inextricably linked. As a result of these physiopathologic observations, a rational basis was provided for the consideration of acid reduction — initially surgically and subsequently by pharmacotherapeutic means — as a definitive intervention in the management of acid peptic disease.*

Rod Gregory of Liverpool announced that he had identified the amino acid composition of gastrin and subsequently demonstrated that the purified agent stimulated acid secretion.

John Edkins died before it became apparent that gastrin was a pivotal agent in the regulation not only of gastric secretion but trophic regulation of the entire gastrointestinal tract. An appraisal of this prescient scientist's later work reveals that he had identified a spiral organism in the gastric fluid of cats. The scientific world may have failed to note that Edkins was twice right. By the middle of the 20th century, Charlie Code, in the United States, had undertaken considerable experimental work on the action of histamine in the stomach and concluded that histamine was the pivotal agent in the regulation of acid secretion. In 1953, Andrew Kay of Glasgow determined that histamine could be used as a physiologic test to determine the level of acid secretion; this level was of clinical relevance in determining the extent of acid peptic disease.

By 1960, I.N. Marks of Cape Town, working with W. Card in Edinburgh, concluded that acid secretion was a function of the parietal cell mass and that acid secretion and peptic ulcer disease were intertwining entities of physiologic and clinical relevance. In 1958, Solomon Berson pioneered the use of radioimmunoassay measure to plasma insulin. Shortly thereafter, Jim McGuigan used this methodologic principle to devise a plasma radioimmunoassay for gastrin. By 1970, Enrico Solcia of Pavia established the source of gastrin as the G cell of the antrum. It appeared that gastric acid secretion and its regulation had been resolved. The subsequent identification of the enterochromaffin-like cell of the fundus and its histamine-secreting capacity was to provide further information in the elucidation of a problem that had taken almost 2000 years to resolve: the nature of acid and the mechanism of its secretory regulation.

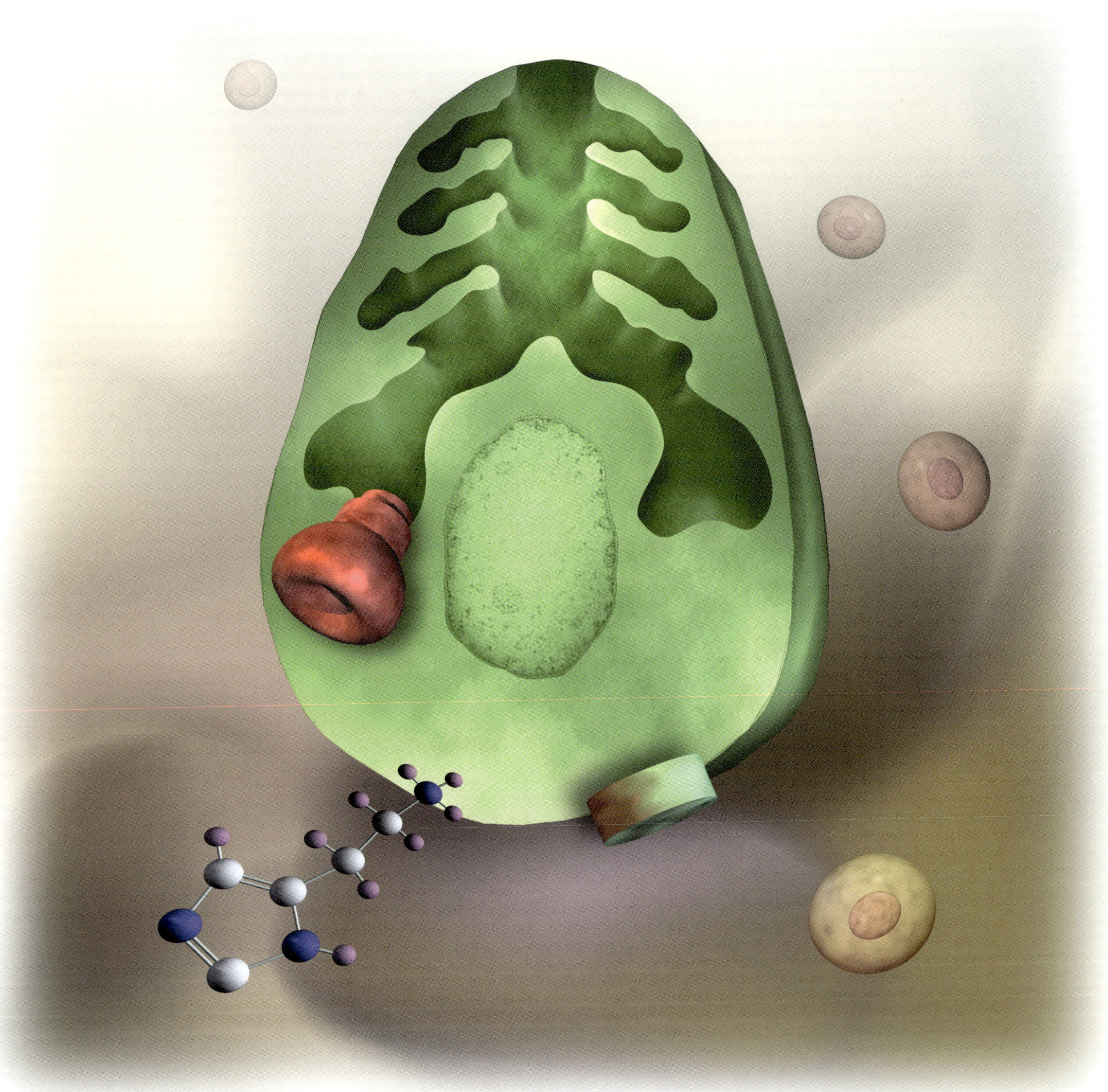

The Parietal Cell

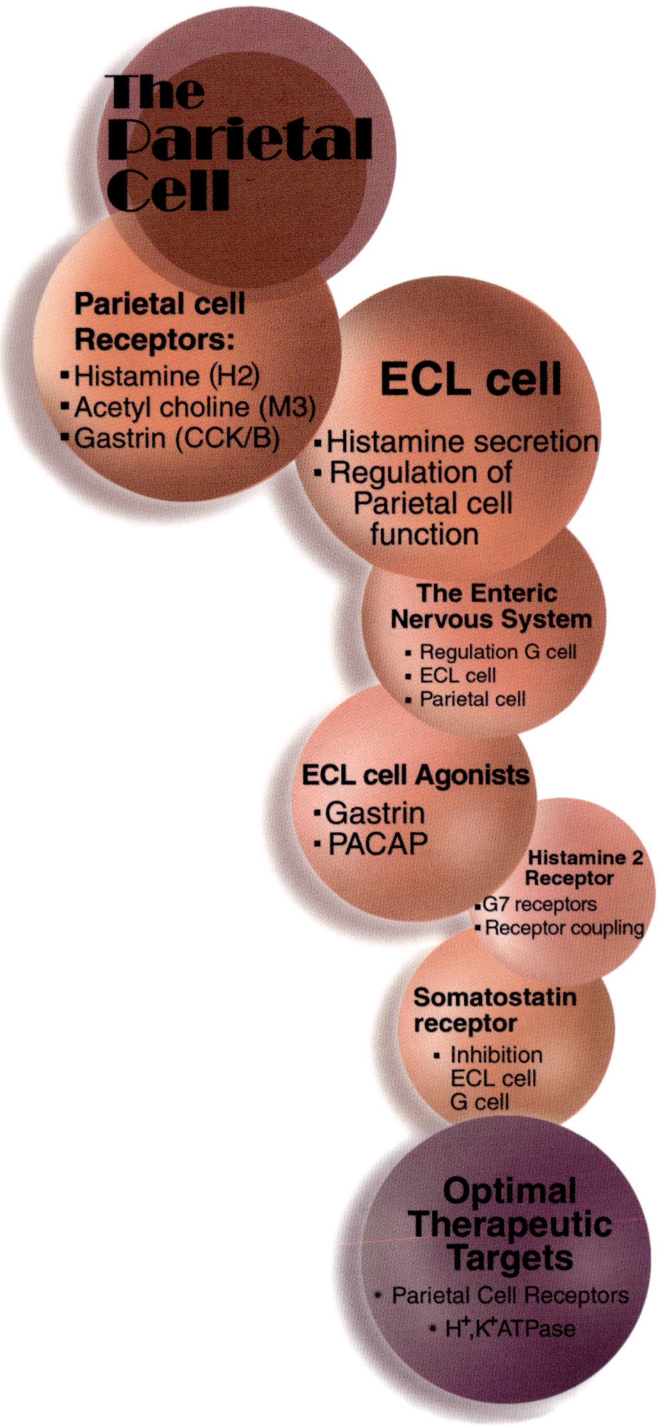

Intragastric pH levels are not indicative of efficacy in healing and/or relief of symptoms.

THE PARIETAL CELL

Introduction

The gastric epithelium is a single-layered epithelium with many columnar infoldings: the gastric glands. In the acid secretory or fundic region of the stomach, these glands contain surface and mucosal neck cells, parietal cells, and chief cells. In addition, they contain several endocrine cells: notably, the enterochromaffin-like cell (ECL) and somatostatin (D) cells. The parietal cells are responsible for acid secretion and B_{12} binding protein, chief cells for secretion of pepsinogen, and the surface and mucous neck cells for the secretion of mucus. Although there is interest in altering the level of pepsinogen secretion and determining the quality of mucus secretion, no drug has been developed that is able to selectively alter these processes, in contrast to the acid secretion of the parietal cell.

Figure 1. — A stimulated rabbit gastric gland in which acidity is shown due to accumulation of acridine orange in the canaliculus of the parietal cell and in the lumen of the gastric gland. The deeper the red color, the greater the acidity. Inset are models of the major endocrine cell of the fundic gland, the ECL cell, and the parietal cell.

Histamine Stimulated Rabbit Fundic Gland

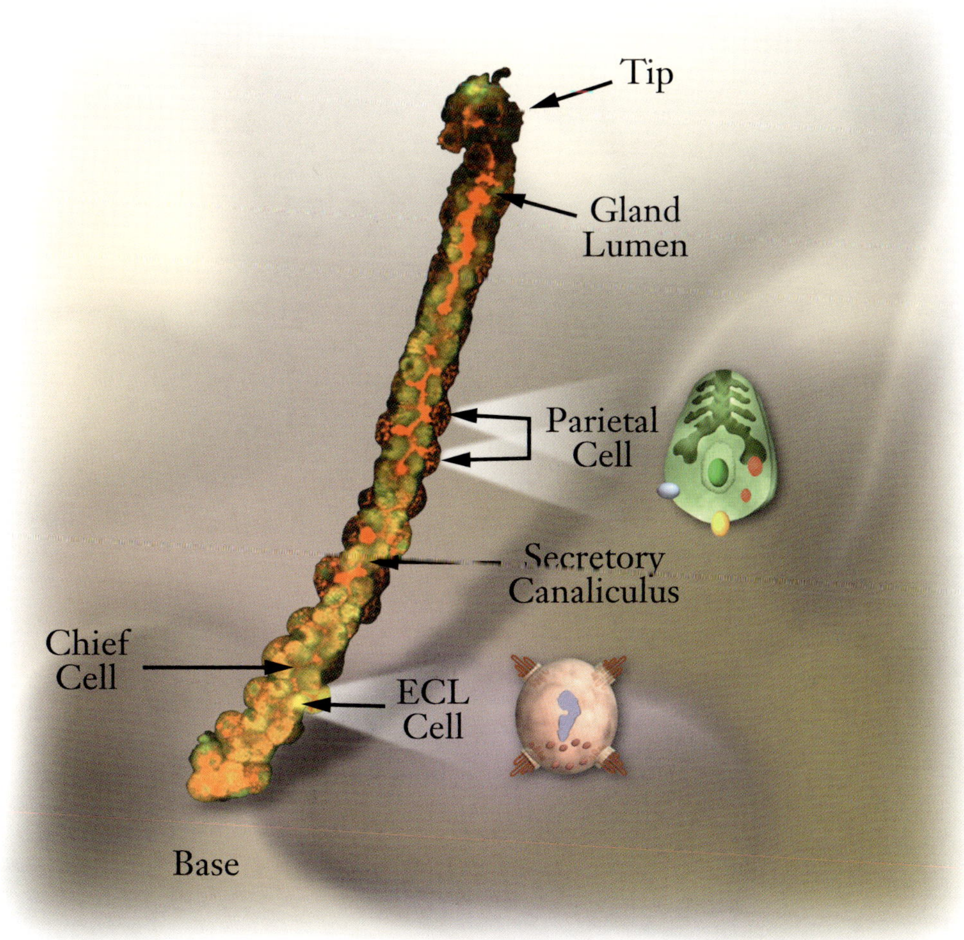

The parietal cell is a conical cell located on the periphery of the column of gastric gland cells. It is morphologically distinctive, containing a very large number of mitochondria (34% by volume), and an infolding of the apical membrane: the secretory canaliculus. Within the cytoplasm of the unstimulated cell, there are abundant membrane tubules or tubulovesicles, that transform into microvilli lining the secretory canaliculus in the stimulated cell. Hence, there is a large morphologic distinction between the resting and stimulated parietal cell, where, in the resting cell, the cytoplasm is filled with the tubulovesicles. In the stimulated cell, there is a large expansion of the secretory canalicular membrane due to arrival of the tubulovesicular membranes and the filling of the canaliculus with acid.

The steps that are thought to occur with this morphologic transformation involve fusion of the tubulovesicular membrane with the canalicular membrane, followed by eversion of the tubules to form microvilli. Some proteins involved in vesicular trafficking have been identified in the parietal cell. These are proteins of the soluble N-ethylmaleimide-sensitive fusion (NSF) protein receptor (SNARE) family, the proteins that are involved in vesicle docking to the plasma membrane and retrieval in many cell types.

Stimulation of Acid Secretion

There is a finely regulated system in the body to ensure that the rate of acid secretion corresponds with the needs of the individual. The final target of this system is the parietal cell of the gastric fundic gland and within the cell, the gastric acid pump: the H^+, K^+ ATPase. There are two major pathways impinging on the parietal cell receptors: a central pathway beginning with the hypothalamus transmitting information to the gastric mucosal plexi through the vagus and muscarinic pathways and a peripheral pathway that has impact on the neuroendocrine cells regulating the release of stimulants or inhibitors. Both activating and inhibitory pathways are present. The stimulatory pathways include those activating histamine release from the ECL cell and gastrin from the G cell, and those having direct impact on the parietal cell such as acetylcholine. The inhibitory pathways include those that activate somatostatin release from either fundic or antral D cell or that affect the parietal cell directly such as EGF, enterogastrone release from the intestine, or substances that inhibit ECL cell function such as galanin or PYY.

Enterochromaffin-Like Cell

The major stimulatory pathway is by stimulation of the release of histamine from the ECL cell that, in turn, stimulates the parietal cell by binding to the H2 receptor on the parietal cell surface, thereby activating the pump to make acid. This ECL cell is stimulated intracellularly either by generation of cAMP or an increase in intracellular calcium. It is situated toward the base of the fundic gastric gland, and the released histamine makes its way to the parietal cell by diffusion along a restricted pathway at the periphery of the gland. The major stimulant for histamine release appears to be gastrin, which is a hormone released from the G cells of the antrum, but there is mounting evidence that pituitary adenylate cyclase activating peptide (PACAP), a neurotransmitter, also stimulates release of histamine from the ECL cell. The major inhibitor of ECL cell function is somatostatin released from the D cell of the fundus.

The histamine in the ECL cell is contained within vacuoles that accumulate the histamine synthesized by the activity of histidine decarboxylase. This accumulation is due to a proton gradient formed inside the vacuoles by a proton pump—the V type ATPase—and exchange of inner protons for outer histamine across a protein transporter, the vesicular monoamine transporter VMAT-2. Histidine decarboxylase is a tightly regulated protein that is synthesized on demand by levels of histamine within the cell. The vacuoles export their histamine by trafficking to the plasma membrane. The released histamine is rapidly broken down by oxidation by an enzyme, diamine oxidase, present in the fundic epithelium. This is therefore a paracrine stimulant of acid secretion.

G Cells

The G cell of the gastric antrum releases gastrin in response to vagal stimulation and to aromatic amino acids in the lumen of the antral gland. The released gastrin, in the form of a 17 or 34 amino acid product-G-17 or G-34-makes its way through the blood to its targets, and therefore this is an endocrine pathway of stimulation. It stimulates the ECL cell to release histamine by activation of calcium release from intracellular stores and calcium entry and also is able to activate calcium signaling directly in the parietal cell owing to the presence on both these cells of a CCK-B G7 receptor. Although the role of gastrin in direct stimulation of the ECL cell is unquestioned, there is some confusion as to the stimulatory role of the CCK-B receptor on the parietal cell as histamine-2 receptor antagonists are able to abolish gastrin-stimulated acid secretion *in vivo* and in isolated fundic gland models.

The G cell has direct connection to the lumen of the antral gland and although it is stimulated by tryptophan, tyrosine, and phenylalanine in the gland contents, it is inhibited when acidity decreases to a pH of 3.0. Much of the latter effect is thought to derive from acid stimulation of the antral D cell.

Gastrin is not only a stimulant of gastric acid secretion but also a trophic hormone for the gastric fundus, stimulating the growth of the gastric mucosa in this region, particularly the ECL cells. However, growth regulation of these and the other cells of the region depends on many factors, so that removal of gastrin by transgenic mice knockouts does not lead to disappearance of the ECL cell. Much has been made of its trophic action on the ECL cell that will be discussed when considering therapy for acid-related diseases.

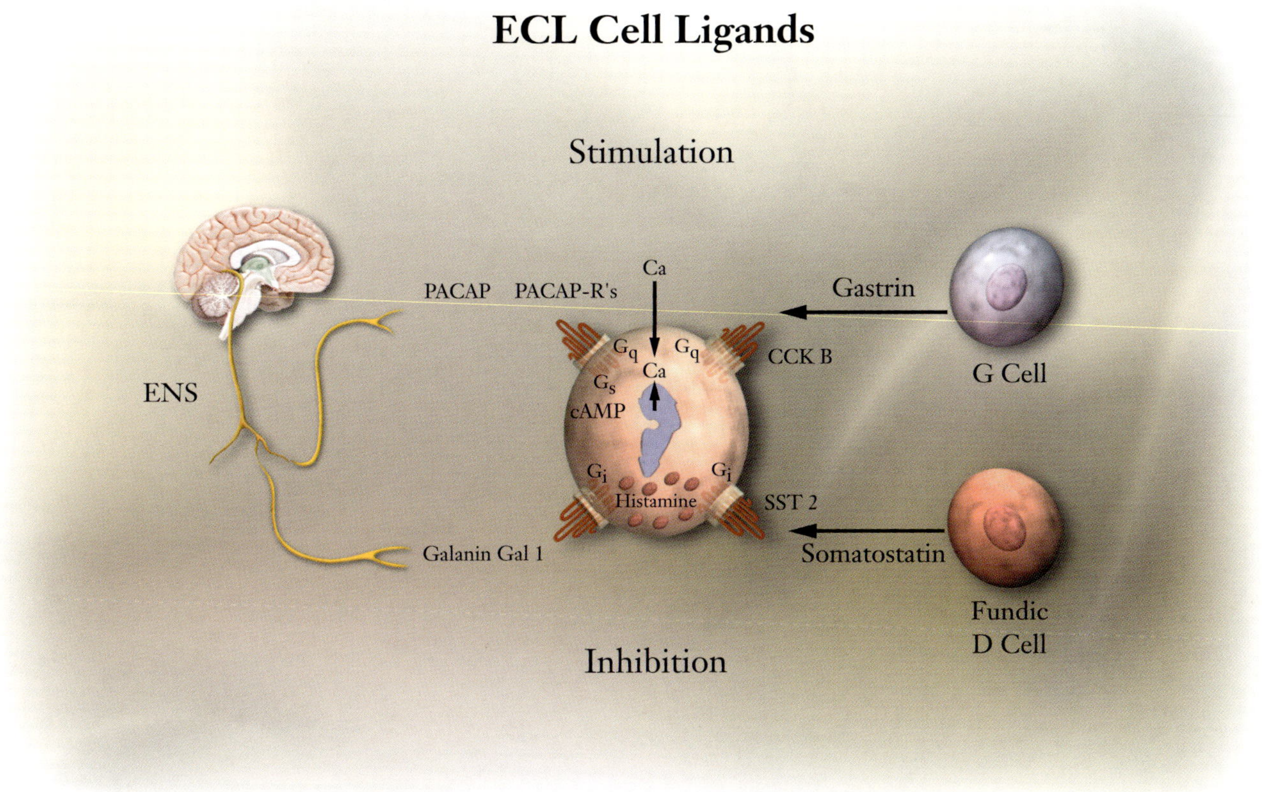

Figure 2. — An illustration of the regulatory pathways of acid secretion involving G and ECL cells as stimulatory relay cells and D cells as inhibitory sites for acid secretion. The large number of ligands and receptors has made unraveling the regulatory pathways difficult in the intact animal, and in vitro results are sometime difficult to fit into an integrated picture of acid secretory regulation. Stimuli leave the brain through the vagus connecting to the enteric nervous system in the myenteric plexus (ENS). Postganglionic fibers leave the ENS to activate the ECL cell, probably by release of PACAP, and may inhibit the ECL cell by release of galanin. PACAP has dual signaling pathways: elevation of cell calcium and cell cAMP. The G cell releases gastrin, which stimulates the ECL cell by elevation of intracellular calcium. The D cell releases somatostatin, which inhibits the ECL cell by inhibiting calcium influx. The calcium activation is due to activation of Gq trimeric proteins; the stimulation of cAMP is due to Gs trimeric proteins; and inhibition by galanin and somatostatin is mediated by Gi trimeric proteins.

D Cells

There are also inhibitory influences on the ECL cell. Somatostatin is a short-lived peptide released from gastric D or somatostatin-containing cells. These cells are found in both fundus and antrum, presumably to regulate ECL-cell function and G-cell function. In the fundus, there is no communication with the lumen of the gland, whereas in the antrum there is direct connection with the lumen. Thus, in the fundus, activation of D cells is only by serosal factors, such as peptides and neurotransmitters. In the antrum, a significant role is played by the pH of the antral gland contents.

Somatostatin inhibits the release of histamine from the ECL cell whether stimulated by gastrin or by PACAP. The D cell is activated by either gastrin or CCK (a peptide released from gastric nerves or the pancreas), is inhibited by vagal stimuli, and plays a major role in the turning off of acid secretion after the stomach has emptied. The antral D cell is activated by a decrease in pH of the antral gland, signaling that digestion has now reduced the buffering action of food. It is thought that this switch-off occurs when the antral gland lumen falls to a pH of 3.0 or less.

Activation of Parietal Cell

The parietal cell is subject to many activating factors that bind to surface receptors and initiate signals within the cell cytoplasm. This activation results in the morphologic transformation of the tubulovesicles to the microvilli of the parietal cell. The acid pump is present in the tubulovesicles, and by dint of its translocation, is placed at the site of acid secretion

The Stimulatory Receptors of the Parietal Cell

That gastric acid secretion is a regulated process in humans was recognized several centuries ago. However, it fell to science of the 20th century to define these receptors and to generate an effective and well-tolerated set of compounds for inhibition of one of these receptors. Selectivity for a given receptor ensures efficacy at that receptor. Selectivity for inhibition of acid secretion depends on the distribution of the receptor in the body as well as on the function of the receptor in the organ where it is present. As will be seen, the H2 receptor is found in the periphery, mainly in the stomach but also in the heart and the uterus. The gastrin receptor (CCK-B) is mainly found in the stomach, on the parietal and ECL cell. Muscarinic receptors are found in virtually every organ.

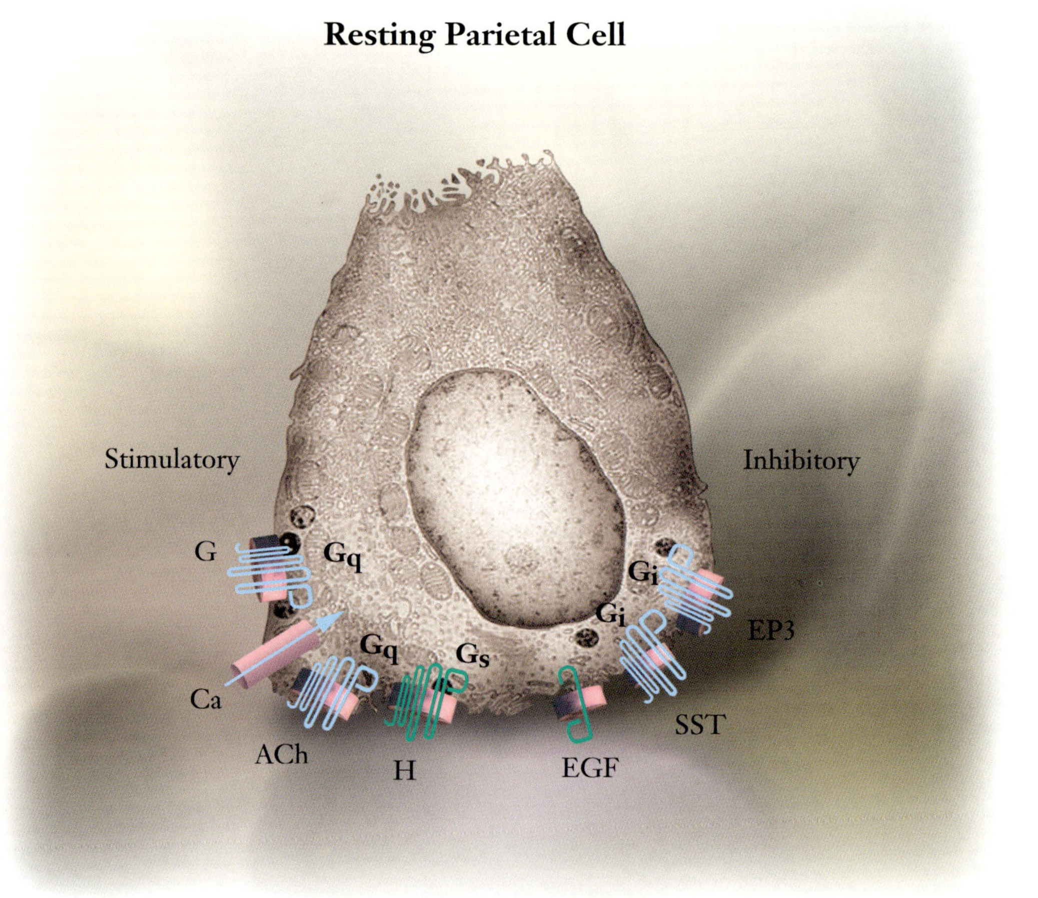

Figure 3. *— Receptors on the parietal cell. On the left are the three major stimulatory receptors on the parietal cell. The G illustrates the CCK-B receptor coupled to increases in cell Ca through coupling to the Gq trimeric G protein, as is the m3 receptor responsible for stimulation by acetylcholine. The major stimulatory receptor is the H2 receptor, coupled to Gs trimeric G protein, coupled to elevation of cAMP. This receptor is also coupled to elevation of cell calcium. On the right are the inhibitory receptors on the parietal cell, the prostaglandin EP_3 receptor coupled to a trimeric Gi protein, and the EGF receptor, which is a receptor-stimulated tyrosine kinase.*

Receptors

Biology is replete with molecules that regulate cell function by generating intracellular signals by binding to proteins on the plasma membrane of the cell or even in the cell nucleus. These proteins—the receptors—fall into many different categories, depending on their structure, localization, and the way that they signal the cell to alter its function. Thus, there are nuclear receptors that bind to specific regions of the genome as a function of binding a molecule that penetrates into the cell. Steroids, retinoids, and vitamin D, for example, bind to nuclear receptors. Activation of these receptors results in binding of the receptor to specific regions of the DNA of the cell, resulting in changes in transcription. Cell-membrane receptors fall into at least two categories: those that signal by altering the arrangement of a trimer of proteins, the G proteins; and those that signal by phosphorylating a specific amino acid, tyrosine, in the receptor protein and other protein substrates. These are then called the G-protein-coupled receptors and the tyrosine kinase class of receptor, respectively.

The receptors that activate acid secretion are all G-protein-coupled receptors. These are integral membrane proteins of about 400 amino acids inserted so that their N terminal part is outside the cell and their C terminal part is inside the cell. The outside loops connecting the membrane segments, and the segments themselves contain the information necessary for binding the various agonists that affect intracellular signaling. The inside loops connecting membrane segments determine the nature of the intracellular signals generated by ligands binding to the receptor.

They are coupled on their inside surface to the G proteins. These are trimers of alpha, beta, and gamma subunits that are tightly bound to the receptor when the receptor is inactive, and in this tightly bound state they are complexed with guanosine diphosphate, which is bound to the alpha subunit. Upon ligand binding to a G7 receptor, the G protein complex dissociates, and GTP displaces GDP on the alpha subunit. The signal terminates, as the alpha subunit is a GTPase, and GDP is reformed resulting in reassociation of the three subunits and binding to the receptor. The binding affinity of the ligand is also altered to a lower affinity state when the trimeric G protein dissociates from the receptor, also helping to down-regulate the effect of ligand. Further, a complex series of reactions can alter receptor properties. For example, the receptor can be phosphorylated by kinases in the cell, again altering affinity. Another effect is internalization of the receptor so that receptor numbers on the cell surface are decreased with trafficking of the receptor to various sites in the cell. This pathway is initiated by phosphorylation of a serine residue on the receptor by a G protein receptor kinase (GRK). This enables binding of one of the arrestin protein families and then interaction with the clathrin-coated vesicles. When the ligand is dissociated inside the cell, the receptor can be trafficked back to the plasma membrane or into a degradative pathway. The cell therefore has several means of becoming relatively refractory to the receptor-binding ligand.

The effect of stimulation of the parietal cell is to change its morphology from a resting to a stimulated state and the acid pump from a resting cytoplasmic to an active microvillus position. Here the cytoplasmic location of the acid pump is moved to the microvilli of the secretory canaliculus, this structure expands greatly, and acid is then transported across this membrane into the canaliculus and then exits from the apex of the conical parietal cell.

Different G proteins result in different intracellular signals. The two major sets of activating cell signals involve changes in intracellular cyclic AMP and changes in free intracellular calcium. The changes in cAMP are brought about when the receptor is coupled to Gs trimeric proteins, the changes in cell calcium when the receptor is coupled to Gq or Go proteins. Quite often, a single receptor is coupled to more than one signaling pathway.

Increases in cAMP are generated when the alpha subunit of the Gs trimeric complex binds to the adenylate cyclase on the membrane. The level of cAMP in the cell is then regulated by phosphodiesterases, of which there are at least five isoforms. cAMP binds to the regulatory subunit of a R_2C_2 complex protein that then dissociates releasing the active C or catalytic subunit. This is a cAMP-dependent protein kinase that is able to phosporylate a variety of serines or threonines on cell proteins. Changes in intracellular calcium occur when the Gq or Go dissociate from the receptor and the alpha subunit activates phospholipase C, of which there are several isoforms. Phospholipase C hydrolyzes phosphatidyl inositol bisphosphate to provide inositol 1,4,5 trisphosphate (IP_3) and diacylglycerol. IP_3 binds to a receptor in the endoplasmic reticulum that results in activation of a calcium release channel. The level of intracellular calcium then regulates the channel itself, inhibiting calcium release, and calcium is reloaded into the endoplasmic reticulum by activity of the Ca ATPase in the membrane. Calcium also binds to calmodulin, and the calcium-calmodulin complex activates the plasma membrane calcium pump, resulting in export of calcium. Diacylglycerol provides a binding site for protein kinase C that results in phosphorylation of intracellular proteins again on serine or threonine residues. Therefore, whether calcium or cAMP is the signaling pathway, protein phosphorylation results from both.

Acetylcholine Receptor

The effect of acetylcholine released from the parasympathetic system is mediated by muscarinic receptors, of which there are five subtypes: m1 to m5. Vagal stimulation stimulates acid secretion, and this effect was exploited surgically by operations such as truncal vagotomy, selective vagotomy, and highly selective vagotomy. Acetylcholine, the mediator released from vagal nerves, was shown to stimulate acid secretion as did its congener, carbachol. Even before this, extract of belladonna, which contains the nonselective muscarinic antagonist atropine, had been used in patients with ulcer disease. The problem with atropine is that this drug inhibits all muscarinic receptors such as those that control salivation, heart rate, and pupil constriction. So when it was administered, patients complained of a variety of side effects such as dilated pupil and visual disturbance (hence the name, belladonna) and dry mouth or palpitation.

In the 1960s it was recognized that there was more than one subtype of muscarinic receptor, and research programs started in order to find receptor-selective muscarinic antagonists and to find the nature of the receptors controlling acid secretion. It was established, both pharmacologically and by using molecular biologic techniques such as reverse transriptase polymerase chain reaction (RT-PCR) that amplifies the presence of a messenger RNA (mRNA) in an organ or cell, that the parietal cell expressed the m3 subtype of muscarinic receptor. The addition of carbachol results in stimulation of acid secretion in isolated fundic glands or parietal cells. This is accompanied by an increase in intracellular calcium but no change in levels of cAMP.

Figure 4. — A stimulated parietal cell showing the coupling of the H2 receptor to cAMP generation and of the gastrin and ACh receptors to Ca signaling by release of Ca from intracellular stores as well as entry of calcium. The inhibitory receptors for Somatostatin and the prostaglandin EP3 receptorsare coupled to Gi trimeric proteins. The change of morphology of the secretory canaliculus associated with relocation of the gastric acid pump is highlighted.

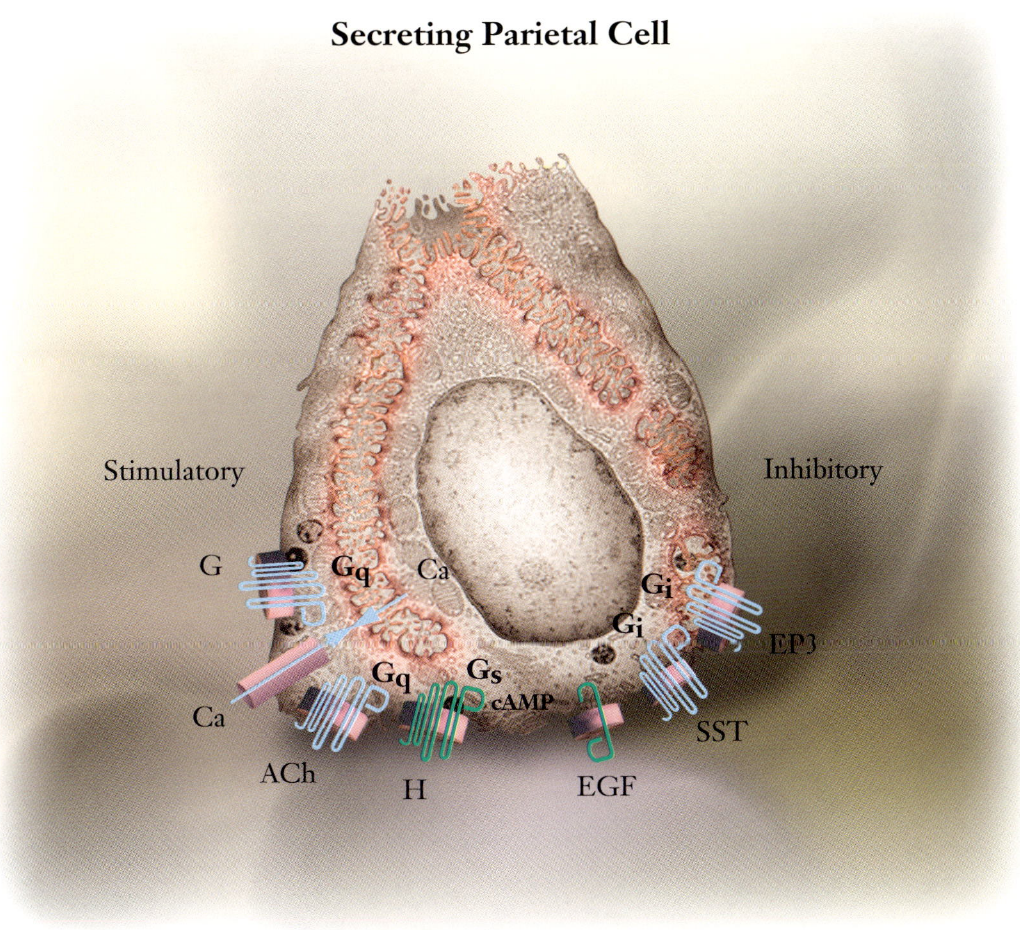

Activation and Shutdown of G7 Receptors

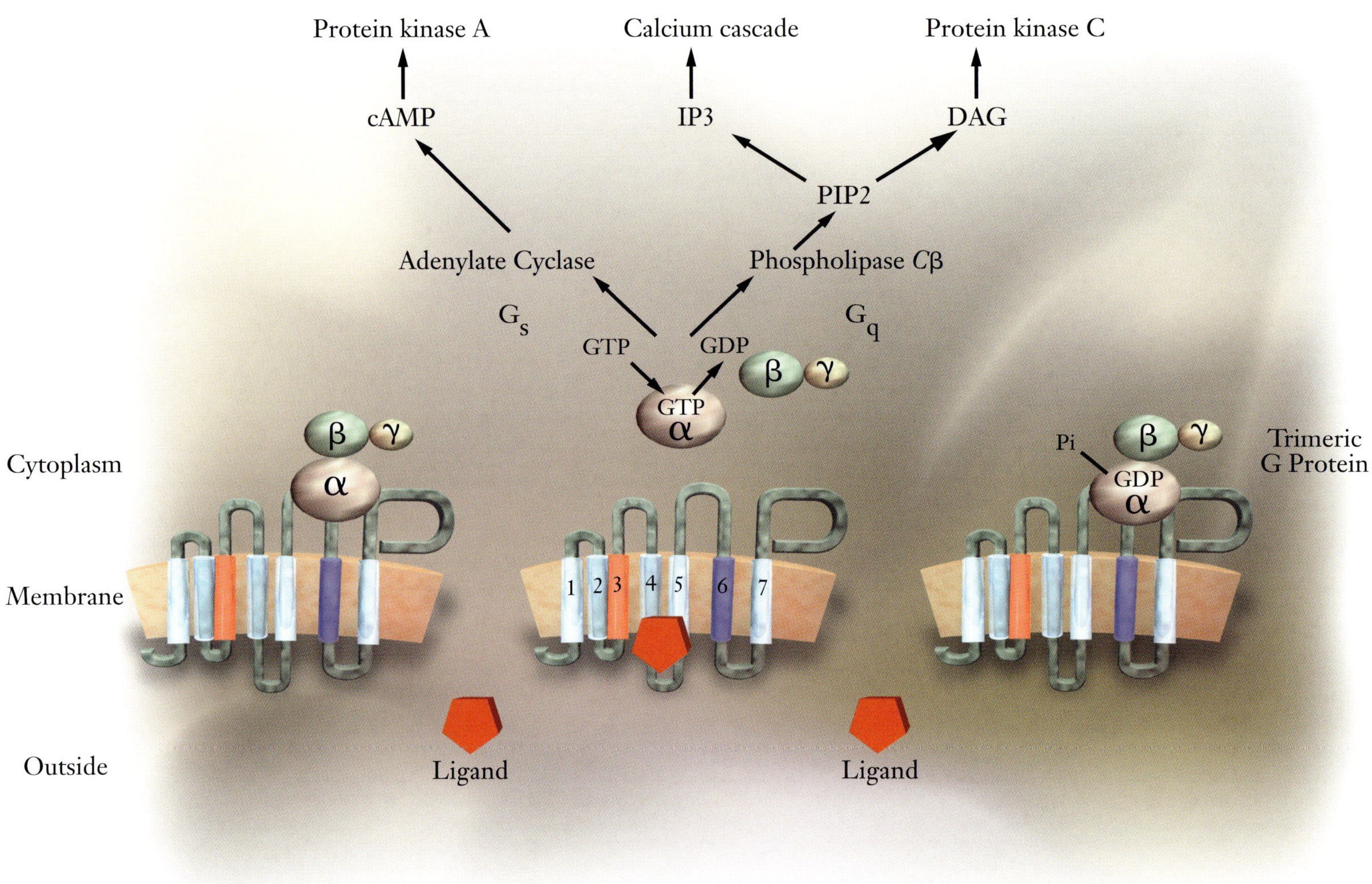

Figure 5. *— Illustration of the many pathways available to stimulatory G7 receptors. On the left below is the unstimulated receptor where the trimeric G protein is firmly anchored to the receptor as the alpha subunit of this trimeric receptor binds GDP. With activation by binding of ligand (center), the trimeric G protein dissociates and GTP displaces GDP. The alpha subunit of Gs activates adenylate cyclase, which produces cAMP and activates protein kinase A. The alpha subunit of Gq activates phospholipase C, which hydrolyses phosphatidyl inositol bis phosphate (PIP2). The inositol trisphosphate (IP3) produced results in calcium release from intracellular stores and activation of calcium entry. The DAG produced binds and activates protein kinase C. The G alpha subunit hydrolyses GTP to GDP, rebinds the beta and gamma subunit, and reforms the inactive ligand-trimeric G protein complex. Termination of cAMP action is brought about by the activity of phosphodiesterase.*

The first muscarinic receptor antagonist after atropine that was introduced into treatment of acid-related disease was a m1 antagonist. Although this was relatively effective in suppression of acid secretion, it continued to have side effects such as dry mouth and visual disturbances. It was not particularly effective in inhibition of diurnal pH but showed benefit in treatment of duodenal ulcer. Hence, it did not achieve widespread use. At this time, there are no m3 receptor antagonists available for medical use, although these would presumably retain the side effects that patients find difficult to tolerate, as other secretory organs have m3 muscarinic receptor subtypes.

Histamine Receptor

Histamine was first isolated by Henry Dale. However, credit for showing histamine-stimulated acid secretion fell to Leon Popielski, a student in the laboratory of Ivan Pavlov, who made his mark in unraveling some of the central nervous system's influence on gastric function in dogs.

The first set of receptor-targeted medications was developed in the 1950s as antihistaminics. The structure of histamine is shown in Figure 6, and these compounds modified the imidazole ring of this natural ligand. The development of these compounds was driven by the demonstration that histamine release is involved in allergic responses and secretion of mucus from nasal or lung mucous membranes.

In that decade, it was realized that these histamine antagonists did not work well against acid secretion, even when stimulated by histamine, and it was suggested that a different type of histamine receptor was responsible for stimulation of acid secretion. However, the ineffectiveness of the then-available histamine receptor antagonists

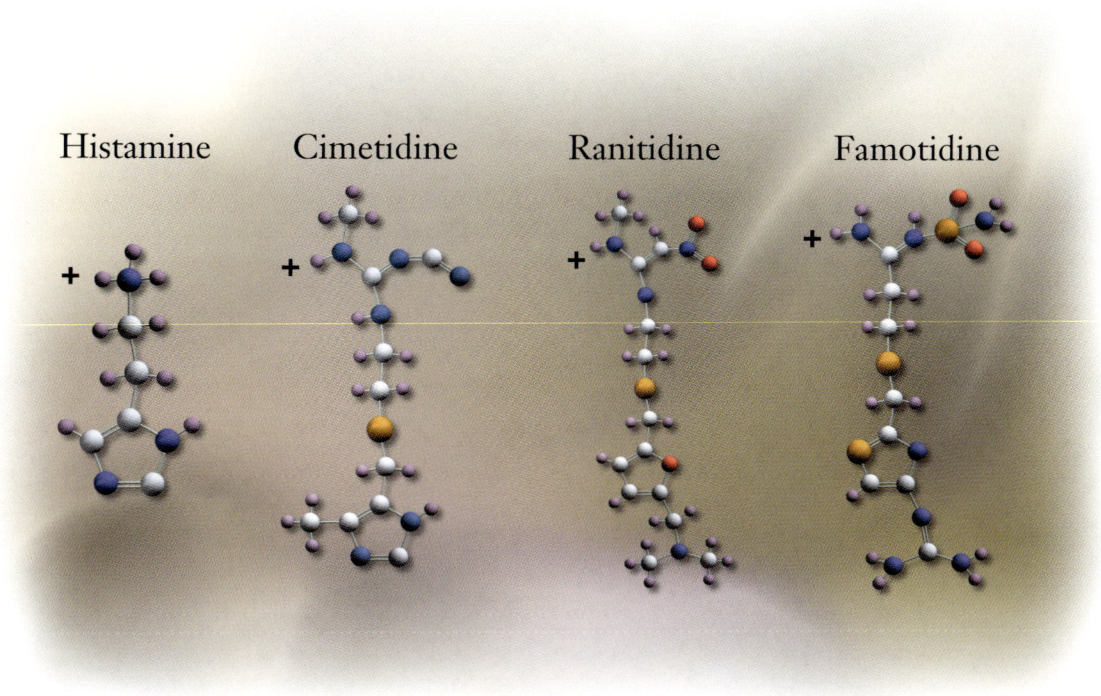

Figure 6. — The structure of histamine and three commonly used H2-receptor antagonists. Nitrogen is ●, Carbon is ●, Oxygen is ●, Sulfur is ●, and Hydrogen is ●.

led to the suspicion among gastroenterologists that histamine was not involved in physiologic regulation of acid secretion.

However, James Black who recognized the separation and clinical usefulness of targeted antagonists for different types of adrenaline receptors, the alpha and beta subtypes—while working for Imperial Chemical Industries—joined SmithKline and French (SK&F) with the express purpose of developing compounds that targeted the histamine receptor responsible for stimulation of acid secretion. The histamine 2-receptor was so named to distinguish it from the histamine 1-receptor that was responsible for allergic reactions.

After some years of research, the pharmacologist and his group were successful in making compounds that were selective for inhibition of histamine stimulation of acid secretion. These differed from the H1 antagonists in that the ring was not modified, only the ethylamine side chain as shown in Figure 6. The product that was finally introduced on the market for acid-related diseases by SK&F was cimetidine. This was effective in the treatment of active duodenal ulcer, active benign gastric ulcer, and gastroesophageal reflux disease (GERD).

Relatively soon thereafter, other companies introduced H2-receptor antagonists such as ranitidine, famotidine, or nizatidine. The advent of these drugs changed the face of acid-related disease therapy, providing, for the first time, a means for the physician to control acid secretion through medical rather than surgical intervention. The advent of these pharmacologic reagents now provided a firm foundation for the recognition of the role of histamine in stimulation of gastric acid secretion.

The receptor on the parietal cell that bound histamine was defined pharmacologically in many different ways. Isolated fundic gastric glands, isolated parietal cells, and isolated parietal cell membranes all provided evidence for selective binding of H2-receptor antagonists or for histamine displacement of H2-receptor antagonists. It was shown in the 1960s, that the second messenger, cAMP, was able to stimulate acid secretion in isolated stomachs and then in the isolated gastric fundic gland and in isolated parietal cells. Finally, the H2-receptor was cloned and its sequence identified. Further, by site-directed mutagenesis, the general localization of the binding site of the receptor antagonists was also explored, as shown in Figure 7.

The membrane receptor consists of 359 amino acids, arranged as shown, as a polytopic integral membrane protein. This means that the chain of the amino acids is threaded in and out of the membrane to make a protein that is sided with a face oriented toward the outside of the cell that binds histamine or the antagonist and a face oriented toward the inside of the cell that responds to binding of histamine by generating intracellular signals.

Binding of histamine to the receptor generates both cAMP and an increase in intracellular calcium. This receptor is therefore coupled to both Gs and a calcium-signaling pathway. There is potentiation between histamine and acetylcholine, showing that these receptor systems use different signaling pathways but share some common mechanism; otherwise, only additive effects would be found.

The histamine molecule and its antagonists bind to regions of the membrane that include the aspartyl and serine residues in the 3rd and 5th transmembrane domains. All currently available H2-receptor antagonists are displaced by histamine and are therefore competitive antagonists. They are effective inhibitors of night time acidity. They are less effective in inhibition of day time acidity.

Histamine 2 Receptor

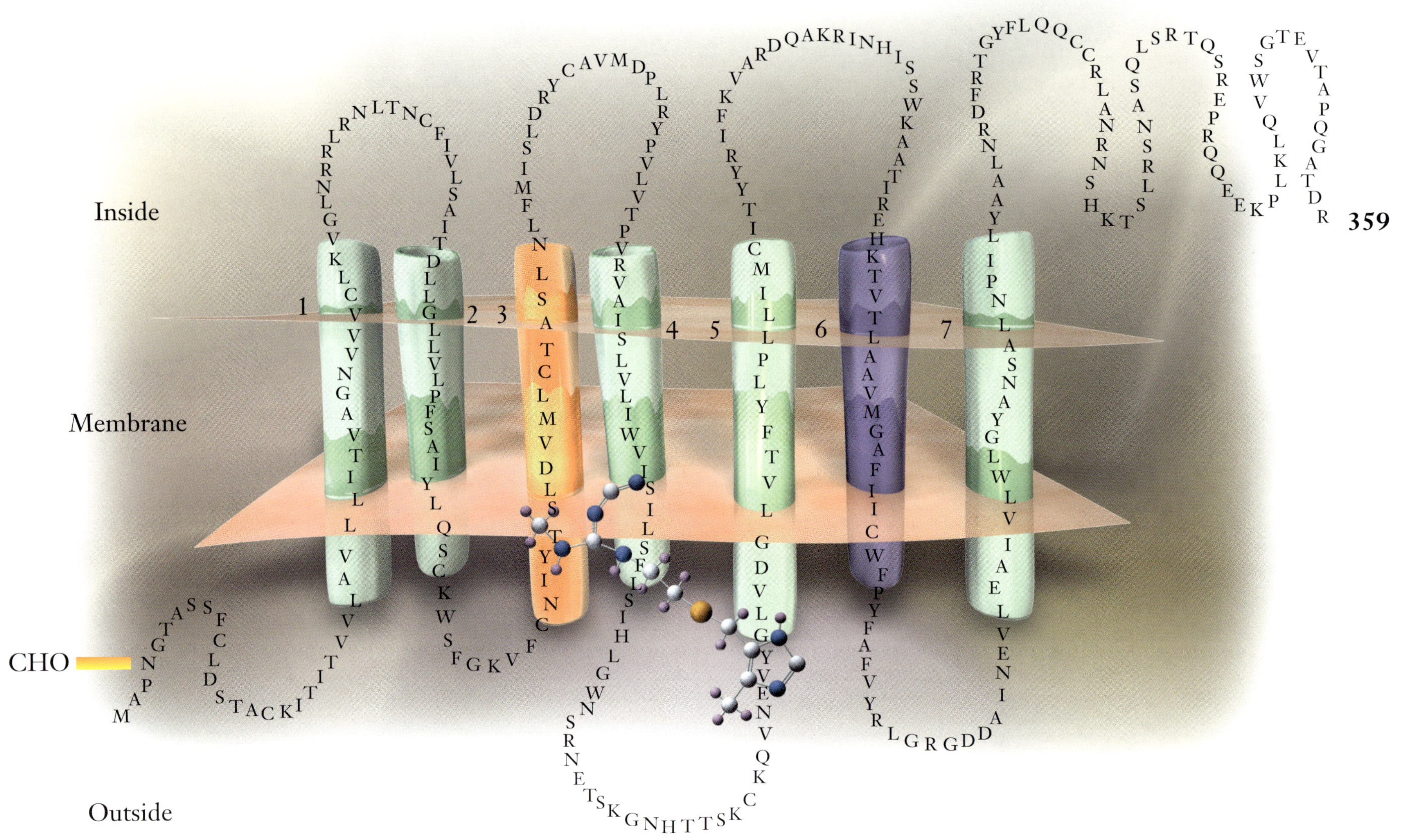

Figure 7. — Illustration of the general structure and the specific amino acid sequence of the H2 receptor. The linear chain of 359 amino acids constituting the receptor is arranged in a typical G7 membrane receptor structure, where the glycosylated N terminal (CHO) faces the outside of the cell and is separated from the C terminal region facing the interior by 7 membrane-inserted segments. Highlighted are membrane segments 3 and 6, which are thought to undergo conformational changes due to binding of the ligand histamine. That also may change with binding of the antagonists (as shown in the model) if they act as inverse agonists, that is, compounds that inhibit the basal activity of the receptor.

Gastrin Receptor

Gastrin was first described by Edkins in 1905 as a stimulatory constituent of an extract of stomach, but his work was not accepted until 1938, when Komarov showed that the effect of a gastric extract was not due to histamine but a peptide. This peptide was purified and sequenced by Gregory and Tracy and for many years was considered to be the most significant stimulant of gastric acid secretion among gastric physiologists.

The peptide is produced in the G cells of the gastric antrum and is released in response to aromatic amino acids in the lumen of the gland as well as by vagal stimulation. Gastrin release is inhibited by acid in the gland lumen and it is considered that this inhibition begins when the pH in the lumen falls to 3.0 or below. Much of that effect is considered to be due to stimulation of the antral D cell by acid and inhibition of the G cell by the somatostatin that is released.

It is synthesized as a large peptide and is progressively processed to a smaller G17 or G34 peptide that then undergoes amidation to form the mature product. Both G17 and G34 are effective stimulants of gastric acid secretion. Their role as a direct stimulant of gastric acid secretion has been somewhat dimmed by the demonstration that H2-receptor antagonists are able to inhibit gastrin-induced acid secretion in animals and people, suggesting that its major role in stimulation of gastric acid secretion is to release histamine from the ECL cell. Nevertheless, through its action on the ECL cell, it is on the major pathway for meal stimulation of acid secretion. Another role for gastrin is that it is a trophic hormone for ECL cells and for the parietal cells of the fundic mucosa. This trophic effect accounts for some of the secondary effects seen with effective doses of H2-receptor antagonists and of PPIs.

Regulatory Pathways of Acid Secretion

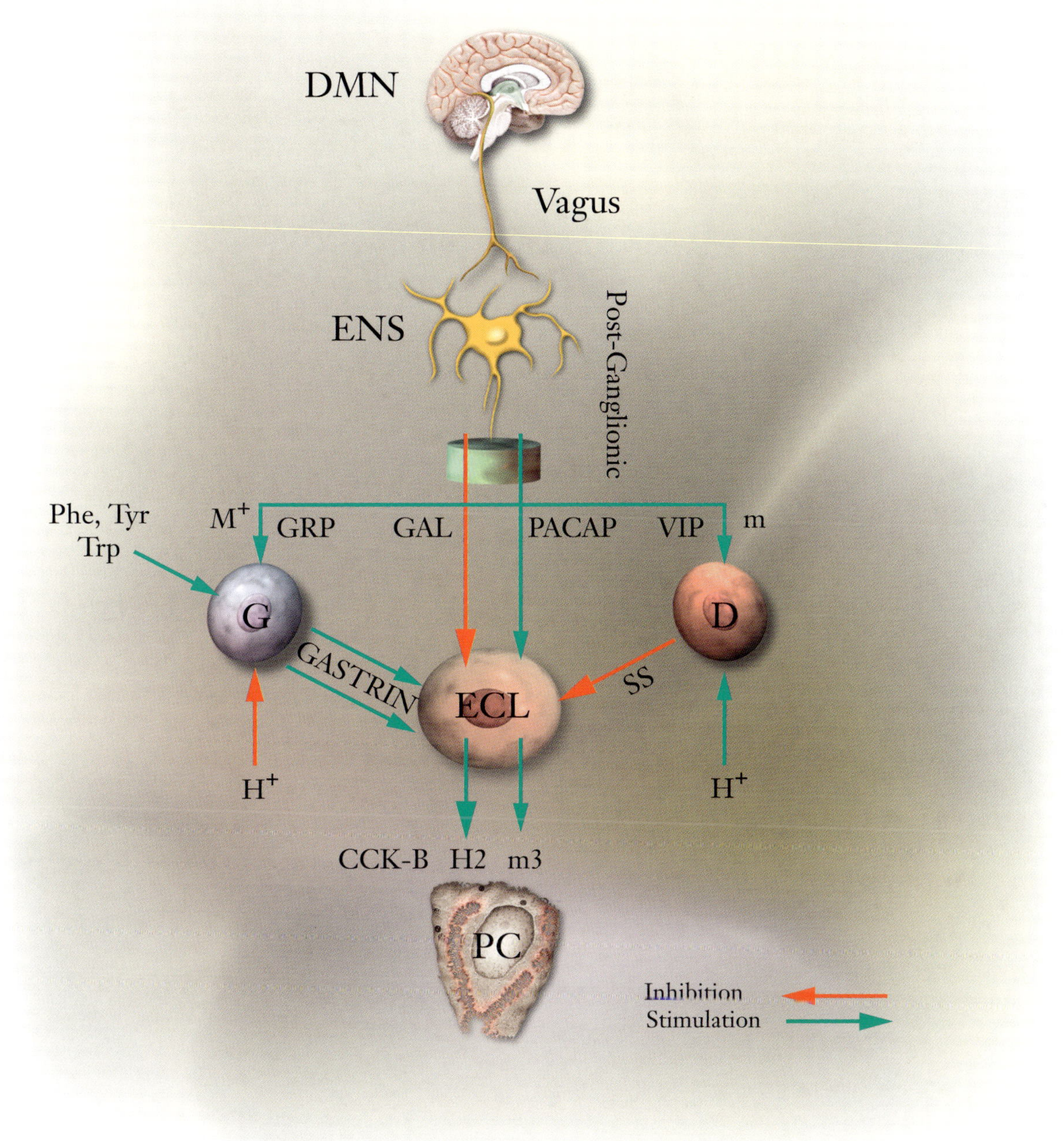

Figure 8. — *The pathways of regulation of gastric acid secretion. The cephalic phase originates in the brain and reaches the dorsal motor nucleus (DMN) of the hypothalamus. The vagus nerve progresses to the enteric nervous system (ENS) to affect the neurons of this "second brain." The postganglionic fibers leave the myenteric plexus and activate G cells by stimulation of muscarinic receptors or by release of gastrin releasing peptide or inhibit fundic D cells by muscarinic pathways and also directly activate the parietal cell by an m3 receptor. The endocrine cells also interact with the parietal cell. The ECL cell releases histamine in response to gastrin released from the G cell, which, in turn, is stimulated by aromatic amino acids present in digested food. It is stimulated by PACAP released from gastric nerves and is inhibited by galanin also released from gastric nerves. The histamine stimulates the parietal cell by activation of the H2 receptor. Acid in the lumen stimulates somatostatin (SS) release from antral D cells, which inhibit G-cell function, which also may be directly inhibited by luminal acidity. Gastrin stimulates the D cells, generating another feedback loop controlling acid secretion.*

The gastrin receptor — the CCK–B receptor—has been cloned and is a member of the G7 family of receptors, as are the histamine and muscarinic receptors. It is coupled to Gq and therefore to calcium-signaling pathways. Nevertheless, in contrast to stimulation by vagal pathways, whether *in vivo* or *in vitro*, gastrin stimulation of acid secretion by the parietal cell is blocked by H2-receptor antagonists *in vitro* and *in vivo*, demoting this receptor from a primary stimulatory role. Gastrin is, however, a primary stimulant of fundic epithelial growth, with differential effects on different cell types that appear to be species dependent. This trophism is mediated by the CCK-B receptor as well but may have different coupling pathways compared to the CCK-B-mediated release of histamine. There are now available several high-affinity CCK-B receptor antagonists that are being evaluated as therapy for acid-related diseases. One aspect of their development is that there is a likelihood, but not a certainty, that the trophic effects of inhibition of acid secretion will be absent with these antagonists in contrast to the effect of H2-receptor antagonists.

Pharmacology of Inhibition of Acid Secretion

The multiplicity of pathways involved in activation of the parietal cell to make acid has resulted in a multiplicity of receptor antagonists designed to regulate acid secretion. However, with this promiscuity among receptors, it has been difficult to design antagonists with the efficacy apparently required to inhibit enough of the acid secretion to optimize treatment of acid-related disorders.

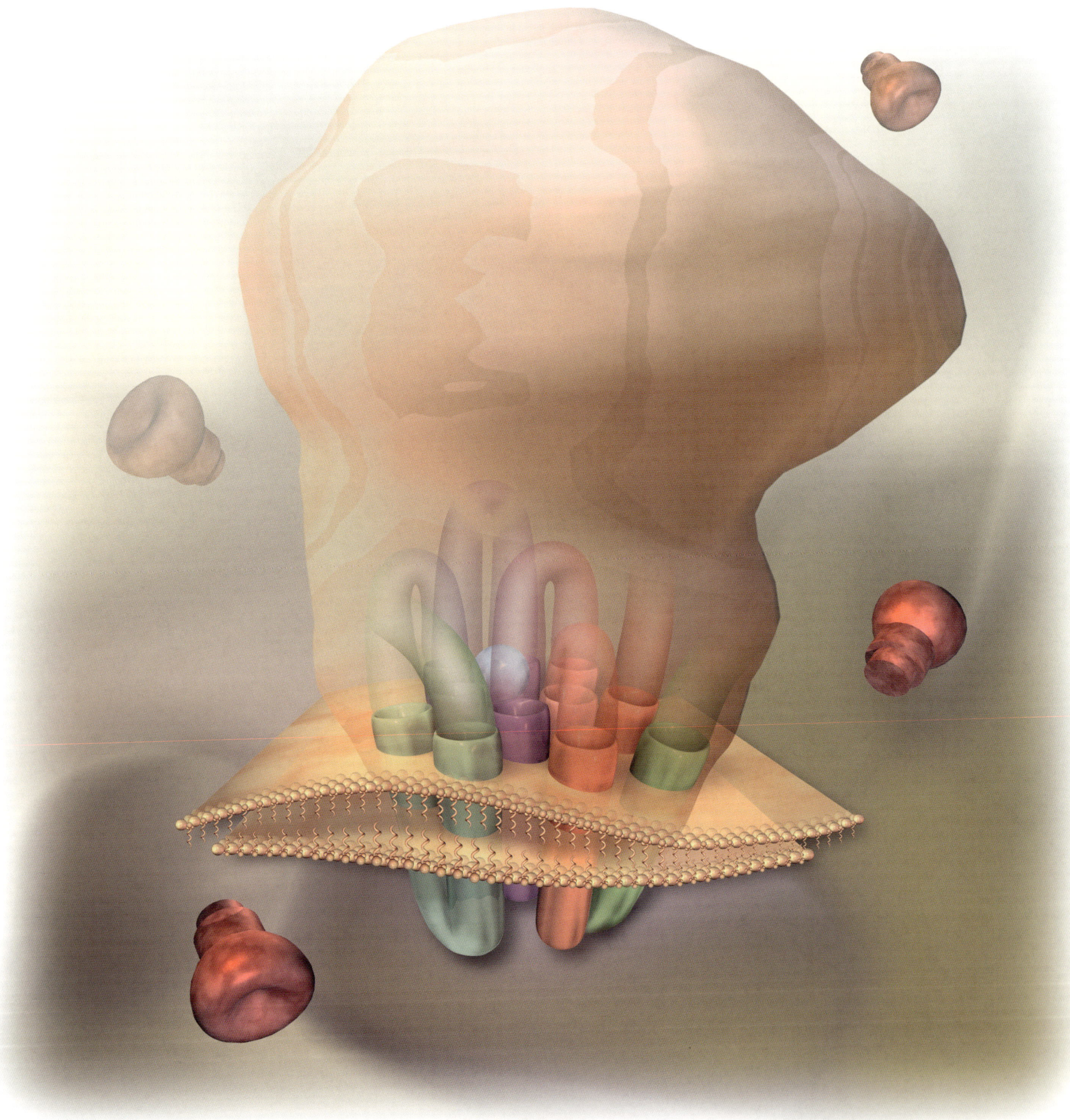

Chapter III

The Gastric Acid Pump

Introduction

H^+, K^+ ATPase

Structure

Mechanism

Activation

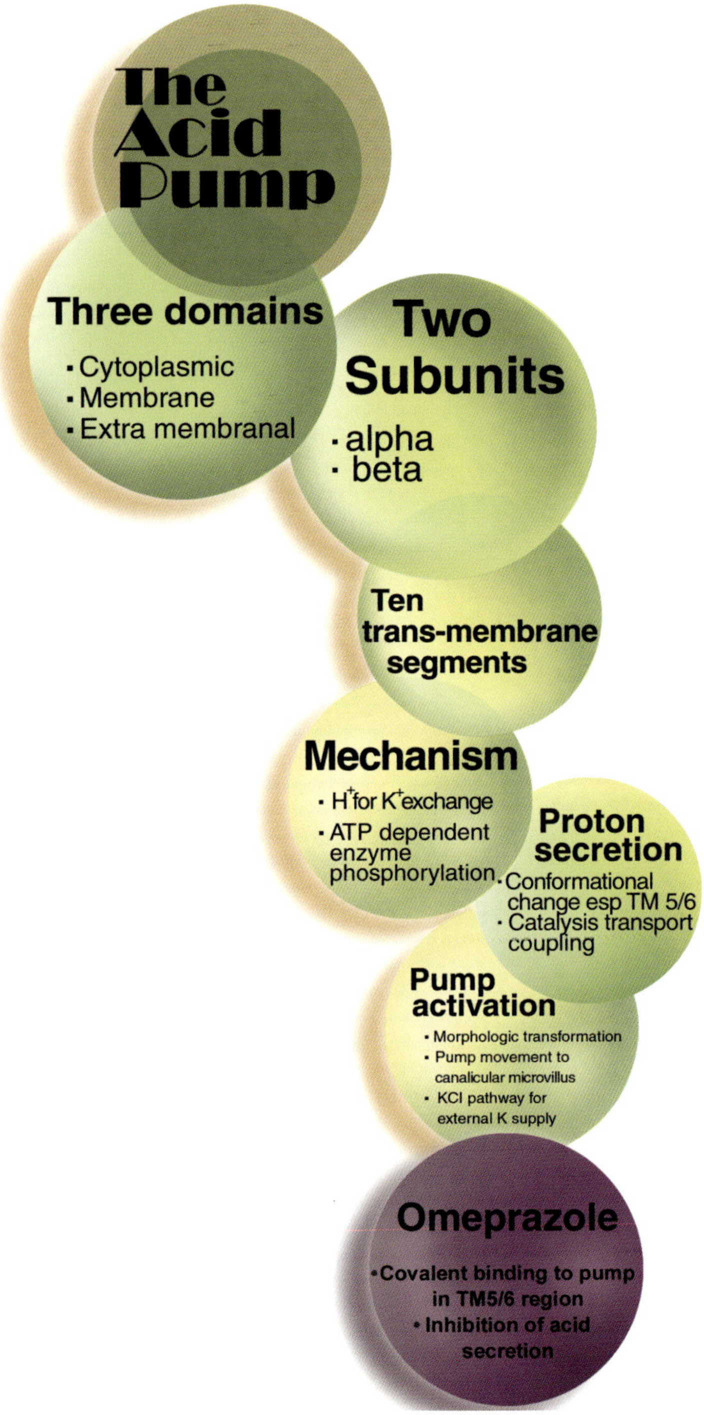
The Acid Pump
Three domains
• Cytoplasmic
• Membrane
• Extra membranal
Two Subunits
• alpha
• beta
Ten trans-membrane segments
Mechanism
• H^+ for K^+ exchange
• ATP dependent enzyme phosphorylation
Proton secretion
• Conformational change esp TM 5/6
• Catalysis transport coupling
Pump activation
• Morphologic transformation
• Pump movement to canalicular microvillus
• KCl pathway for external K supply
Omeprazole
• Covalent binding to pump in TM5/6 region
• Inhibition of acid secretion

The Gastric Acid Pump

Introduction

The role of acid secretion in relation to diseases such as active duodenal ulcer or active benign gastric ulcer, as well as erosive gastroesophageal reflux disease, was further emphasized by the effectiveness of the H2-receptor antagonist, cimetidine. It still seemed possible to further improve acid inhibitory therapy. This belief stemmed from the better understanding of the mechanisms of acid secretion and from an understanding of the biochemical basis for acid secretion by the stomach. Gastric acid is composed of hydrogen ions, and chloride ions, and the gradient of hydrogen ions between the blood and the lumen of the stomach is more than one millionfold. This means that energy must be supplied for acid secretion to occur.

The universal currency for energy in mammals to pump ions, such as hydrogen ions or chloride ions, is adenosine triphosphate (ATP). In the 1950s, the pump that creates gradients of sodium ions, Na^+, and potassium ions, K^+, was discovered and called the Na^+,K^+ ATPase. Mammalian cells need internally high concentrations of K^+ in order to maintain a resting transmembrane potential. They also use the inward gradient of Na^+ to help accumulate nutrients such as glucose and amino acids.

After this discovery came the realization that the intracellular concentration of calcium ions, Ca^{2+}, was used by mammalian cells as a signaling device for muscle contraction. A pump, the Ca^{2+} ATPase was found that was able to accumulate Ca^{2+} in stores in muscle cells that were released upon stimulation of the muscle. A similar pump was found on the surface of red cells responsible for moving Ca^{2+} out of these cells. This type of pump was also found on the surface of other cells. Subsequently, it was realized that changes of free calcium in many cells was used as a signaling device for initiation or termination of many cell processes.

__Figure 1.__ — A general model of an ion pump showing the cytoplasmic, membrane, and extracytoplasmic domains. The ions pass through the membrane domain energized by changes in the cytoplasmic domain induced by the breakdown of ATP.

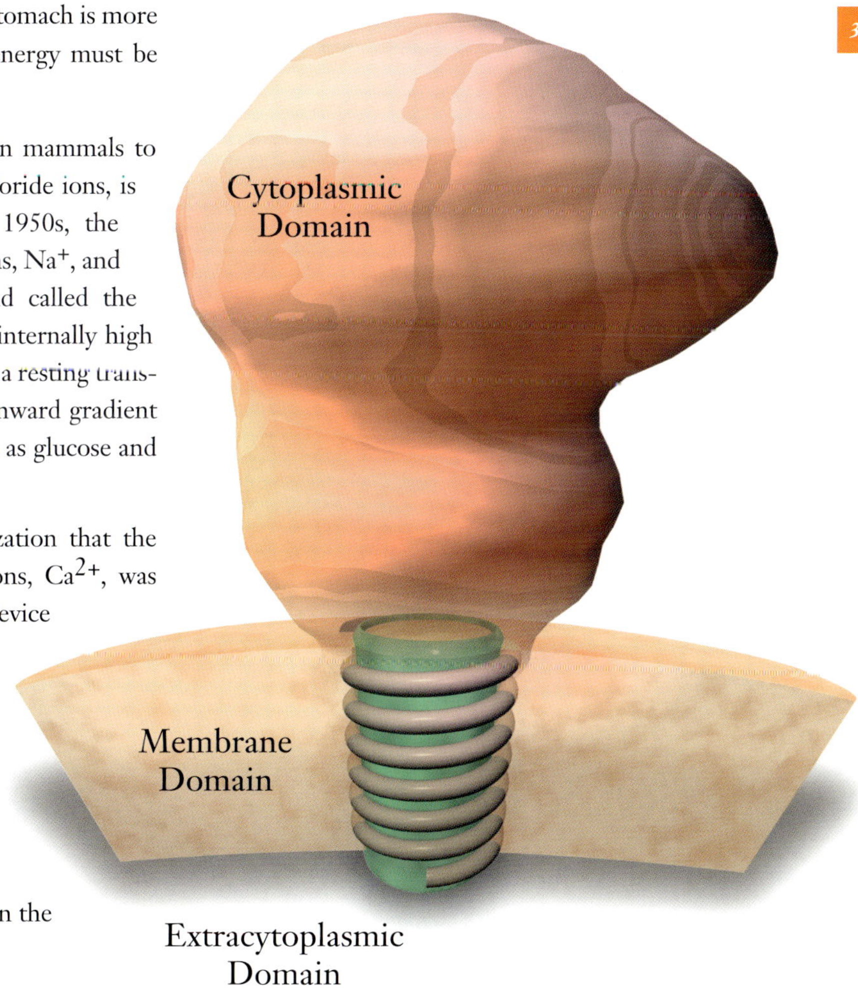

Gastric H,K ATPase

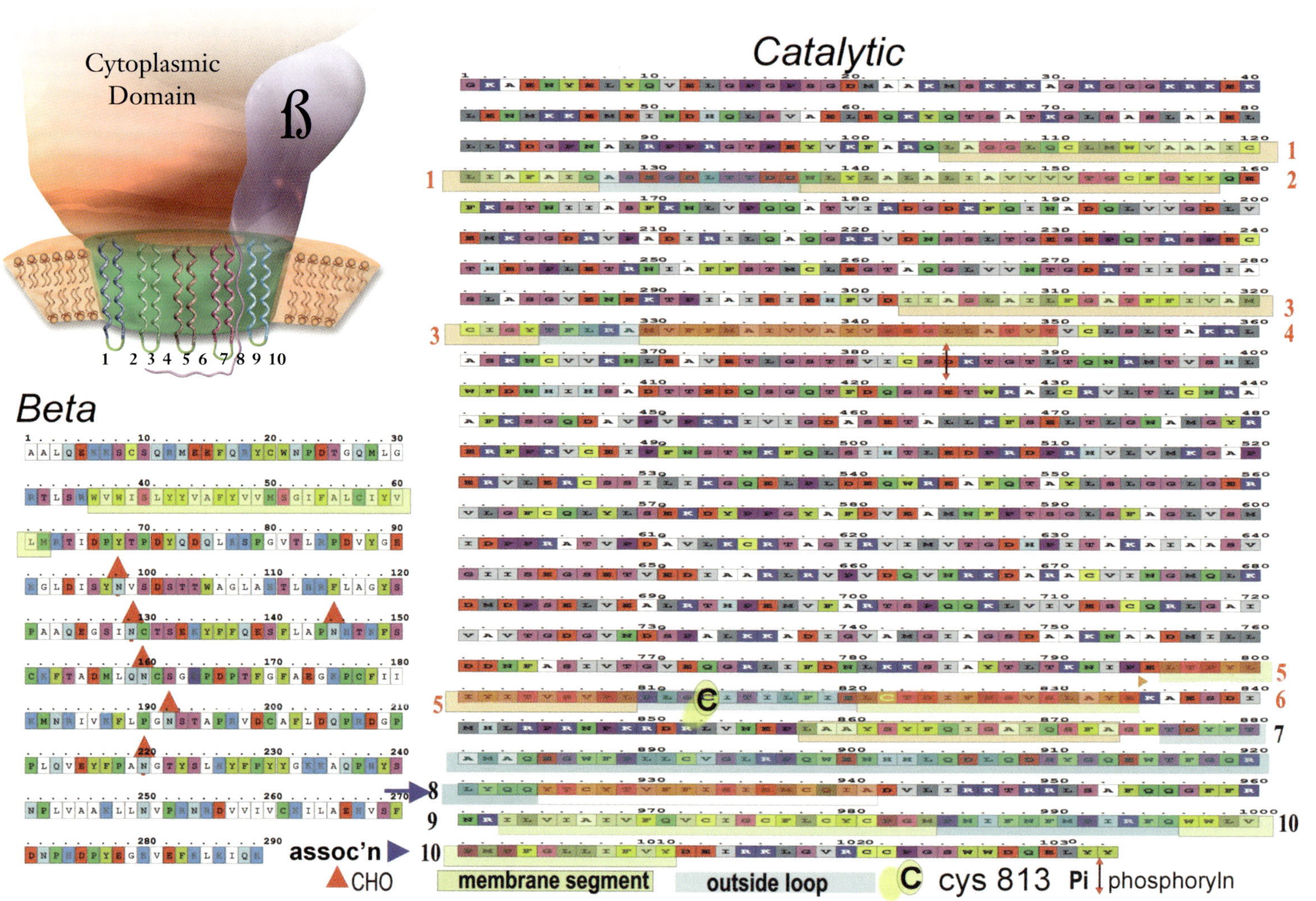

Figure 2. — *The amino acid sequence of the catalytic subunit of the gastric acid pump, illustrating different catalytic and structural aspects known about this enzyme. The phosphorylation site and the membrane segments with their connecting loops are illustrated as well as the phosphorylation consensus sequence common to this family of ion transport ATPases. The amino acids are color coded according to hydrophobicity, hydrophilicity, and charge. The membrane segments contain a preponderance of hydrophobic amino acids. The cysteine later shown to be involved in inhibition by omeprazole is highlighted in yellow.*

This figure also shows the amino acid sequence of the beta subunit of the gastric H^+,K^+ ATPase with the single transmembrane segment and the sites of glycosylation. Most of the subunit is extracellular, and only about 35 amino acids are cytoplasmic. The amino acids are color coded according to hydrophobicity, hydrophilicity, and charge.

H^+, K^+ ATPase

It seemed logical to think that gastric acid secretion was also dependent on ATP as the energy source, and in the 1970s it was shown that gastric acid secretion depended on counter-transport of hydrogen and potassium ions, H^+ for K^+, by a pump quite similar to the Na^+,K^+ ATPase, called the gastric H^+,K^+ ATPase. The gastric acid pump is very similar in structure to the sodium pump and is composed of two proteins — the catalytic or alpha subunit and the beta subunit — that are placed very close together in the apical membrane of the acid-secreting cell of the stomach: the parietal cell. The employment of molecular biologic methods has allowed the amino acid composition and sequence of the gastric acid pump's subunits to be elucidated. From such knowledge, we can derive understanding of the way this pump works. From a mechanistic viewpoint, we can then understand how to design inhibitors of this pump.

Because there is only one acid pump in the stomach, inhibition of this pump would be expected to be an extremely effective way of inhibiting acid secretion and thereby treat acid-related diseases. To comprehend how to inhibit the pump, we have to be able to describe how the pump works and where, in its mechanisms do we have to insert a compound that prevents the pump from working.

For ion transport to occur across a biologic membrane, it has to be shielded from the hydrophobic fatty acids in the interior of the membrane. The building block of a membrane is phospholipid. Glycerol, which has three hydroxyl groups, is the fundamental brick. The first hydroxyl group is bound by an organic molecule that is relatively hydrophilic, such as choline, serine, or ethanolamine, the head group of the phospholipid. The second two hydroxyl groups are esterified with fatty acids. Hence, the building block has two sides: a side that orients toward water and a side that orients away from water. The actual membrane is made up of a bilayer of the phospholipids, so that both sides of the membrane facing the cytoplasm or outside the cell consist of the head groups and the interior of the membrane contains the fatty acids that are bound to glycerol. The bilayer thus has a hydrophilic surface and a hydrophobic core. For ion transport to occur across a membrane bilayer, a protein must span the bilayer and provide a hydrophilic surface for ions to be able to cross the membrane. For ATP-driven transport, there must also be binding of ATP on the cytoplasmic surface of the pump in the cell membrane and breakdown of the ATP at that location to transmit energy through the protein to the ion. Perhaps the simplest way to start to build a picture of the acid pump is to describe what the acid pump looks like at various levels of resolution.

The acid pump is a polytopic integral membrane protein. Proteins are made up of chains of amino acids that are folded in specific ways, depending on the actual sequence of the natural twenty amino acids that are the components of proteins. These amino acids have a common structure — R-CH (NH_2)-COOH — that is linked by peptide bonds

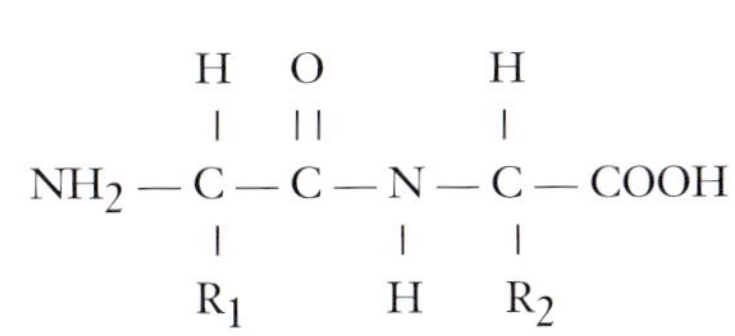

The important difference between the different amino acids is in the nature of the R group. It can even be hydrogen, as in the simplest amino acid: glycine. Based on differences of the R group, amino acids can be classified into those which are relatively neutral in terms of partition between water and octanol, those that prefer octanol or are hydrophobic, and those that prefer water. For example, those with hydrophilic side chains, and especially the positively and negatively charged amino acids—such as lysine, arginine, glutamate, and aspartate—prefer water.

Structure

There are 1033 amino acids in a linear chain that make up the catalytic subunit, and 292 amino acids make up the beta subunit. An analysis of the role of sections of these sequences of these amino acids is the basis of describing structure-function of the pump itself. Based on this, it is possible to assign mechanism to an inhibitor of the pump.

The protein of the two subunits of the pump has sequences that contain largely hydrophobic amino acids that span the membrane in the form of alpha helices. These sequences are about 20 amino acids in length. There are 10 such sequences in the catalytic subunit of the gastric acid pump and one in the beta subunit. The transport of protons in exchange for potassium occurs across these sequences that comprise the membrane domain of the protein. The loops connecting the membrane segment constitute the external or extra-cytoplasmic surface of the protein. There are therefore about 250 amino acids in the membrane and external domains. The membrane segments and the loops connecting them have been defined in various ways such as analysis of hydrophobicity of the amino acid sequence, the presence of membrane peptides after cleavage of the cytoplasmic domain, *in vitro* translation of sequences of the pump, and analysis of two-dimensional crystals. From such analyses, the catalytic subunit has 10, and the beta subunit 1, membrane-inserted segment.

From Figure 2 defining the amino acid sequence of the pump and from the beta sequence, it is possible to present a general view of the gastric acid pump.

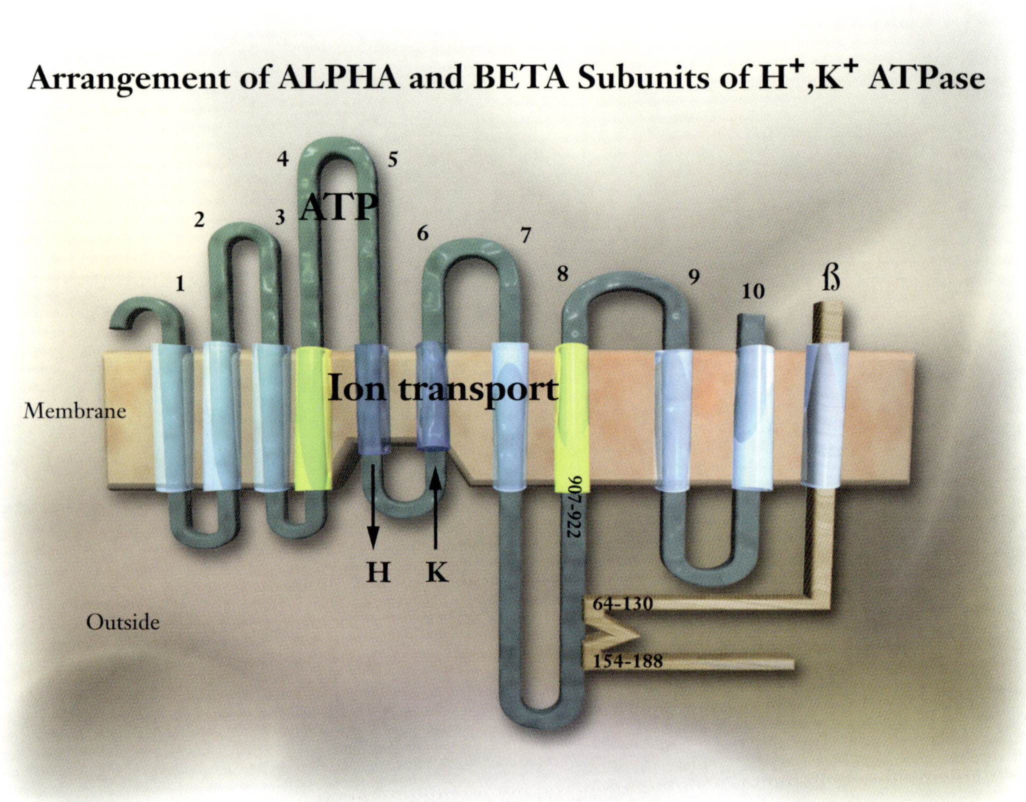

Figure 3. — *An illustration of the two-dimensional arrangement of the gastric H^+,K^+ ATPase, showing the 10 membrane segments of the catalytic subunit and the single membrane subunit of the beta subunit, with the sites of strong association in the region before the 8th transmembrane segment of the catalytic subunit and two regions of the beta subunit with number of the positions of the amino acids in these regions. The H^+ and K^+ transport pathways are colored to illustrate the role of the 4th ,5th ,6th, and 8th membrane-inserted segments.*

Mechanism

The helices of the membrane domain bind the hydrogen ion with high affinity, and there is a gate made up of interacting amino acids within these helices, preventing the ion from moving out of the cell. With phosphorylation, the gate opens by changes in the tilt of the helices, the binding affinity for the hydrogen ion falls, and the ion moves out of the cell. This occurs because of a change in conformation of the phosphorylated enzyme: for convenience, classified as E1 in the high-affinity state for hydrogen ions and E2 in the low-affinity state for hydrogen ions. The binding site for hydrogen ions enlarges, so that the binding for the small hydrogen or hydronium ion is weakened, and now there is room for the larger potassium ion.

The possible conformational change in the cytoplasmic domain with phosphorylation and binding of the hydrogen ion and changes of tilt in the membrane domain are illustrated in Figure 5.

The pump, after binding ATP, breaks it down in two steps: first transferring the terminal phosphate to the protein and then hydrolyzing the phosphoprotein bond. This occurs within the part of the protein facing the cell interior: the cytoplasmic domain. The amino acid that is phosphorylated and dephosphorylated is an aspartyl carboxylate in the cytoplasmic loop connecting the 4th and 5th transmembrane segments. As a function of phosphorylation and dephosphorylation, the cytoplasmic domain undergoes a change of shape or conformation that is transmitted to the membrane helices. The gastric acid pump exports hydrogen ions in strict exchange for potassium ions: hence, the name, the gastric H^+,K^+ ATPase.

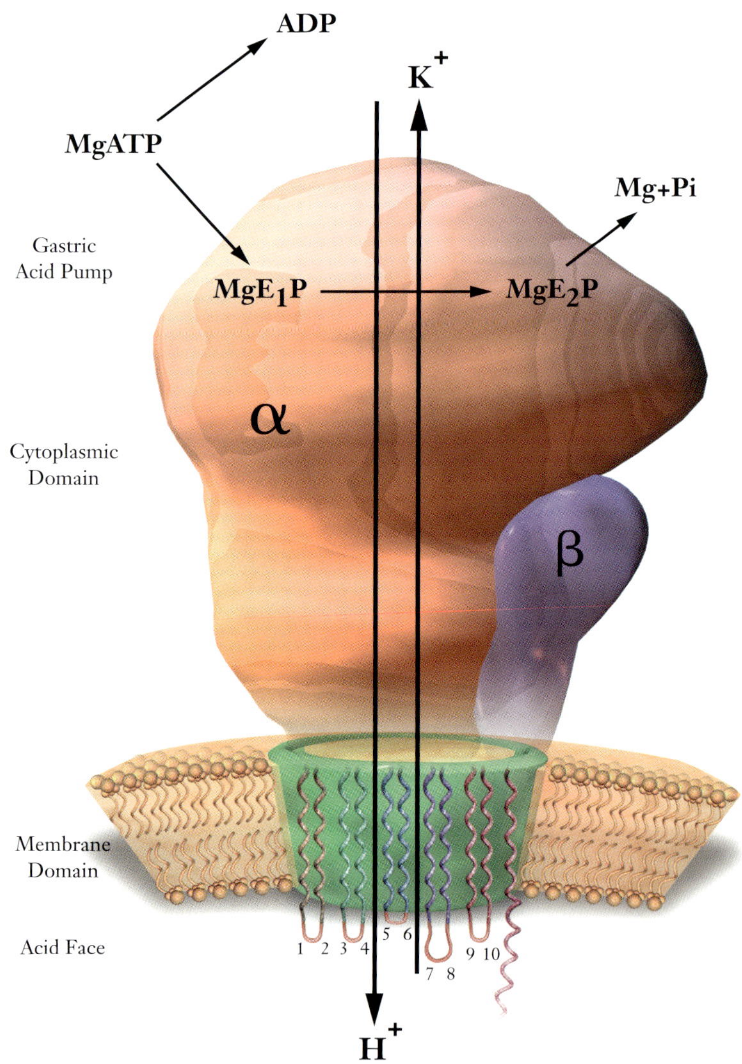

Figure 4 — *A more realistic representation of the gastric acid pump, showing the two subunits, the 10 membrane segments inserted into the phospholipid bilayer, and the H^+ for K^+ exchange resulting from ATP-dependent enzyme phosphorylation and dephosphorylation.*

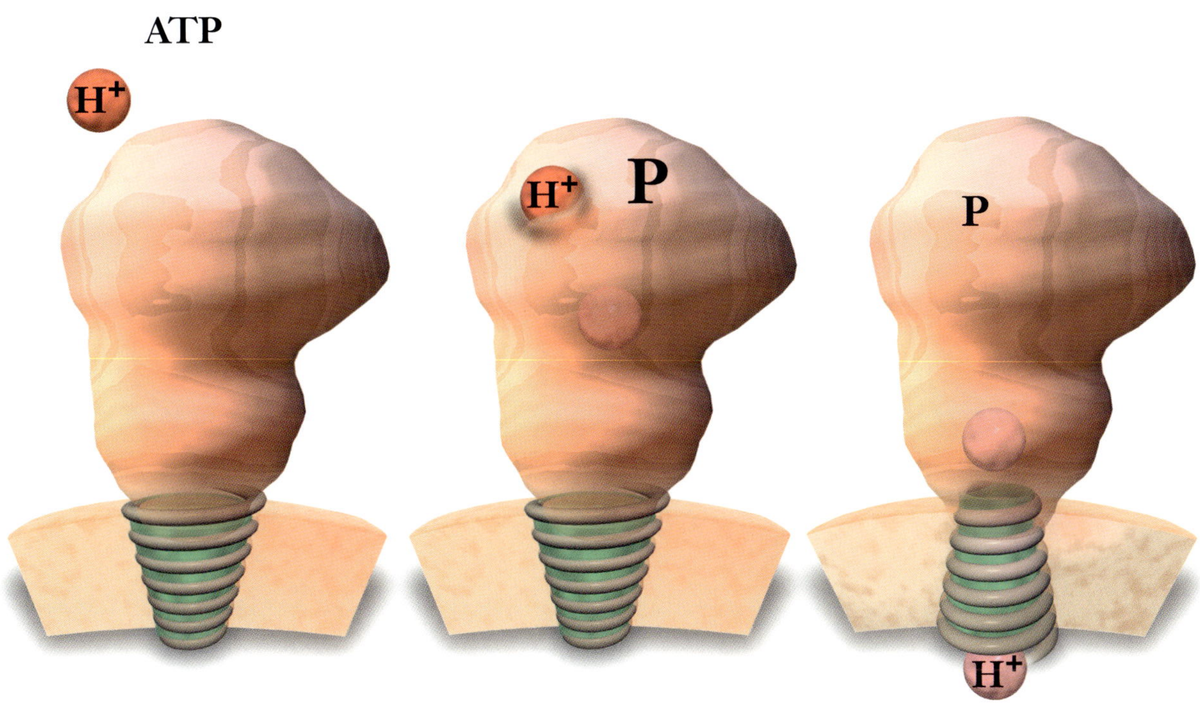

Figure 5. — An illustration of the effect of enzyme phosphorylation and entry of the hydrogen ion into the pump with conformational changes in the cytoplasmic domain transmitted to the membrane domain. H^+ enters a crevice in the cytoplasmic domain, and, with phosphorylation, this domain changes shape, moving the H^+ through the membrane domain.

Therefore, as hydrogen ions leave, the site that bound hydrogen ion in the outward direction now binds potassium in the inward direction, and as the enzyme dephosphorylates and achieves its original conformation, potassium is transported inward. Without potassium binding on the external face of the enzyme, the enzyme is stuck in the E2-P conformation, and only one half cycle of transport can occur.

A series of studies have been carried out to find which of the 10 membrane segments actually are involved in ion transport. Most of these involve site-directed mutagenesis of this enzyme and the Na^+,K^+ and Ca^{2+} ATPases, as they have common ancestry in the hydrogen ion pump present in yeast. From such work, it is established that membrane segments 4,5,6, and 8 contain amino acids essential for transport.

Furthermore, it appears from other work that segments 5 and 6 have mobility within the protein, being readily extractable after removal of the cytoplasmic domain and showing positional sensitivity to the presence of bound molecules on the outside face of the membrane pair. Other studies have investigated the relative position of the different helices by cross-linking studies and by measurement of interactions between the alpha and beta subunits. A three-dimensional crystal has been reconstructed of the yeast hydrogen ion and sarcoplasmic reticular calcium pumps that visualizes the membrane domain and the overall shape of the cytoplasmic domain. By analogy, it is possible to construct a hypothetical three-dimensional model of the gastric H^+,K^+ ATPase and to consider mechanisms of inhibition of this pump using this model.

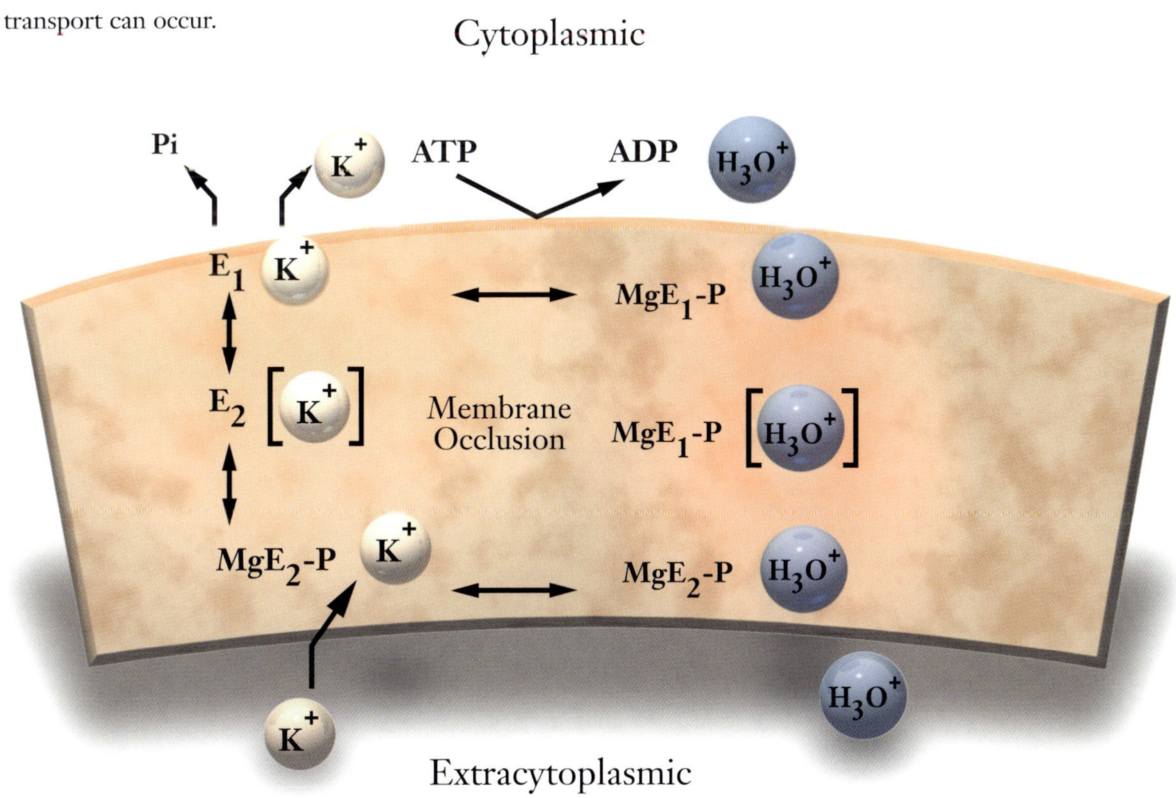

Figure 6. — A representation of the chemical steps involved in outward transport of hydrogen ion and uptake of potassium. Transport occurs by a cycle of protein phosphorylation and dephosphorylation: the phosphorylation step energizing secretion of hydrogen ions, the dephosphorylation step energizing reuptake of potassium.

Three Dimensional View of Gastric ATPase

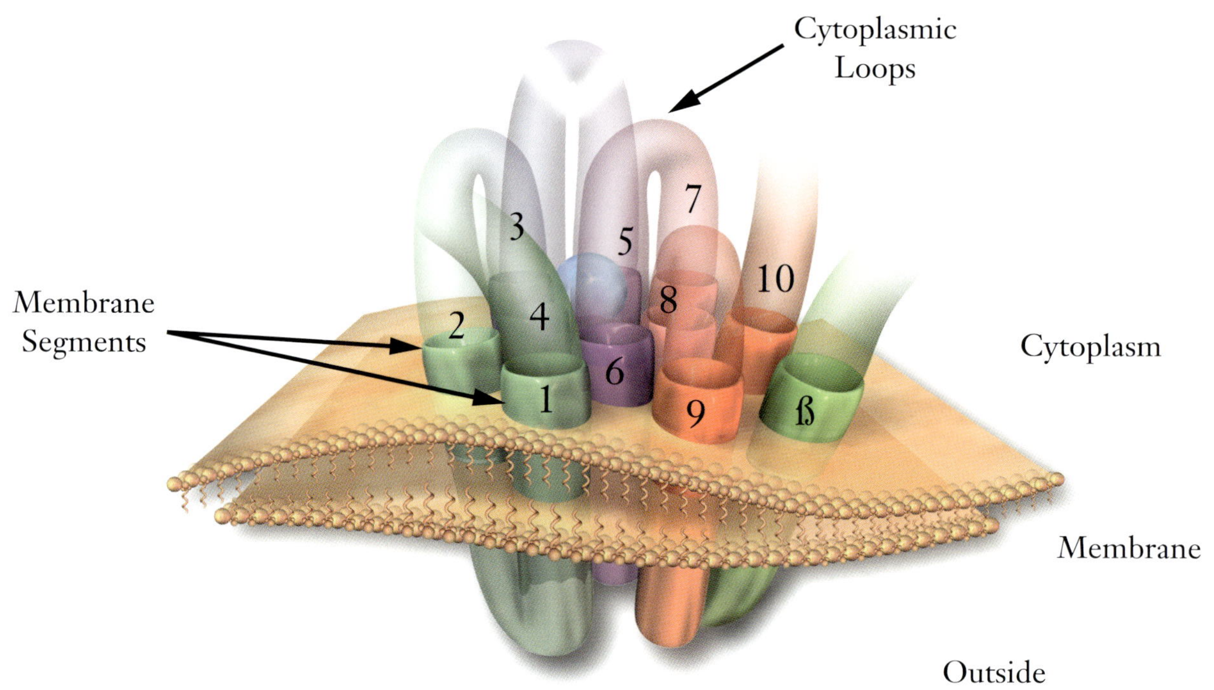

Figure 7. — *A three-dimensional model of the gastric acid pump viewed at an angle, cytoplasmic side up. The cytoplasmic loops connect segments 2,3 and 4,5 and 6,7 and 8,9. The N terminal sequence is before 1, and the alpha subunit ends after 10. The beta subunit has a single transmembrane segment and is tightly associated with transmembrane sequence 8 of the catalytic subunit. The ion transport region includes TM 4,5,6, and 8. Conformational changes are largely in TM5 and 6.*

As discussed, ion transport, the process we want to inhibit, occurs across the membrane domain. Therefore, the inhibitor should be designed to bind to the membrane domain. The region of the membrane domain carrying out the transport is the space enclosed by membrane segments 4,5,6, and 8. Within this region, segments 5 and 6 are mobile as if they were the pumping segments. If a molecule binds to the outside of this membrane pair, mobility and pumping would stop.

We will see that omeprazole does exactly that: namely, bind covalently to the loop between M5 and M6, stopping the pump from moving hydrogen ions into the canaliculus of the parietal cell.

Catalysis-Transport Coupling

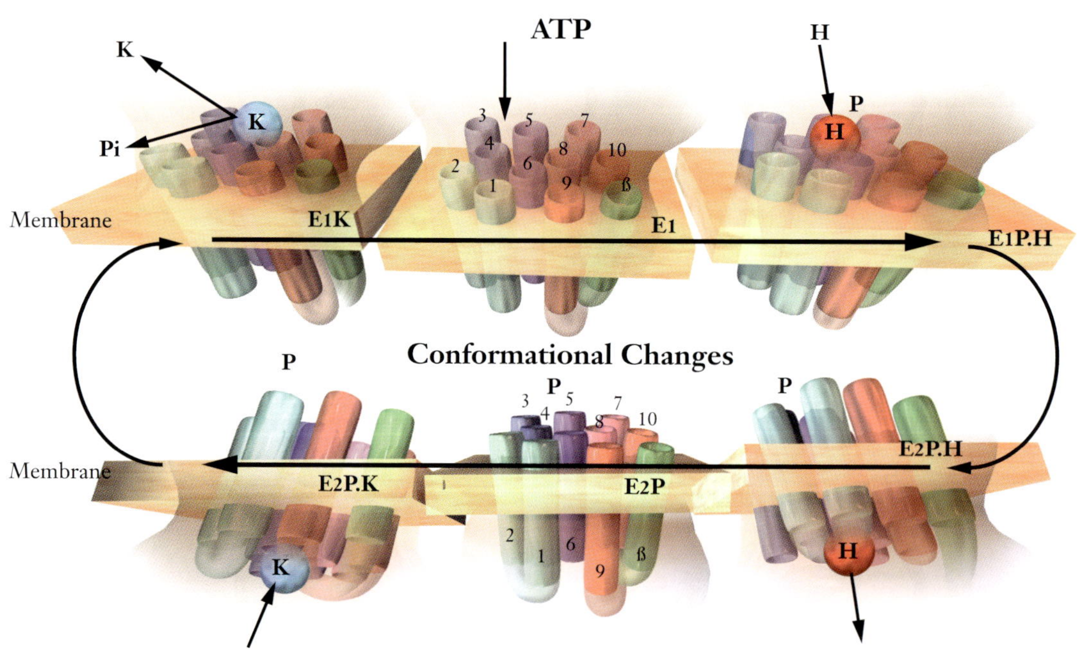

Figure 8. — *A three-dimensional representation of the steps involved in transporting H^+ ion outward and K^+ ion inward by conformational changes in the cytoplasmic domain induced by phosphorylation. These changes are transmitted to the membrane domain — in particular, M5 and M6 — which are mobile in the membrane and contain ion-binding sites. Binding of the hydronium ion (H_3O^+) occurs from the cytoplasmic surface. Motion of the membrane domain moving this site to outward exposure induced by phosphorylation results in outward hydrogen ion secretion. A change in the size of the site during this motion reduces H^+ ion affinity and increases K^+ ion affinity. K^+ ion can then bind to this site and induce motion inward associated with dephosphorylation of the protein.*

Activation

The gastric H^+,K^+ ATPase is found in two locations in the parietal cell: either the tubulovesicular membranes or the microvilli of the secretory canaliculus. The former location signifies a resting pump condition, the latter an activated pump. The movement or transformation of the tubulovesicles to the canalicular membrane is regulated by the various signaling systems such as changes in cAMP or intracellular calcium. The sodium pump—the Na^+,K^+ ATPase—is confined to the basal lateral membrane.

For activity of the pump, K^+ ion is required on the outside surface of the pump. Activation of the enzyme is therefore accompanied by a large increase in the KCl permeability of the membrane containing the ATPase, enabling H^+ for K^+ ion exchange. This KCl permeability is as yet ill defined but is essential for acid secretion. The steps involved in activation are triggered by protein phosphorylation following activation of cAMP dependent protein kinase A and perhaps a calcium-dependent protein kinase.

Trafficking of the ATPase to the apical membrane or eversion of the tubulovesicles is apparently dependent, at least in part, on the presence of a tyrosine in the N terminal domain of the beta subunit of the H^+,K^+ ATPase, which appears to be phosphorylated as part of the stimulatory pathway. Removal of this tyrosine apparently leads to permanent residence of the pump in the secretory membrane.

Selective localization of the H^+,K^+ ATPase to the apical as compared to the basal lateral surface is altered by mutations in the 4th transmembrane segment but is apparently due to conformation of the loop immediately following this transmembrane segment. This results in the differential localization of the acid pump to the apical membrane and the sodium pump to the basal membrane.

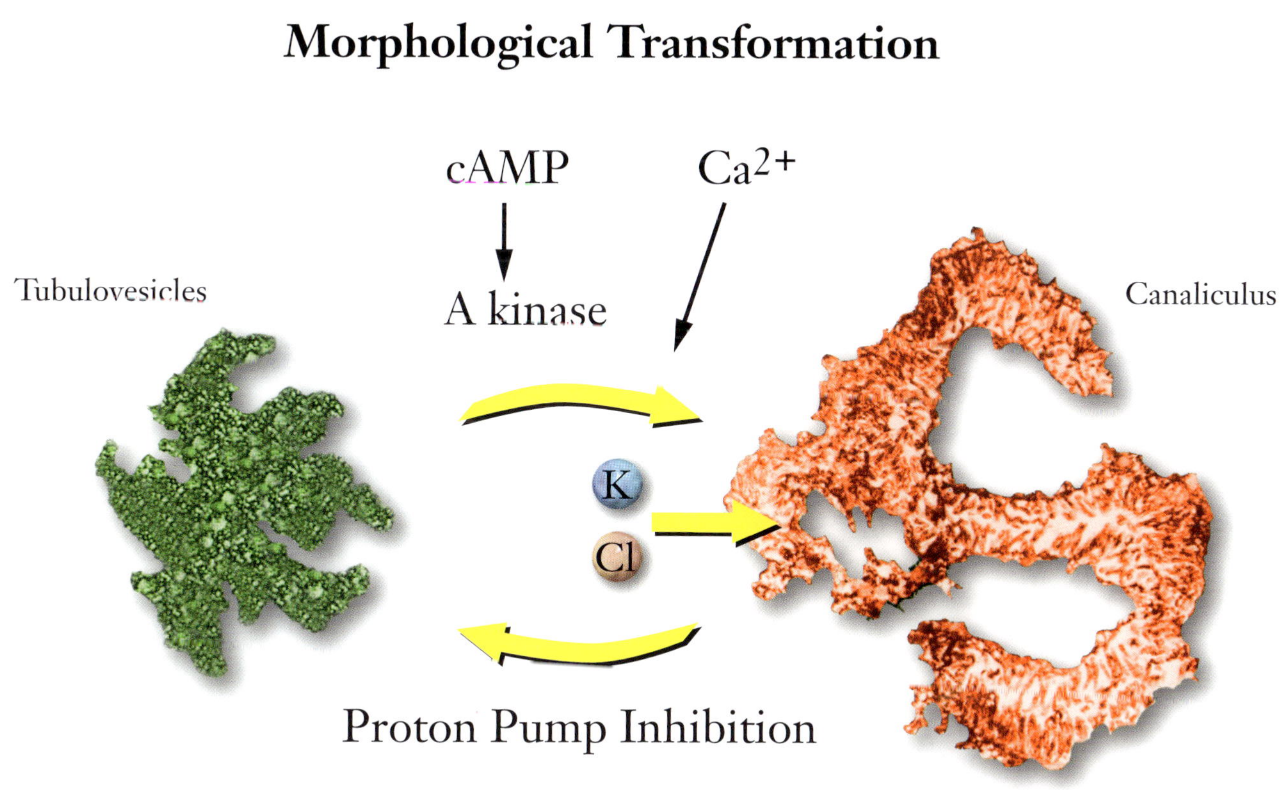

Figure 9. — *A model of the activation of the acid pump by movement into the microvilli of the canaliculus of the parietal cell and association with a KCl pathway.*

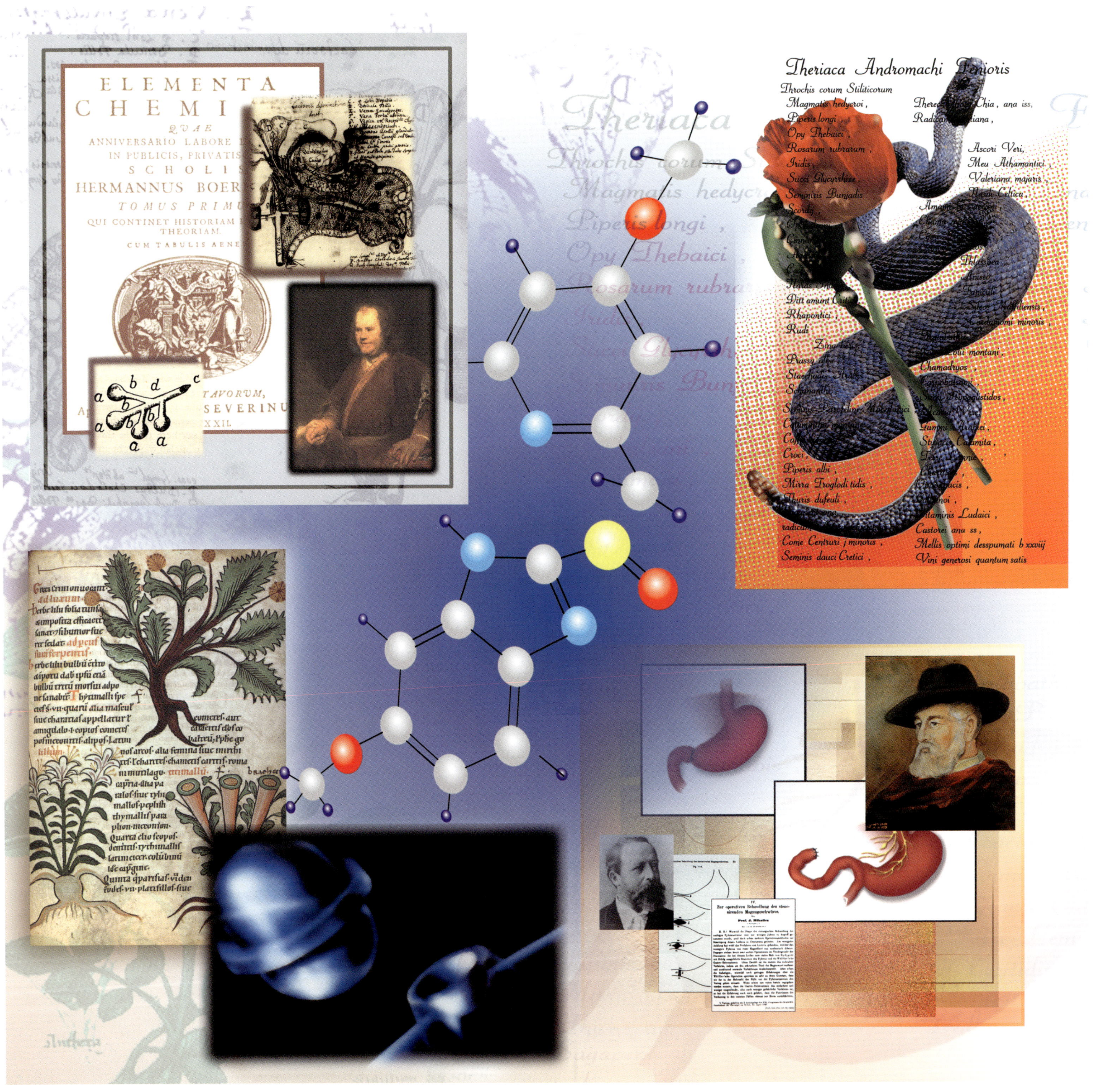
ELEMENTA
Theriaca Andromachi
Throchis corum Stiliticorum
Magmatis hedycroi,
Piperis longi,
Opy Thebaici,
Rosarum rubrarum,
Ascori Veri,
Meu Athamantici,
Valeriana majaris,
Rhapontici,
Piperis albi,
Mirra Troglodi tidis,
Come Centruri j minoris,
Seminis dauci Cretici,
Castorei ana ss,
Mellis optimi desspumati b xxviij
Vini generosi quantum satis

Chapter IV

Therapy Failure to Success

Concepts

Remedies

Ulcers and Acid

Cytoprotection

Anticholinergics

Prostaglandins

The H2-Receptor Antagonists

Proton Pump Inhibitors

Novel Agents

Surgery

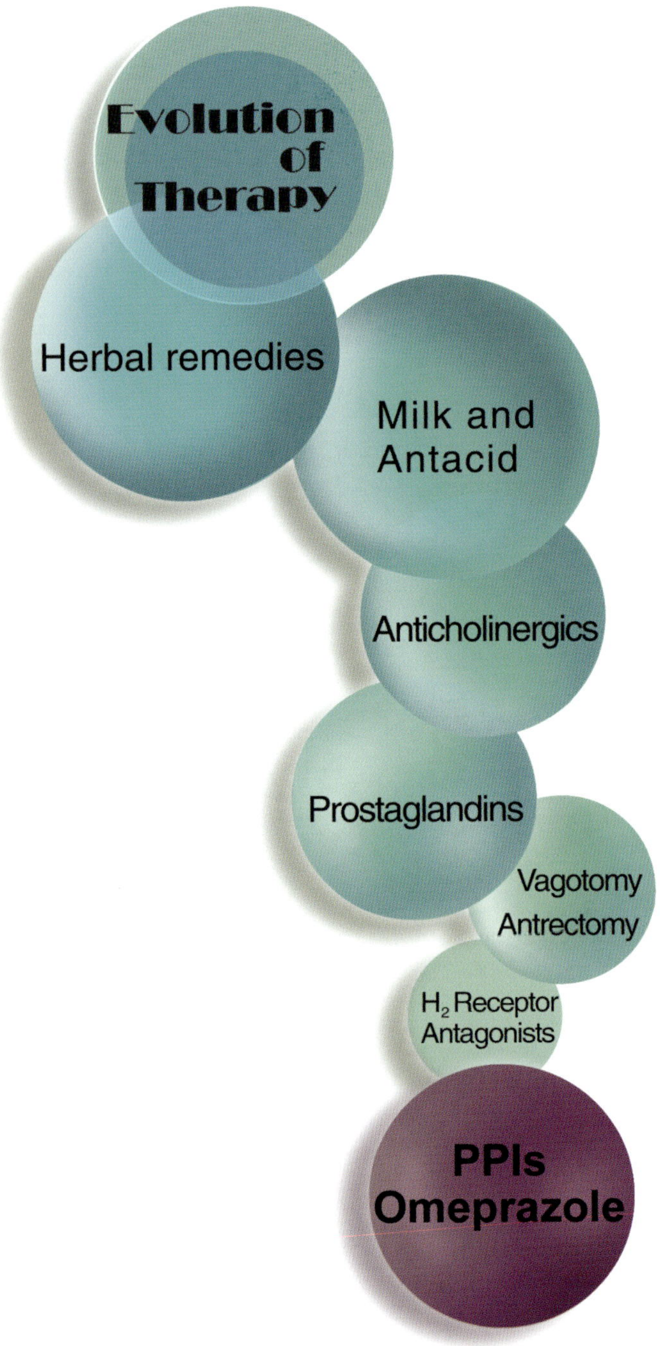
Evolution of Therapy
Herbal remedies
Milk and Antacid
Anticholinergics
Prostaglandins
Vagotomy Antrectomy
H2 Receptor Antagonists
PPIs Omeprazole

Chapter IV

THERAPY
FAILURE TO SUCCESS

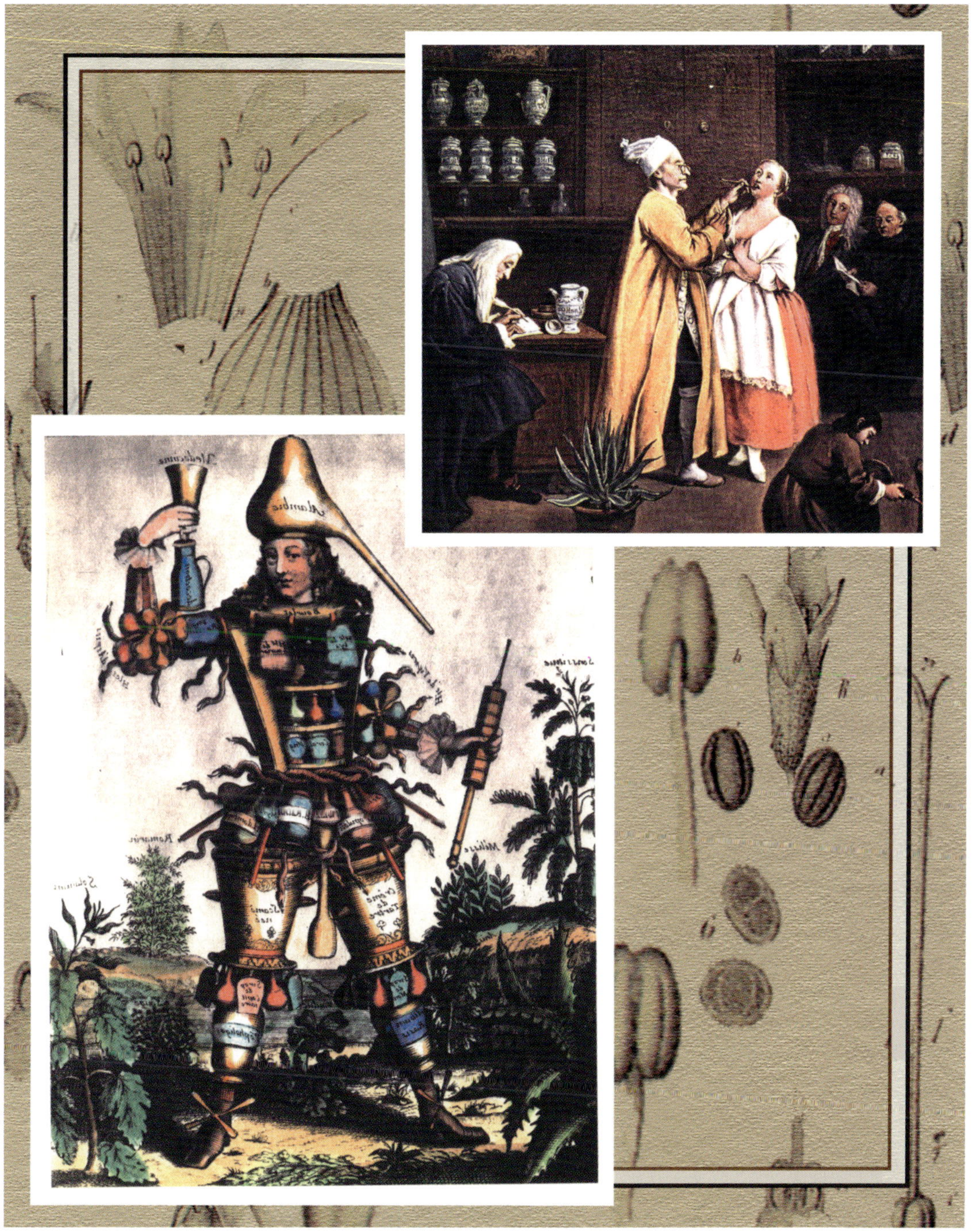

Figure 1. — The dubious success of early pharmacotherapeutic remedies led to considerable skepticism. Physicians were considered to often have ulterior motives in treating patients, particularly when those who sought their help were women. Thus, pictures of persons in odd garb and full of "puffed" learning were cynically depicted (top right). *An obsession with substances derived from various plants that had persisted from the earliest of times was reinforced by the overt sexuality of the floral taxonomy proposed by Linnaeus* (bottom right). *Issues of potency, vigor, and reproductive strength thus became closely aligned with stamens, pistols, seeds, and concepts of good health and physical vigor. The ludicrous notion of pharmacists and physicians proposing multiple and bizarre remedies, each of which claimed to cure a multiplicity of sundry ailments, was vividly captured by the French caricature of polypharmacotherapy* (left). *In much the same way as a process had been sought to transmute all base metals into gold, so did the medical fraternity seek a remedy that would transform all illness into health.*

Concepts

The pursuit of good health has been an age-old preoccupation. The universal salutation of greeting and conviviality almost always includes words directed toward the maintenance of health. The concerns of the human race have always been focused on the stomach and heart. In this respect, the relationship of mental well-being to physical health extends as far back as the commentaries of the ancient Roman and Greek philosophers. The loss of balance between a sound mind and a healthy body was long considered to generate illness in its many and varied forms. Among the most common concepts well-being was engendered by gastric satisfaction or satiety. Thus, from the earliest yearnings of a child for maternal milk and its benefits, humans remain obsessed with the need for oral and digestive comfort, the lack of which often leads to symptoms. So linked are these processes of pleasure and satisfaction that failure to satisfy the latter may often culminate in disturbances of the former with dyspepsia, heartburn, and a variety of disorders that significantly alter health and well-being. The earliest well-being of a child relates to breast milk. Milk, for thousands of years, has been the universal panacea for digestive disorders including those related to peptic acid disease. If it is true that *homo est quod est* (man is what he eats), then consideration of acid peptic diseases of the mucosa of the esophagus, stomach, and duodenum leads to the conclusion that the problem is acquired. Earliest texts address disorders of digestion and remedies.

Sufi mystics, Sephardic sages, philosophers of the Tang dynasty, and the Odes of the Mantuan Bard all examine the fundamental issues of food, the stomach, and digestion: a matter of concern to physicians and their patients for as long as records exist. From the Ebers Papyrus to the reflux symptoms of Einstein, the failed management of dypepsia has been documented.

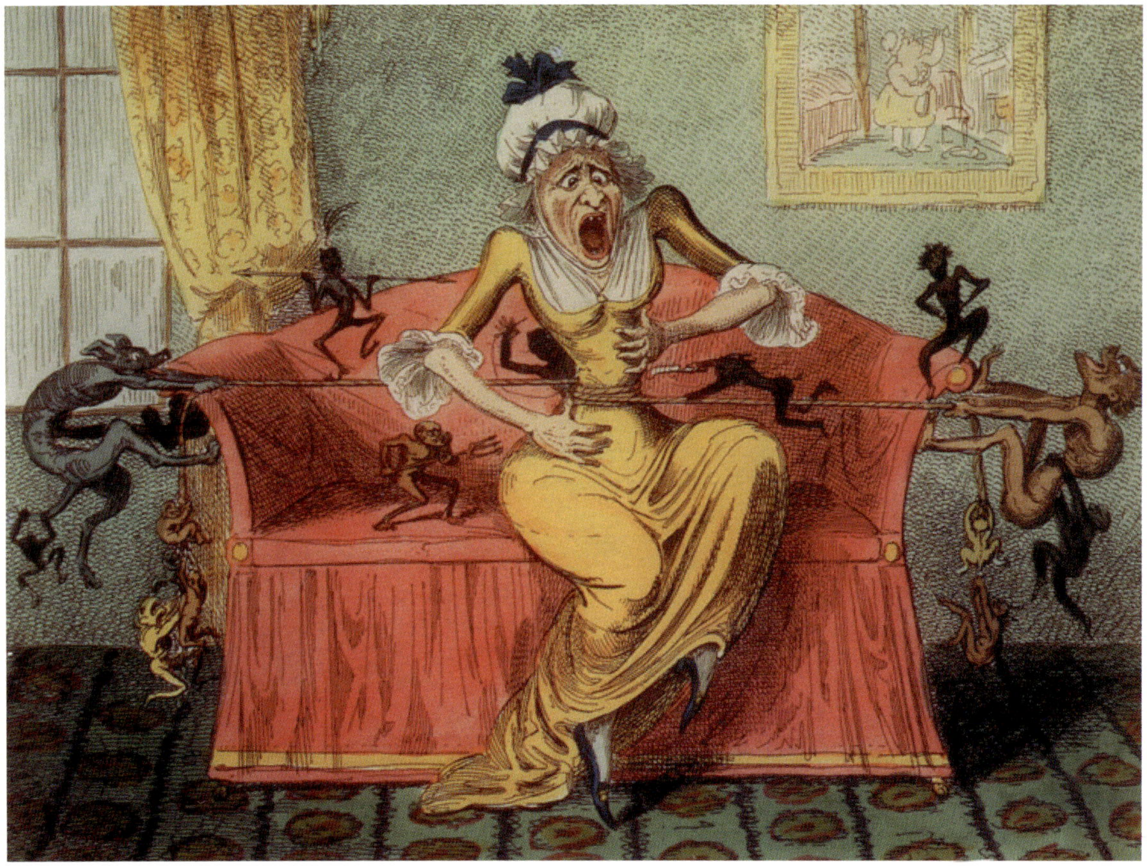

Figure 2. — *The treatment of unremitting dyspepsia and indigestion was a continued source of comment and caricature during the 18th and 19th century. Whether the cause was deemed to be hysterical due to a wandering uterus or melancholy due to a disorder of the spleen, no reliable remedies were available. This lampoon depicts a woman at her wits' end and is best summarized by Matthew Blunderhead's reminisces with regard to a doctor's visit to himself and his sister:*

I'm bilious, I find, and the women are nervous;
Their systems relax'd and all turn'd topsy turvy,
With hypochondriasis, obstructions and scurvy,
And these are distempers he must know the whole on,
For he talked of the peritoneum and colon,
Of phlegmatic humours oppressing the women,
From feculent matter that swells the abdomen;
But the noise I have heard in my bowels like thunder,
Is a flatus I find in my left hypochonder,
So plenty of med'cines each day does he send,
Post singules liquidas sedes sum end
Ad crepitus vesper' et man' promo vend,
In English to say, we must swallow a potion,
For driving out wind after every motion;
The same to continue for three weeks at least,
Before we may venture the waters to taste;
Five times have I purged yet I am sorry to tell ye,
I find this same gnawing and wind in my belly...

Clearly there was little relief available from dyspepsia and its symptomatology!

Remedies

Despite the preoccupation with dyspepsia, there was little rational therapeutic intervention for the treatment of gastric disorders. Until the late 19th century, the stomach was often not clearly recognized as a source of symptoms nor was it known that the problem was acid related. Early folk medicine noted that chalk, charcoal, and slop diets provided symptomatic relief from dyspepsia. The ancient Romans and Greeks, including Celsus and Praxigoras, had advised against eating "acrid" food. In the 17th century, chalk and pearl juleps were used for infant gastric disorders, but little rational comment was available in regard to adult problems. Jan Heurne, the first proponent of bedside teaching, left a posthumous pamphlet on the diseases of the stomach in 1610, and Martin Harmes and Ferriol, in 1684 and 1668, respectively, produced books on diseases of the stomach and intestines. These contributions offered dietary advice and superstition. In 1664, Swalbe published a long satire on "the quarrels and opprobria of the stomach," and Cullen and his Edinburgh colleagues espoused a nervous basis for problems affecting the digestive system.

A widely held opinion of 17th century physicians was that dyspepsia was due to gastric atony, as in the term *de imbecilitate ventriculi*. This term continued into the 18th century, when it was associated with "hectic stomach" (Arnold, 1743) and later with *embarras gastrique*. Throughout the 18th century, there were various descriptions of gastric and intestinal diseases, but no specific remedies were recorded. Treatment ranged from hydrotherapy to magnetism, and quack medicines, theriacs, and superstitions were common. Nevertheless, the general doctrine of acidity was prevalent. In a treatise on *Dyspepsia and Other Rearrangements of the Stomach*, Wright emphasized the importance of "...cerebral dyspepsia or those distressing symptoms associated with worry and the overtaxed brain, occasioned by the close

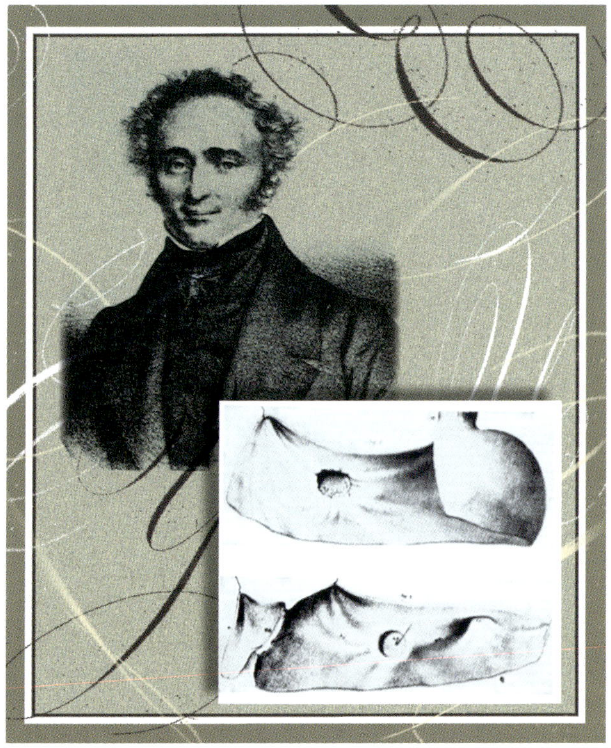

Figure 3. — *Jean Cruveilhier (1791-1873) was born in Limoges and studied with Dupuytren in Paris. In 1836, he attained the Chair of Pathology in Paris and became one of the foremost authorities on stomach ulcers in France, where his name was so closely linked to gastric ulcer that it was referred as Cruveilhier's disease. Although a brilliant clinician and pathologist, Cruveilhier abjured the use of microscopy and preferred illustrated pathologic anatomic text. It was a source of considerable interest to Cruveilhier as to why an ulcer of the stomach might occur in a single place when the rest of the stomach was as he put it "in a state of perfect integrity." This early consideration of a locus minoris resistentiae has yet to be elucidated. The gastric specimen* (bottom) *is that of an unfortunate carpenter with a deep ulceration "six lines in dimension" upon whom Cruveilhier undertook an autopsy. "A stylus introduced into the coronary artery of the stomach pushed a clot out of the center of the ulcer and entered the gastric lumen." The 29-year-old patient, a carpenter, had been admitted on April 15, 1830, to the Charité Hospital, Paris, with a history of recurrent epigastric pain and hematemesis. Initially, mustard plasters were applied to the feet, and venesection undertaken. A repeat hematemesis was treated with the application of 20 leeches to the epigastrium and mustard plaster to the calves while rice and eau d' Kabel were administered orally. The subsequent development of severe melena was treated with the application of 20 leeches to the anus and further applications of mustard plasters to the legs. Accepting the treatment as worse than the disease, the patient died of a further hemorrhage and was at autopsy noted to have a gastric ulcer with a visible vessel* (bottom right).

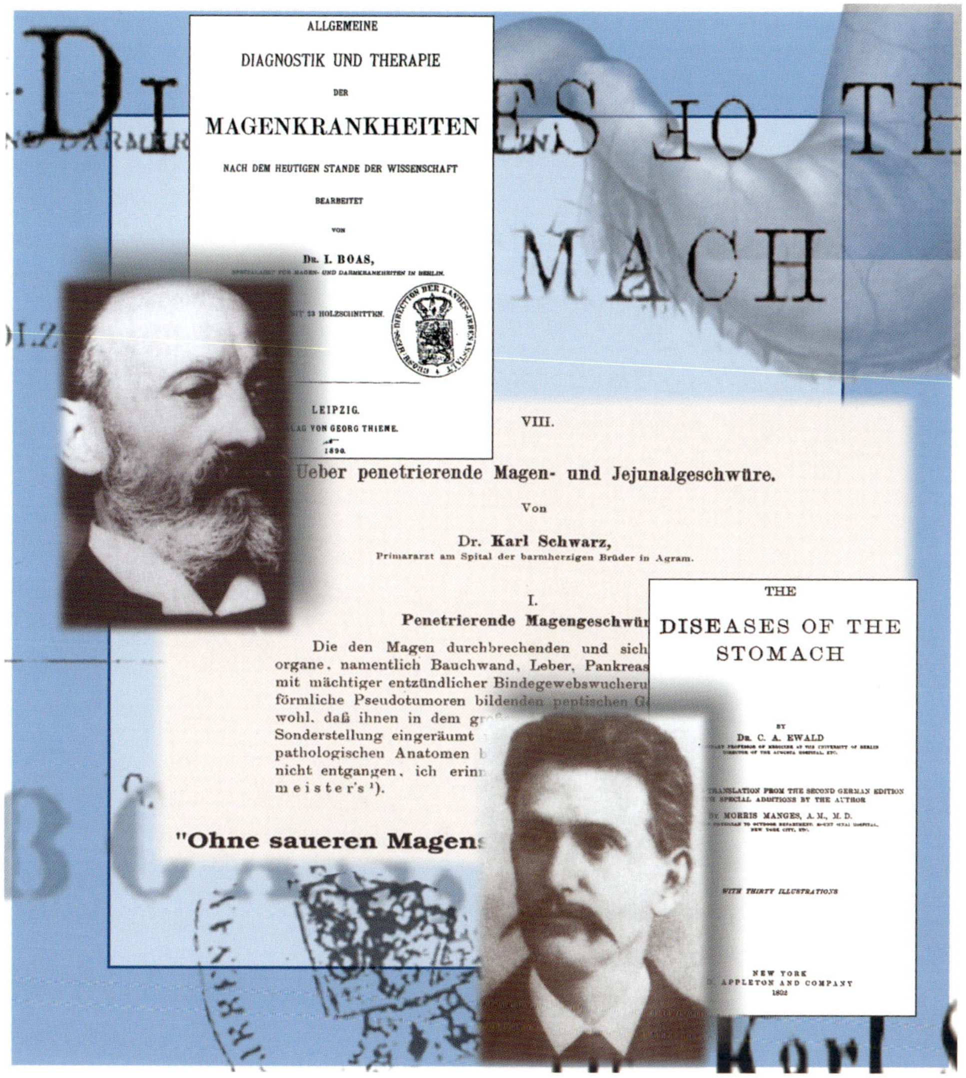

Figure 4. — Ismar Boas (1858-1938) (top left) *was the founder of the specialty of gastroenterology and the editor of the first medical journal for digestive diseases. From 1885 to 1910, he directed a clinic in Berlin, where he trained numerous physicians from many countries. In 1895, he founded and thereafter edited, until 1933, the first medical journal for digestive diseases Boas' Archive fur Verdauungskrankheiten. Although he was a founder of the German Society for Gastroenterology and Metabolic Diseases, he was hounded from the country and committed suicide in Vienna in 1938 as a result of the Nazi Anschluss. As the author of several text books and the founder of a clinic devoted to gastroenterology, Boas and his colleague, Carl Anton Ewald (1845-1915), were the established authorities on ulcer disease at the turn of the century. Ewald (bottom right) was not only a pioneer in gastroenterology but together with Boas developed the first gastric function test (the Ewald Boas test meal). His monographs on diseases of the stomach and intestine (1886) and the gallbladder and biliary tract in 1904 defined the state of the art. In 1914, he was the president of the First Congress of Gastroenterology in Germany.*

In 1910, Karl Schwarz published his classic article that contained the now-famous Schwarz's dictum "no acid, no ulcer" (center). *Although his discussion of penetrating stomach and duodenal ulcers and their relationship to acid had been considered over the previous two decades by Riegel, Ewald, and Boas, it was Schwarz who definitively drew the conclusion that acidity was a prerequisite for gastric or duodenal ulcers.*

sympathy existing between the cerebral and gastric functions..." Joseph Black, in 1754, writing on the subject of carbon dioxide, commented on *de humore acido a cibo orto*, thus recognizing the issues of food, acid, and the stomach.

Ulcers and Acid

In 1835, in Paris, Cruveilhier had written extensively on the pathology of peptic ulcer and so widespread was recognition of the condition that it was referred to as Cruveilhier's disease. However, little specific therapy — apart from bizarre suggestions of applying leeches to the anus, peculiar dietary adjustments (quinces in brandy), or odd homeopathic remedies — were suggested.

In 1875, Drewry, in his book entitled *Common Sense Management of the Stomach*, regarded dyspepsia and its management as so complex as to require division into four kinds in the "first division" and nine in the "second division." Each of these groups required different food, behavior modification, and a variety of herbal and proprietary remedies.

Although Prout had initially identified gastric acid as hydrochloric acid in 1823, it was only in the late 19th century that hyperchlorhydria was recognized as contributing to generation of ulcers. The recognition in this first part of the century that mucosal damage was caused by acid, and that this acid could be decreased by luminal neutralization, resulted in a wave of enthusiasm for antacid preparations, bland diets, and milk as therapeutic options.

Thus, although treatment had not changed over centuries, as pathogenesis and regulatory pathways emerged, therapeutic targets and surgical and medical therapy became more focused and effective.

Early management strategies focused chiefly on the avoidance of acid-containing foods and substances containing capsaicin-related compounds or the intake of neutral foods to ameliorate discomfort. Bland diets were then augmented with neutralizing compounds and antacids.

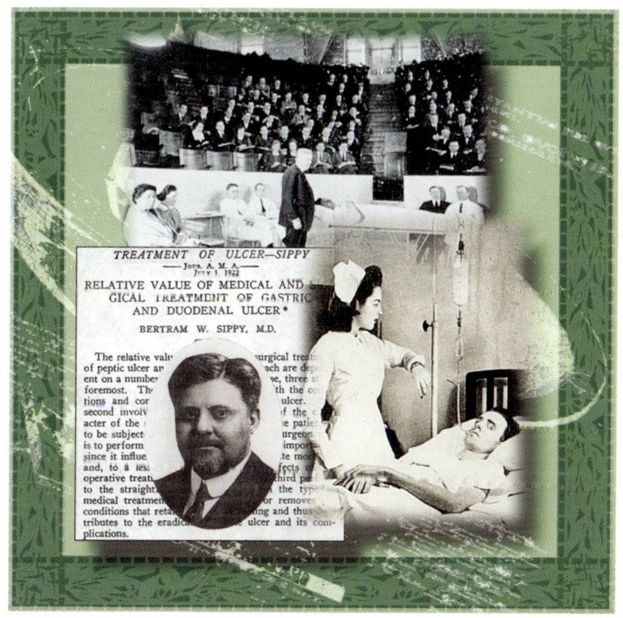

Figure 5. — Dr. Bertram Sippy of Chicago (bottom left) *devised a complex dietary regimen of bland food that included hourly feedings of milk, eggs, and puree as well as the administration of large quantities of calcium and sodium bicarbonate. In addition, he proposed that particularly severe nocturnal dyspepsia could be relieved by regular gastric aspiration. Although cumbersome and likely to generate obsessive-compulsive disorders, this strict regimen was of some benefit and particularly efficacious when compared with the outcome of current surgical intervention for acid peptic disease. Many physicians* (top center) *enthusiastically attended lectures by Sippy to learn more of his novel therapeutic techniques. An alternative dietary therapy developed by Richard Doll proposed hospital admission for up to 3 weeks with continuous nasogastric milk infusion with and without alkali. Although this therapy promoted ulcer healing and relieved pain, the prolonged hospitalization and use of resources as well as loss of productive work time generated a less than optimal solution for the management of acid peptic disease. Cynics proposed that the excessive use of milk accelerated coronary artery disease and that any putative therapeutic benefit was actually derived from the bed rest, the charm of the nursing staff, and the Freudian benefits of the acquisition of milk. This treatment soon fell into disregard except among unusual sects of medical practice.*

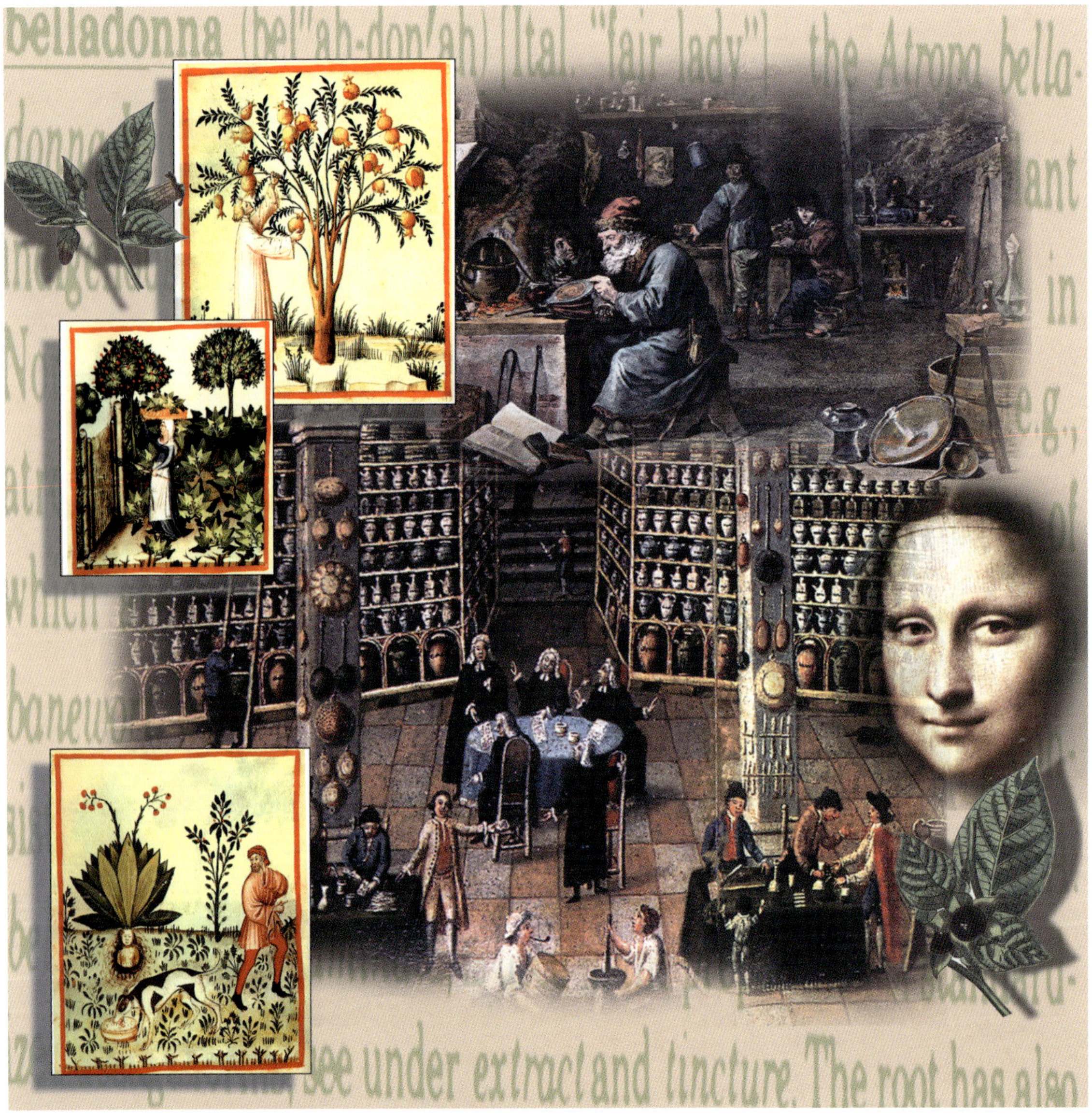

Figure 6. *— The development of modern chemical technology has considerably advanced drug design and the development of rational pharmacotherapeutic strategy. Nevertheless, many of the compounds initially used had their origin in the active principles of herbal remedies. Apothecaries developed mystical techniques* (top right) *for the isolation of the active and pure principles necessary for the cure of disease. Their secrets were closely guarded and handed down from generation to generation. Most treatments were prescribed by physicians who practiced both as alchemists and apothecaries* (center). *In many instances, the remedies themselves were mystic and their effects based on spiritual and magical concepts. Thus, Mandragora* (bottom left) *was known to promote soporific qualities that would induce well-being. The roots, however, were believed to harbor the souls of departed spirits whose release would result in insanity for those who unearthed them. To forestall this devastating possibility, harvesting was accomplished by tying a starving black dog to the plant and offering it food, thus inducing it to tear the plant from the earth and enabling its safe acquisition. Belladonna* (bottom right) *contained an atropine-like substance. This not only dilated the pupils and was used for cosmetic purposes but inhibited acid secretion and was thus favored for the management of dyspeptic problems. The dangers of excessive use of the agent resulted in the nomenclature atropine after Atropos, the Fate, whose responsibility it was to cut the thread.*

The evolving trend to use less invasive management of peptic ulcer disease resulted in a significant interest in antacids in association with diet modification and bed rest. Numerous preparations with different concentrations of alkali or buffers were developed to remove the pain of peptic ulceration and to facilitate healing. Their widespread availability and relative safety resulted in broad popular acceptance. Such agents required four- to six-times-daily administration and could result in side effects including constipation, diarrhea, and decreased absorption of concomitantly administered medications. Large doses of baking soda have led to gastric rupture. Other side effects (diarrhea, milk/alkali syndrome) were associated with the use of excessive alkali and cation-containing agents.

In 1915, Dr. Bertram Sippy advocated hourly feedings of milk, eggs, and purees from 7:00 AM to 8:00 PM. Between these hourly feedings, and every half hour for 2 ½ hours after the last feeding, Sippy powder (calcium and sodium bicarbonate) was administered. In addition, to relieve dyspepsia, the patient's stomach was aspirated at regular intervals each night. This regimen provided a challenge for the patient and the nursing staff. Although this therapeutic strategy seemed to improve the nutritional status of his patients, the obsessional need for dietary management and regulation of alkali intake so interfered with the life style of patients and so often failed to prevent complications from developing, that even surgery became a reasonable option.

An alternative dietary therapy developed by Dr. Richard Doll involved the use for up to 3 weeks of continuous milk drips through a nasogastric tube with or without alkali. Whether the benefit of this procedure was related to the bed rest or the Freudian power of milk was never resolved, but the therapy soon fell into disregard.

Cytoprotection

A consideration of the possibilities of agents that might confer protective properties on the mucosa resulted in the use of glycyrrhizic acid as a therapeutic tool. This constituent of liquorice had long been used as a component of folk remedies for peptic ulcer disease. The oleandane derivative of glycyrrhizic acid was used to treat peptic ulcers, but its cardiac and renal toxicity precluded its use. Subsequently, a sulfated polysaccharide, sucralfate, was developed as an antiulcer agent for treatment of active duodenal ulcer and maintenance therapy after healing of acute ulcers. It is claimed that antiulcer activity is the result of formation of an ulcer-adherent complex that covers the ulcer site and protects it against further attack by acid.

Anticholinergics

As it became recognized that secretion of acid depended on stimulation by a variety of ligands, such as acetylcholine, gastrin, and histamine, a more logical approach to pharmacotherapy evolved. In this respect, the ancient awareness of the efficacy of the atropine family of plants was of initial interest. Extract of belladonna had been used in the latter half of the 19th century for treatment of peptic ulcer disease.

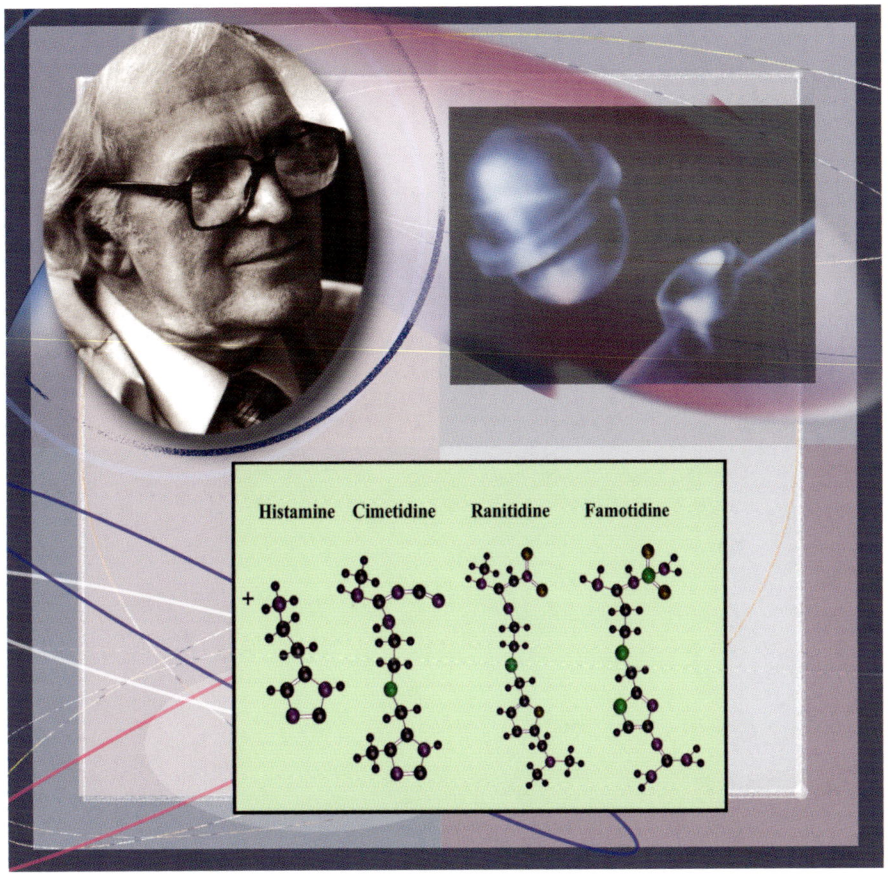

Figure 7. — In 1973, a team of scientists led by James Black, (left) produced the first clinical H2-receptor antagonist cimetidine and introduced the age of acid suppression. This and the subsequent development of additional H2 receptor antagonist agents reformed the treatment of acid-related diseases and provided a highly attractive and safe alternative to surgical therapy, which was associated with a significant morbidity and mortality. Although relatively free of adverse effects, H2 receptor antagonists have nevertheless proved to have some drawbacks. In particular, their action as competitive inhibitors of the H2 receptor-binding site did not block or inhibit other parietal cell stimulatory mechanisms. Such problems became particularly evident in patients undergoing long-term maintenance therapy, particularly in the management of reflux esophagitis or gastrinoma.

The active principle, atropine, is a nonselective muscarinic antagonist able to block transmission in the enteric nervous system. This medication was administered 1 hour before each meal and at bedtime, but the evening dose was high in an attempt to control nocturnal symptoms. As a result of the widespread distribution of muscarinic receptors, unpleasant side effects, such as blurred vision, dry mouth, and bladder dysfunction, limited its use. The development of a relatively selective muscarinic M1 receptor antagonist failed to obviate the side effects and had relatively low efficacy. The subsequent introduction of an even higher-affinity M1 antagonist failed to have an impact on ulcer treatment, as the relevance of the histamine-2 (H2) receptor assumed therapeutic dominance.

Prostaglandins

The discovery of prostaglandins in the 1960s and their cytoprotective and acid-reducing properties engendered a wave of enthusiasm. Naturally occurring substances, they are derived from arachidonic acid, which is released from phospholipids or diacyl glycerol by the action of phospholipase A2. There are two enzyme cascades responsible for generation of prostaglandin, based on cyclooxygenase I (constitutive) and cyclooxygenase II (regulated). After the initial conversion of arachidonic acid into the prostaglandin core structure, several modifications generate various prostaglandins with specific affinities to different prostaglandin receptors. Prostaglandins of the E class are potent inhibitors of acid secretion by action at a Gi coupled EP3 receptor. These were natural lead compounds for development of antiulcer agents. Because natural prostaglandins have a short half-life, the concept driving development of these compounds was prolongation of their half-life. The currently available compound, misoprostol, is not particularly receptor-subtype-selective and can result in stimulation of intestinal secretion and diarrhea in some patients. It was introduced as therapy for prevention of nonsteroidal anti-inflammatory drug (NSAID)-based gastric ulcers, and can increase bicarbonate and mucus production that is depleted by administration of Cox 1 inhibitors such as aspirin or indomethacin through inhibition of prostaglandin synthesis. The acid antisecretory property of misoprostol may contribute to its gastric mucosal protective effect.

The H2-Receptor Antagonists

The first series of H2-receptor antagonists was synthesized at a site of a stately house that had previously been used for development of diving gear during WWII; there was a deep pond on the property. Cimetidine reformed the treatment of acid-related diseases by introducing effective pharmacotherapy with a safety profile that was considerably different from that of the anticholinergics that were commonly used. During the 1980s, the H2-receptor antagonists became first-line therapy in peptic ulcer disease and led to improved clinical management for a large number of patients. At the time, this class of drugs was a clear step forward and provided good inhibition of nocturnal secretion although somewhat lesser inhibition of daytime secretion of acid.

Although the introduction of the H2-receptor antagonist class of agents improved the management of acid peptic-related disease, some issues still required consideration. Tolerance was a problem as well as the inability to adequately control erosive esophagitis or hypersecretors such as in patients with gastrinoma. It was possible that further improvement in the regulation of the acid secretory process would yield better clinical results.

The identification of the molecular mechanism of acid secretion-the proton pump-resulted in the development of a new class of therapeutic agents: the proton pump inhibitors (PPIs). By defining the pump as the therapeutic target, an almost complete inhibition of acid secretion and consequent therapeutic efficacy can finally be achieved.

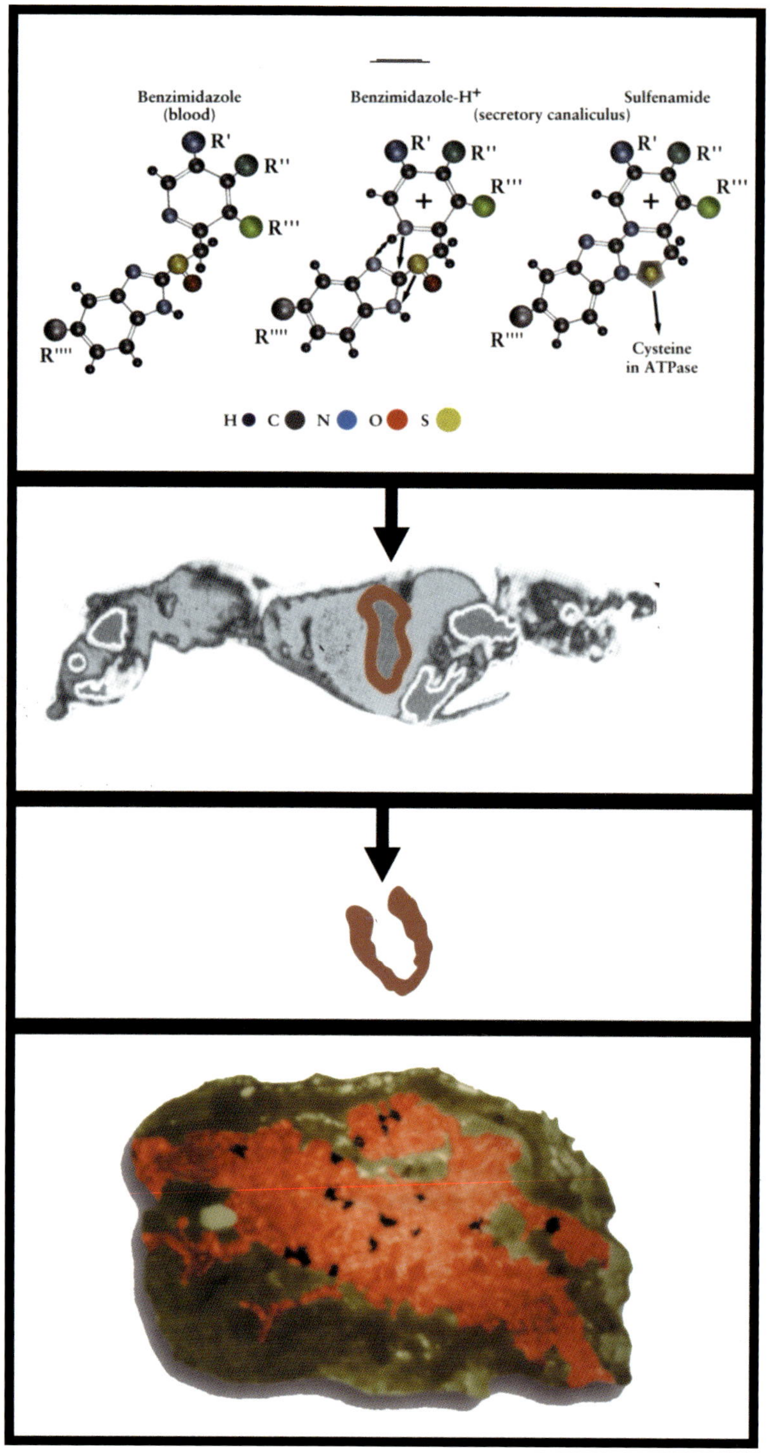

Figure 8. — The development of the substituted benzimidazole class of drugs (PPIs) revolutionized the management of acid peptic disease. The concept of a prodrug that would selectively target the acid pump of the parietal cell of the gastric fundus was epitomized by the development of the first agent in its class: omeprazole. The top panel demonstrates a benzamidazole molecule, which, on accumulation in the acid space of the secretory canaliculus of the parietal cell, becomes protonated and then converted to a sulfenamide. The subsequent covalent binding to a cysteine residue of the H^+,K^+ ATPase inhibits the proton pump of the parietal cell. The second image is of a transected mouse that has ingested omeprazole, which targets only the acid secreting cells of the gastric fundus, as indicated in the third panel. Panel four is an autoradiograph of an isolated parietal cell from the same stomach, demonstrating the isotopically labeled benzimidazole molecule covalently bound to the proton pumps of the secretory canaliculus of a parietal cell.

Proton Pump Inhibitors

The concept that drove the development of alternatives to H2-receptor antagonists was the recognition that such agents had limited efficacy, especially in patients with erosive esophagitis. It seemed that inhibition of the pump itself would be a more effective way to control acid secretion. Although work towards this end had been initiated at the US site of SK&F, it was terminated with the launch of cimetidine. The identification of the proton pump as the final step in the pathway of parietal cell acid secretion provided a unique opportunity for better control of parietal cell secretion. The synthesis of timoprazole, the forerunner of omeprazole, was a novel therapeutic approach to acid control and a novel drug design.

The PPIs have a unique mechanism of action; they are acid-activated prodrugs. They covalently inhibit the gastric H^+,K^+ ATPase based on their accumulation in the acid space generated in the secretory canaliculus of the parietal cell. This accumulation is followed by acid activation and covalent inhibition of the function of the acid pump. Because of the safety and clinical efficacy profile of omeprazole, within a decade, it superseded H2-receptor antagonists in the United States as the most prescribed antisecretory.

Novel Agents

Despite the widespread use of PPIs, a novel class of agents — the acid pump antagonists — have been developed to generate a more rapid onset of inhibition and stability that will allow more flexible formulations. Whereas the PPIs have a unique mechanism of action based on their chemistry, acid pump antagonists have a structural specificity for their target: the K^+ binding region of the H^+,K^+ ATPase. Although they have been actively pursued for almost 15 years, to date no such compounds have reached the marketplace.

The central role of gastrin in stimulation of ECL cell release of histamine has resulted in significant effort being applied to development of gastrin antagonists. For many years after the definition of the structure of gastrin, gastrin antagonists were sought in the form of peptide analogs of pentagastrin, but without success. More recently, nonpeptide antagonists of both the CCK-A and CCK-B receptors have been synthesized, based on a benzodiazepine core structure. Some of the more recent compounds are potent and highly selective for their receptor subtype and may be introduced clinically, although clinical evaluation will be necessary to determine if they are superior to H2-receptor antagonists.

Surgery

Although the management of acid peptic disease and its consequences were extremely limited at the turn of the 20th century, the advent of anesthesia and antisepsis facilitated the approach to the abdominal cavity, and the stomach became a viable surgical therapeutic target. Before Lister and Morton, surgery of the stomach had been confounded by mortality associated with sepsis and technical considerations contingent upon lack of adequate anesthesia. By the late 19th century, Naunyn described abdominal surgery as "an autopsy *in vivo*." By 1881, however, Billroth in Vienna, Péan of Paris, and Rydiger of Chelmo had all resected the human stomach, although only Billroth met with success. Wolfler in Vienna had successfully developed the procedure of gas-

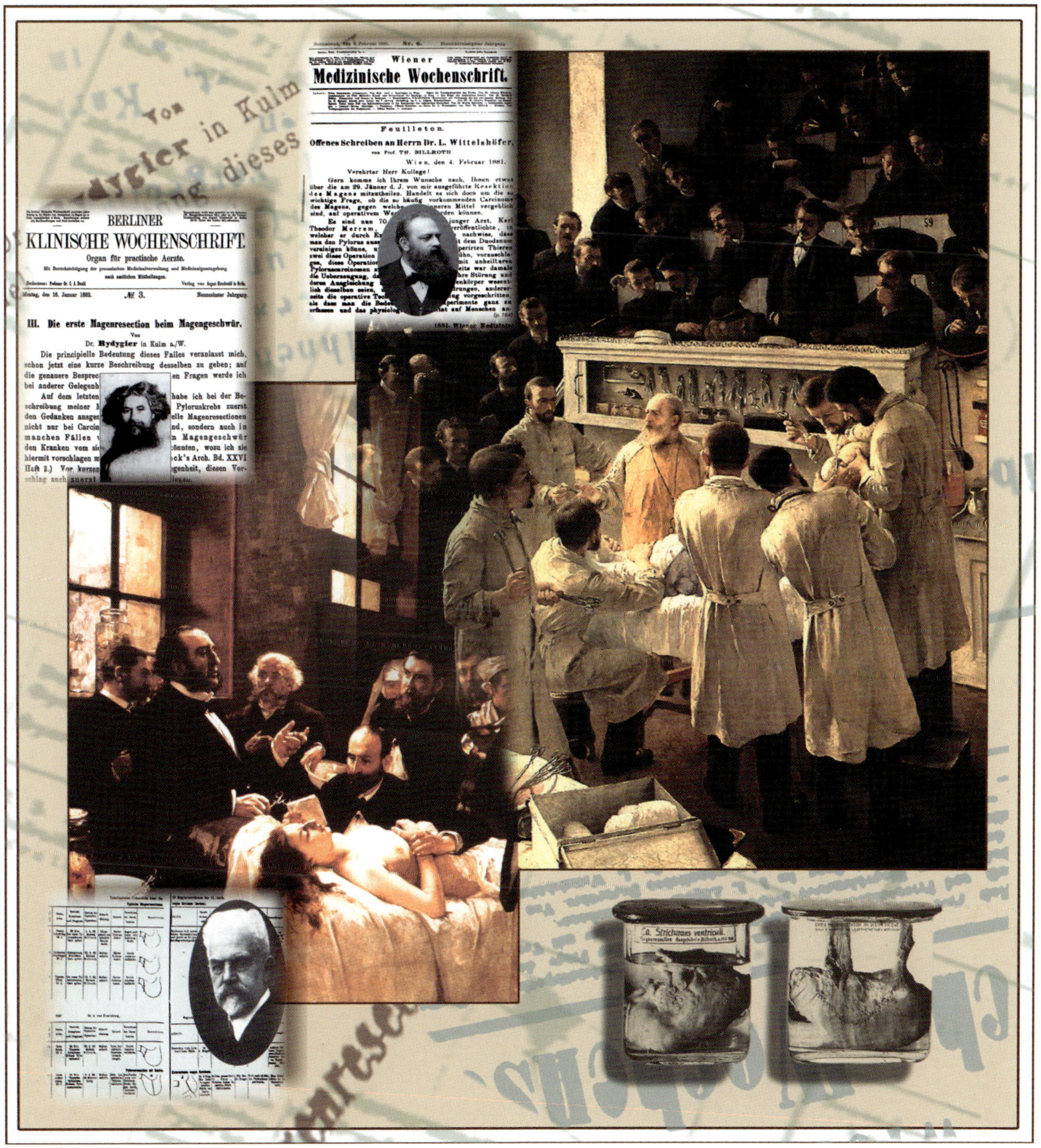

Figure 9. — The concept of removing the stomach was almost too quixotic for consideration until Theodore Billroth in Vienna, on January 29, 1881, removed a pyloric tumor from a 43-year-old patient, Theresa Heller. Although she successfully recovered from the resection of the obstructed pyloric antrum (bottom left specimen) *she died 31/2 months later of hepatic metastases. At autopsy* (bottom right specimen), *it was evident that the gastroduodenal anastomosis was intact. Billroth reported this success in a letter to a medical journal claiming the first successful gastrectomy* (top center). *The editor commented at the bottom of the page: "and hopefully the last." In 1879, Jean Péan had also successfully resected a pyloric gastric cancer in an operation that lasted 2 hours. Although the patient initially successfully recovered, he underwent a blood transfusion and died on the fifth postoperative day (Landsteiner would only describe blood groups some 50 years later.) Péan often operated in a dress suit en route to the Paris opera* (left image). *On November 16, 1880, Ludwig Rydygier of Chelmo* (top left) *performed the second documented unsuccessful gastrectomy. By his success, Billroth thus achieved the reputation as the Father of Gastric Surgery. The central picture painted by A.F. Seligmann is of the opening of Billroth's new operating room at the Vienna General Hospital in 1890. Billroth is being handed a scalpel by Dr. Bottecher while the anesthetic is delivered by Dr. Anton Eiselsberg. Eiselsberg would later become a leading surgeon and contribute substantially to a wide a variety of modifications of the Billroth gastrectomy* (lower left). *Karl Theodore, the Duke of Bavaria, at the far left in the lowest front row, commonly attended Billroth's lectures and surgical demonstrations, deeming them more entertaining than other current Viennese pastimes. The operation depicted is that of a neurotomy for trigeminal neuralgia and allows consideration of the possibility of prescience in art. The next major surgical advance in the treatment of acid peptic disease was to be the development of neurotomy of the vagus (vagotomy). It is possible to consider that a future surgical therapeutic option may embrace identification of the precise central regulatory center for acid secretion and microcellular ablation of the source of acid secretion.*

troenterostomy, and Jaboulay of Lyons had, in addition to gastroenterostomy, severed the vagal nerves at the hiatus as well as resected the celiac ganglion.

The recognition that the ulcer was the crux of the issue led to the development of techniques to resect the area. By the second decade of the century, Moynihan of Leeds had transformed the treatment of peptic ulcer disease and initiated a unique surgical discipline as endless permutations of gastric resection and anastomosis were introduced. Gastric surgery was dangerous. Peptic ulcer disease is complicated and its associated morbidity produced mechanical and metabolic postgastrectomy syndromes. In addition, there was often a rapid recurrence of the lesions. Alternative strategies to decrease the secretion of acid were evaluated.

Advances in physiology led to the elucidation of the role of the vagus in the secretion of acid and the development of peptic ulcer. As a result, vagotomy, which had been initiated in Lyons by Raymond Latarjet in 1922, and then rediscovered in Chicago by Lester Dragstedt in 1943, became the surgical vogue, as it decreased gastric acid output without entailing gastric resection and the likelihood of anastomotic leakage. Although the decreased postoperative gastric emptying dampened initial enthusiasm, this difficulty was obviated by the construction of a variety of pyloroplasties to facilitate drainage. The modest 20% to 30% decrease in acid secretion and problems with stasis culminated in high rates of recurrence of ulcers. As a result of these difficulties, as well as the consequences of denervating

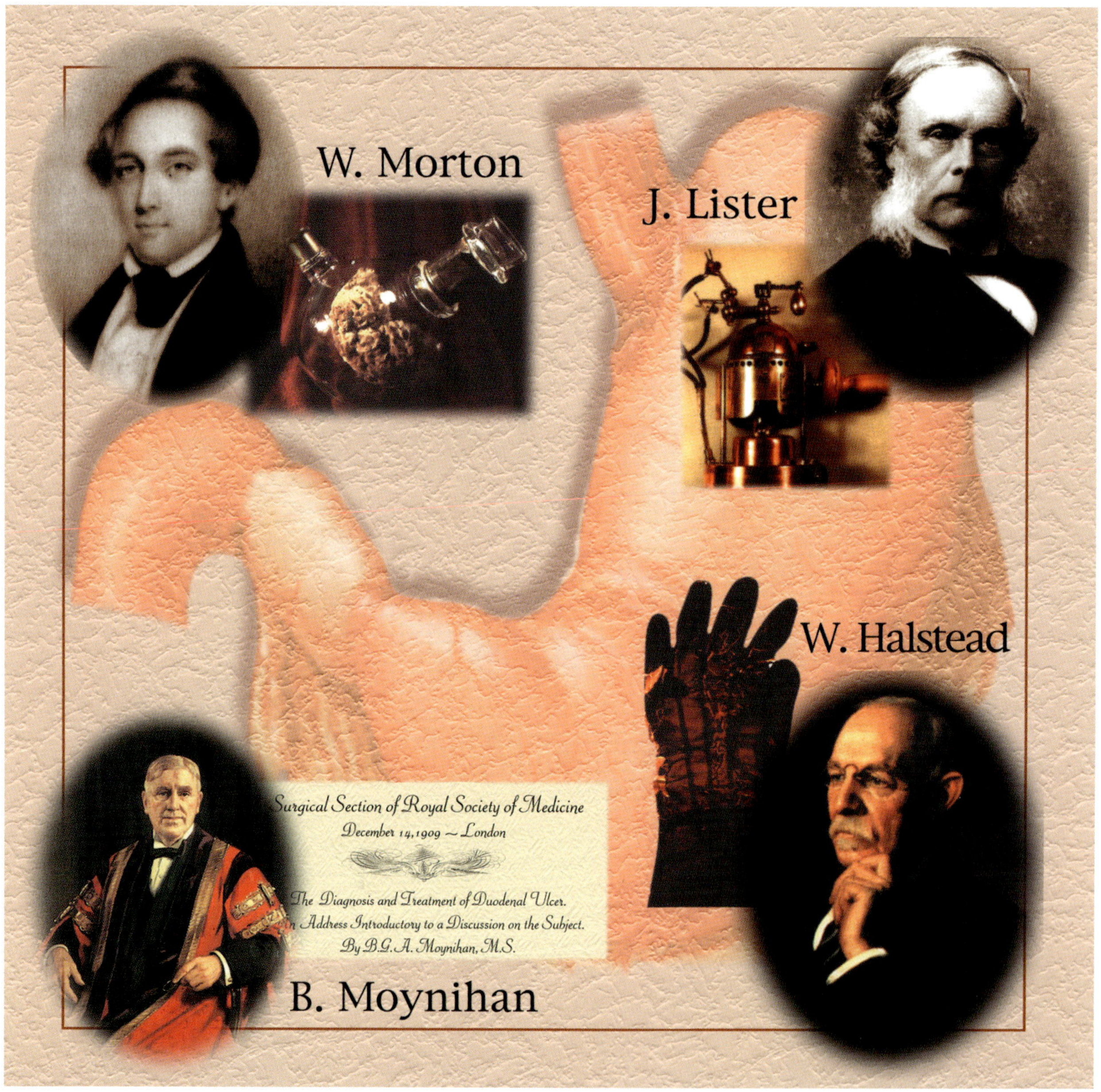

Figure 10. *— In the era before the introduction of acid suppression, chronic peptic ulceration resulted in considerable morbidity and mortality. The only effective remedy for intractable pain and complications, such as perforation, bleeding, and gastric outlet obstruction, was surgery. The results, however, were so terrible that many eminent physicians (Naunyn) regarded surgery as little more than an autopsy in vivo. The introduction of anesthesia (inhaler) by William Morton allowed for surgery to be performed in an unhurried fashion on a patient protected from pain. The subsequent advent of antisepsis (carbolic spray), as introduced by Lord Joseph Lister, significantly decreased infectious complications and facilitated the performance of cautious and meticulous surgery. In addition, advances in hemostatic technique (the first-time use of gloves) as instituted by William Halstead of Baltimore, and technical efficiency as promulgated by Berkley Moynihan of Leeds, facilitated the development of relatively safe gastric surgery. Nevertheless, the morbidity of postgastrectomy syndromes engendered by such operations resulted in patients being cured of their peptic ulcer only to acquire a series of lifetime disabilities. Thus, the consequence of the anatomic and physiologic derangement attendant upon gastric resection, pyloric ablation, and a variety of gastrojejunal and duodenal anastomoses were as debilitating if not worse than the original disease.*

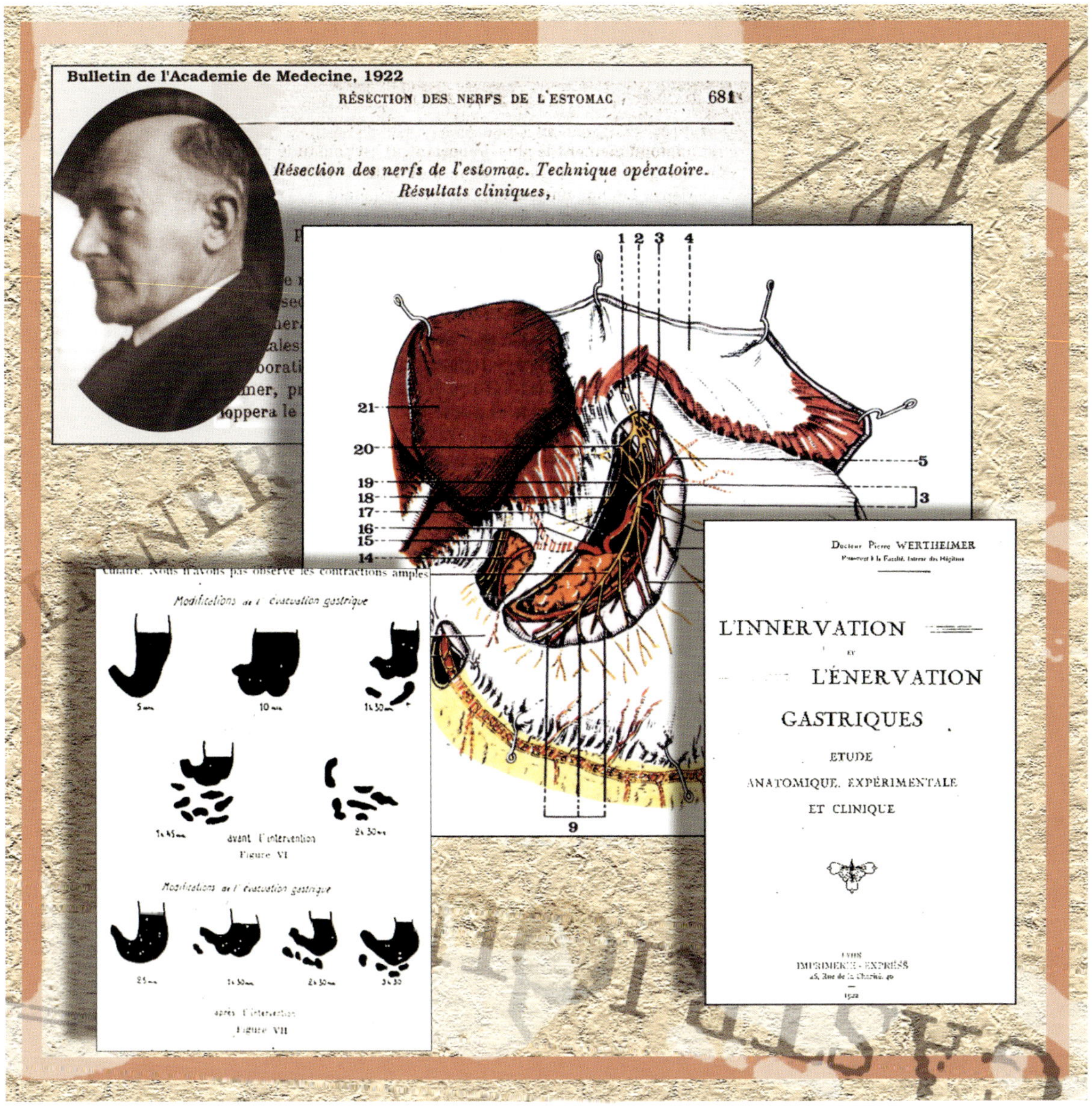

Figure 11. — *Andre Latarjet (1877-1947) was born in Dijon and studied medicine in Lyons. In collaboration with Pierre Wertheimer, he defined the neural innervation of the stomach in detail and recognized that the vagal nerve supply to the lesser curve was critical in the regulation of gastric acid secretion. In 1923, he published the results of a series of operations in which he had severed the vagal nerves to the stomach and demonstrated not only a decrease in gastric acid secretion but also a resolution of acid peptic disease. A rigorous scientific thinker, he documented the associated significant delay in gastric emptying consequent upon vagal denervation and described the need to add a drainage procedure to the operation. Lester Dragstedt introduced the vogue for vagotomy in the United States, on January 14, 1943, in Chicago at the Merritt Billings Hospital. As a transmogrified physiologist, Dragstedt was able to provide experimental evidence that gastric denervation decreased acid secretion and facilitated ulcer healing and relief of pain. It has taken almost 50 years for the surgical community to recognize that Latarjet's original decision to abandon the operation was well founded on scientific fact. The long-lasting dramatic postvagotomy symptomatology consequent upon denervating large portions of the gastrointestinal tract far outweighed the modest advantages achieved by a 20% to 30% decrease in acid secretion. Further debate on the merits and demerits of the innumerable permutations and commutations of vagotomy were swept away by the introduction of H2-receptor antagonists in 1976. The subsequent availability of PPI therapy considerably decreased the use of vagal resection, which should now only be considered in rare clinical circumstances.*

most of the abdominal viscera with resultant abnormalities in motility, alternative procedures were sought. Further recognition that the fundus of the stomach contained the acid-secreting cells, and the antrum, a major component of the regulatory mechanism, led to the development of an extraordinary variety of permutations and combinations of antral and fundic resection.

Such operations were devised with the view to variously removing the ulcer, decreasing gastrin stimulation, ablating neural stimulation, and decreasing the parietal cell mass.

Unfortunately, these procedures were associated with considerable morbidity and mortality. Post-gastrectomy syndromes often resulted, as the gut failed to accommodate to the loss of neural innervation, pyloric function, and the severe neuroendocrine aberrations consequent upon resective intervention. An array of selective, superselective, and highly selective vagotomies were then introduced to ameliorate postvagotomy dysfunction, with varying degrees of success. Although technical problems and recurrence of ulcer continued to mar the use of this procedure, the development of further refinements was obviated by the introduction of cimetidine and subsequently PPIs.

The identification of the H2–receptor subtype, and the development of agents specifically capable of blocking acid secretion by antagonism at this receptor, significantly improved the management of the disease process and considerably decreased the need for surgery as a therapeutic option for peptic ulcer except in cases of emergency. Within a decade, the use of elective gastric or vagal surgery in the management of this disease had declined to the extent that it constituted a rare event.

Surgery has, for the most part, become obsolete for the treatment of peptic ulcer disease, as methods of decreasing acid secretion have evolved into more targeted and precise pharmacologic options. Nevertheless, the early surgical remedies were based upon a reasonable grasp of the pathophysiology and the recognition of the need to effect relief of ulceration and pain, bleeding, perforation, and stenosis. At this time, it is rare to consider surgical intervention in acid peptic disease for anything less than a major complication such as bleeding or perforation. Furthermore, the incidence of surgery for intractable pain, penetration, or stenosis has dramatically decreased with the introduction of omeprazole and the PPI class of drugs.

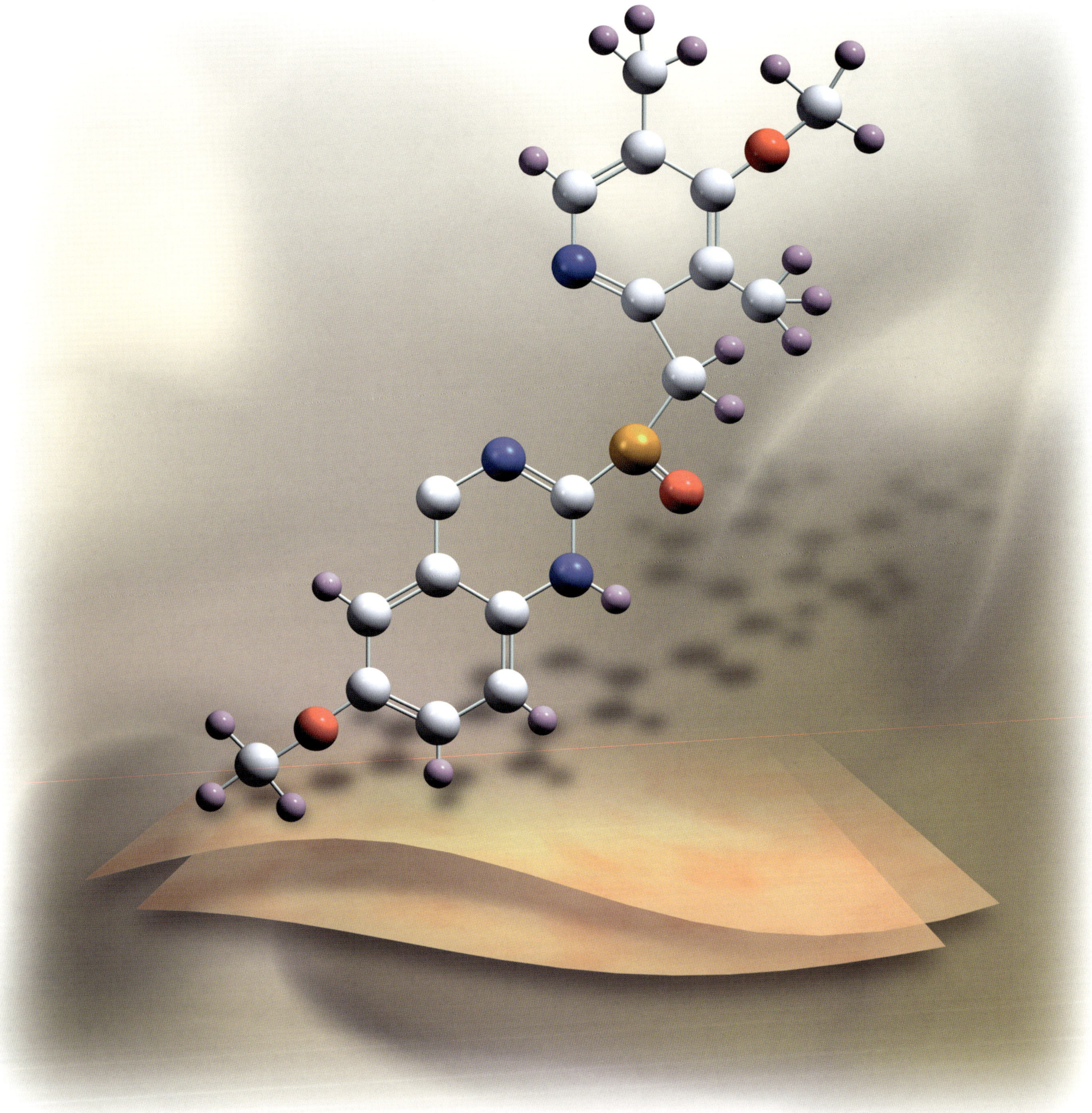

Chapter V

The Story of Omeprazole

Discovery

Mechanism of Action of Omeprazole

Chemistry

Biology

Acid-Catalyzed Activation

Principles of Omeprazole Therapy

The Selectivity of Omeprazole

The Effects of Inhibition of Acid Secretion

The Rise of Omeprazole

The Effectiveness of Antisecretories

Omeprazole

- The first proton pump inhibitor
- Novel class of anti-ulcer drug
- Specific parietal cell targeting

- Substituted pyridyl methyl sulfinyl benzimidazole
- Protonated in the secretory canaliculus
- Forms sulfenamide

- Binds to outer cysteine in H^+,K^+ ATPase
- Blocks H^+ secretion

- Pump half life ~50 hours
- Long duration of action

- Restoration of acid secretory capacity ~24-48 hours

- Once daily dosing

- pH elevation to >3 +/- 18 hrs/day

Intragastric pH levels are not indicative of efficacy in healing and/or relief of symptoms.

The Story of Omeprazole

Discovery

In the early 1970s, Astra-Hassle in Göteborg, Sweden, was investing in compounds with possible antiviral activity. However, as was the case with many drug companies of that era, compounds were tested in a variety of animal models, such as those for measuring acid secretion. The compound of interest was pyridine 2-acetamide, which proved of little use as an antiviral agent but appeared to inhibit acid secretion. This compound was modified to the thioacetamide derivative for increased antiviral activity but proved no better. However, it still inhibited acid secretion. Sparked by the announcement of cimetidine, a benzimidazole was added, as the imidazole ring moiety mimicked histamine. This compound was now tested against acid secretion and proved still to inhibit acid secretion. A minor modification, the introduction of the sulfoxide, retained antisecretory activity. This compound was timoprazole, the forerunner, or core structure of omeprazole and all subsequent PPIs.

Figure 1. — *The steps toward omeprazole. The two compounds on the left inhibited acid secretion, but their mechanism remains mysterious. The compound in the middle was designed to mimic H2-receptor antagonists and led to the synthesis of timoprazole: the basic structural template for all PPIs. This resulted, after 4 years, in the synthesis and then development of omeprazole as an antiulcer medication.*

Development of Omeprazole

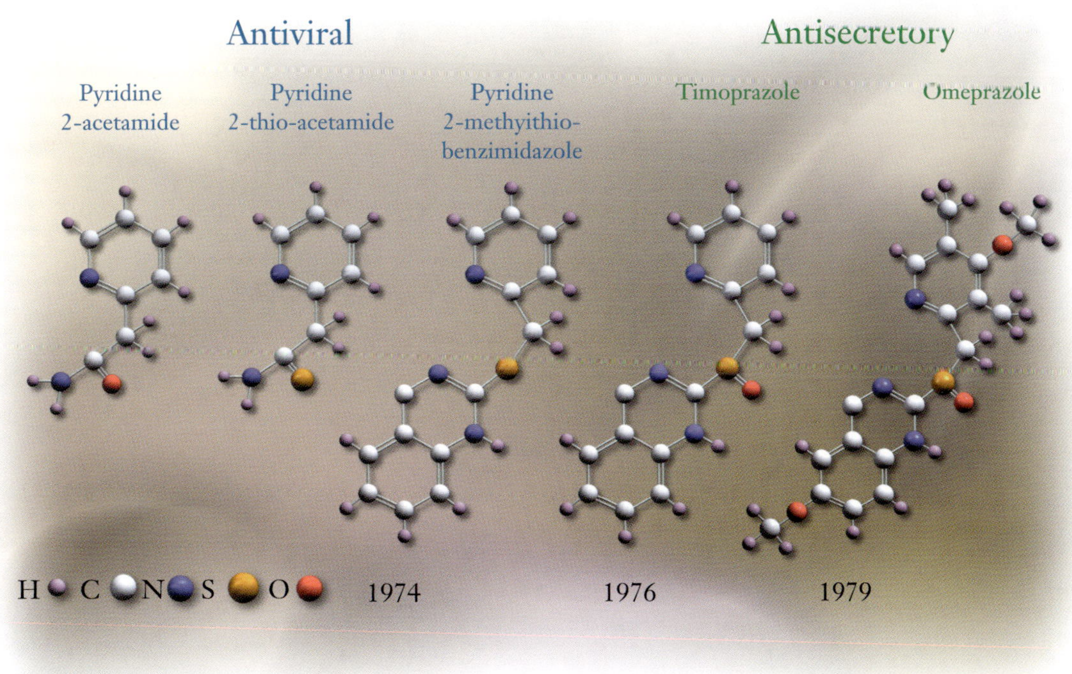

This compound had properties that distinguished it from the H2-receptor antagonist cimetidine. First, it inhibited acid secretion irrespective of stimulus *in vivo*, including histamine or gastrin or carbachol, whereas H2-receptor antagonists were only able to inhibit histamine or gastrin stimulation but not carbachol. It also inhibited cAMP-stimulated acid secretion in isolated rabbit gastric glands. Clearly, it was not simply a H2-receptor antagonist. But what was its target?

There were two chemical properties of note: It was acid unstable, and it was a protonatable weak base with a pK_a of about 3.0. This pK_a implied that it would accumulate in the acid space of the parietal cell and perhaps, being acid unstable, would become reactive in the acid space. The acid instability extended into the neutral pH range.

Experiments were then carried out on the isolated proton pump ATPase and it was found that this and a similar compound was inactive under standard assay conditions, which required the addition of nigericin, a H^+ for K^+ exchanger, to supply K^+ to the inside surface of the inside-out vesicles and that also collapsed the proton gradient.

If, however, the same experiments were carried out using the K^+-selective ionophore, valinomycin, to supply internal K^+ that allowed the development of a proton gradient acidic inside, the compound was an effective and covalent inhibitor of the isolated functioning gastric acid pump. It was then realized that this chemical was a weak base accumulating in acid spaces and then underwent a rapid acid catalyzed conversion to a thiol-reactive species. At first, it was thought that a sulfenic acid was the reactive intermediate, but later the sulfenamide was isolated from solution. It became the accepted intermediate although more recent data do not support conclusively that the sulfenamide is the intermediate that is on the surface of the pump. This compound, timoprazole, and a closely related molecule, picoprazole, were therefore pump-targeted drugs. A later compound, omeprazole, then became the first of a new class of antiulcer drugs named PPIs.

In order to improve neutral pH stability of timoprazole, a methoxy group was added in order to donate electrons into the pyridine ring, elevating the pK_a to 4.0 and reducing neutral pH reactivity. Two additional methyl groups were added to help stabilize the compound further. A methoxy group was added to decrease the thyrotoxicity and thymotoxicity that had been found in animal tests with timoprazole. This was the compound omeprazole.

Mechanism of Action of Omeprazole

Although it was clear that this compound was a weak base that accumulated in the acid space of the parietal cell and was acid activated and therefore presumably a prodrug, neither its chemistry nor its biology had been worked out at the time of synthesis.

Chemistry

The chemistry of omeprazole is intriguing. As a weak base, it is 50% protonated at pH 4.0. Below that pH, the degree of protonation increases. Because the protonated form is positively charged and is relatively impermeant across biologic membranes, the compound will accumulate in acidic spaces with a pH less that its pK_a of 4.0. Given that the canalicular pH of most parietal cells is about 1.0, theoretically, omeprazole would be predicted to accumulate 1000-fold as the protonated form at its target region.

In acid, omeprazole rapidly forms a new compound, a tetracyclic planar cationic sulfenamide, which is highly reactive with free -SH (thiol) groups. As it is a cation, it is also relatively membrane impermeable and stays that way even when the level of acid decreases to pH>4.0. The hypothesis is therefore that the omeprazole sulfenamide will react with available cysteines on the gastric acid pump to form disulfide derivatives. This, in principle, should inhibit the pump if the SH groups are in critical regions and the inhibition should be covalent, depending on de novo protein synthesis for restoration of acid secretion.

The formation of the sulfenamide is interesting in relationship to optimization of the reactivity and accumulation of the prodrug. With too low a pK_a, the unshared free electron pair on the pyridine N is able to react spontaneously with the 2C of the benzimidazole ring, accounting for the neutral pH instability of timoprazole. With a higher pK_a, the reactivity of the pyridine N decreases, improving the neutral pH stability of the compound, as there has to be deprotonation of the N to enable cyclization. In fact, it may well be that, in acidic solution, there is intramolecular transfer of the pyridine N proton to the benzimidazole N. This would in turn increase the electrophilic reactivity of the 2C position. Hence, increasing the pK_a of the pyridine N, enabling intramolecular proton transfer, also leads to neutral pH instability. It appears that a pK_a of 4.0 is optimal for generation of compounds of this type with reasonable neutral pH instability.

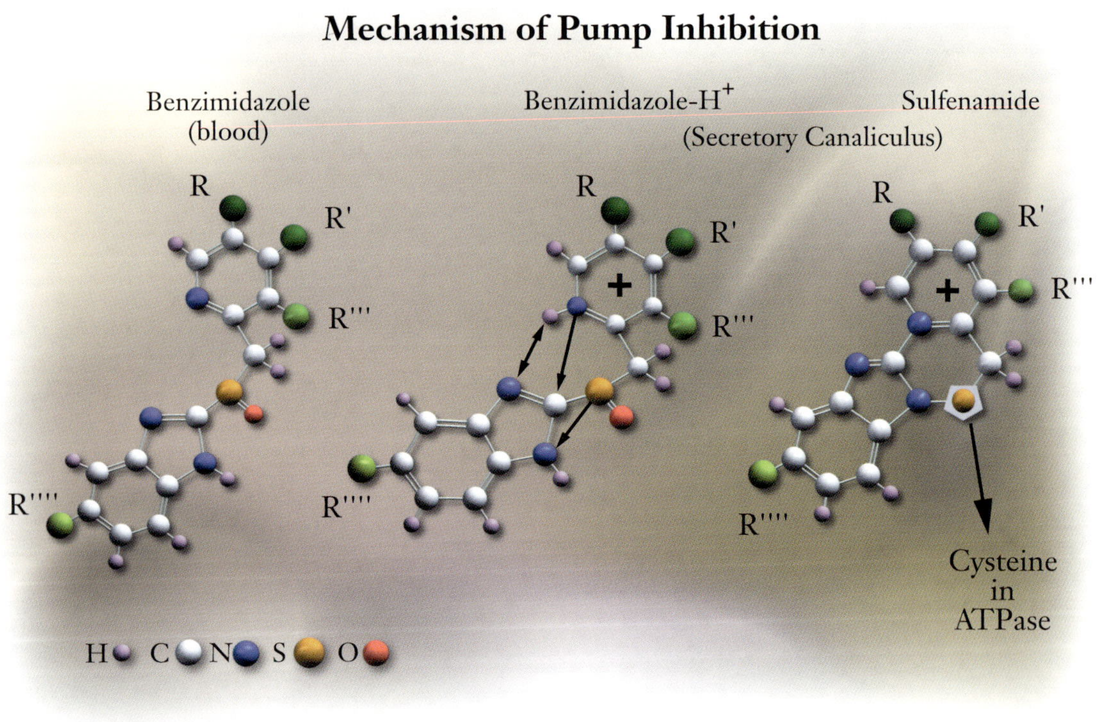

Figure 2. — The general mechanism for PPI-driven inhibition of the gastric H^+,K^+ ATPase. The parent compound is on the left. In the middle is the protonated form that accumulates in the acid space, and on the right is the reactive sulfenamide that is postulated to react with one or more cysteines in the acid pump. In the case of omeprazole, R and R''' are CH_3, and R' and R'''' are CH_3 0 groups. The critical reaction is the attack on the 2C position by the pyridine N. Electron withdrawal by the S=O group results in an electrophilic center on the 2C, and this results in reaction with the unshared pair of electrons in the pyridine N.

Targeting of Omeprazole

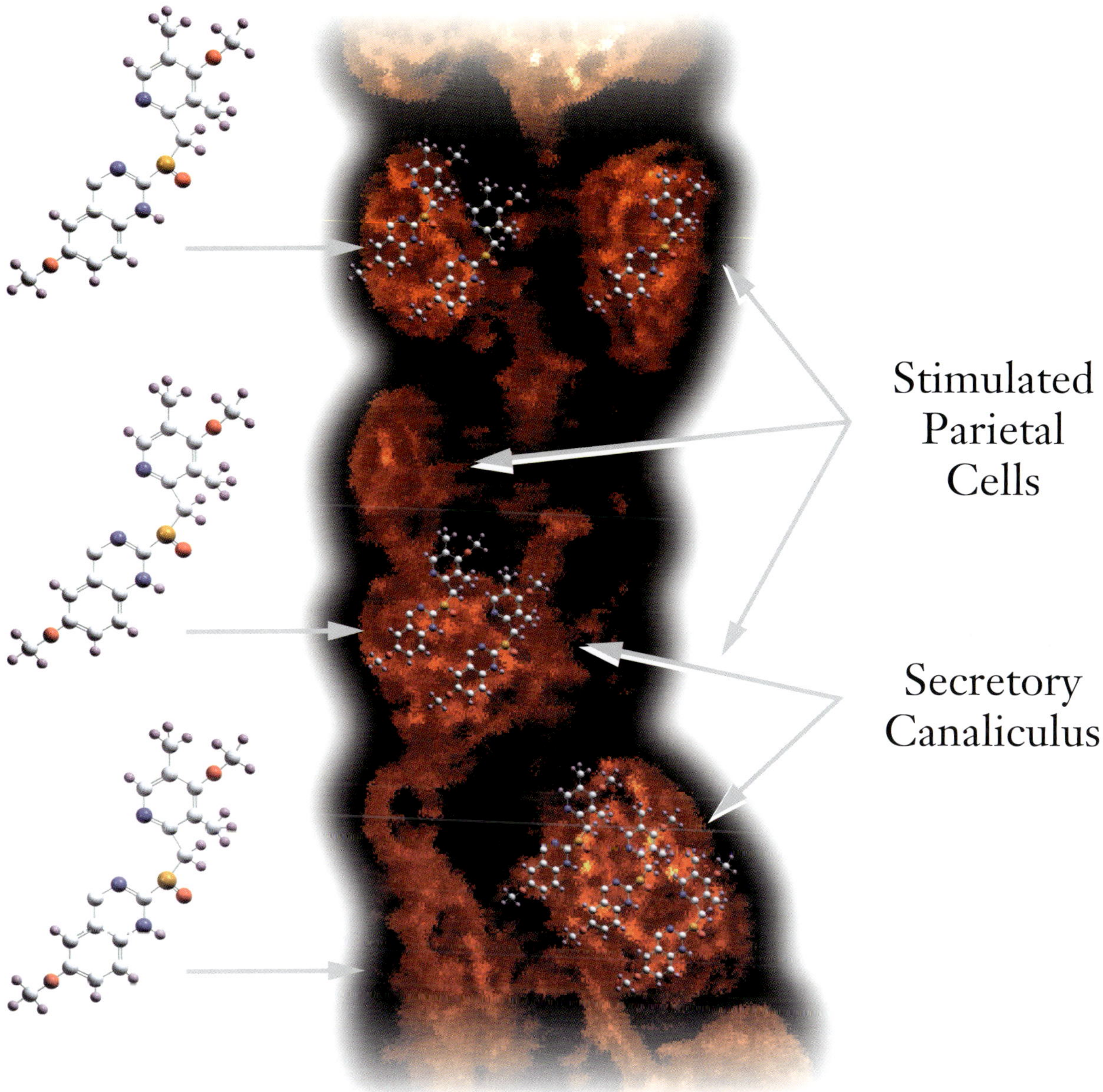

Figure 3. — A conceptualization of the targeting of omeprazole. After duodenal absorption, the drug passes from the blood into the interstitial spaces of the gastric epithelium. Thence, it diffuses into the parietal cell and is accumulated in the active secretory canaliculus of those parietal cells that are active. The theoretical distribution into this space at a pH of 1.0 is about 1000-fold higher than that found in blood.

Biology

Acid-Space Targeting

Autoradiographic studies *in vitro* and *in vivo* have shown a remarkable specificity of omeprazole labeling. It is found initially only bound in the secretory canaliculus that contains microvilli, indicative of active pumps. With cycling of the pump back to the resting state, labeling later appears in the cytoplasm on the tubulovesicles. No other cell in the stomach is labeled, and after washout of the compound by metabolism and excretion, no other organ retains the label. Therefore, the compound is extremely selective for the active parietal cell, as chemistry would predict. There have been no measurements of the accumulation of the compound before activation because, with the high acidity of the parietal cell, there would be rapid conversion of the compound to the sulfenamide. However, there can be little doubt that with a pK_a of 4.0, there is an optimal therapeutic concentration index: that is, the concentration of the compound in its target organ as compared to the blood.

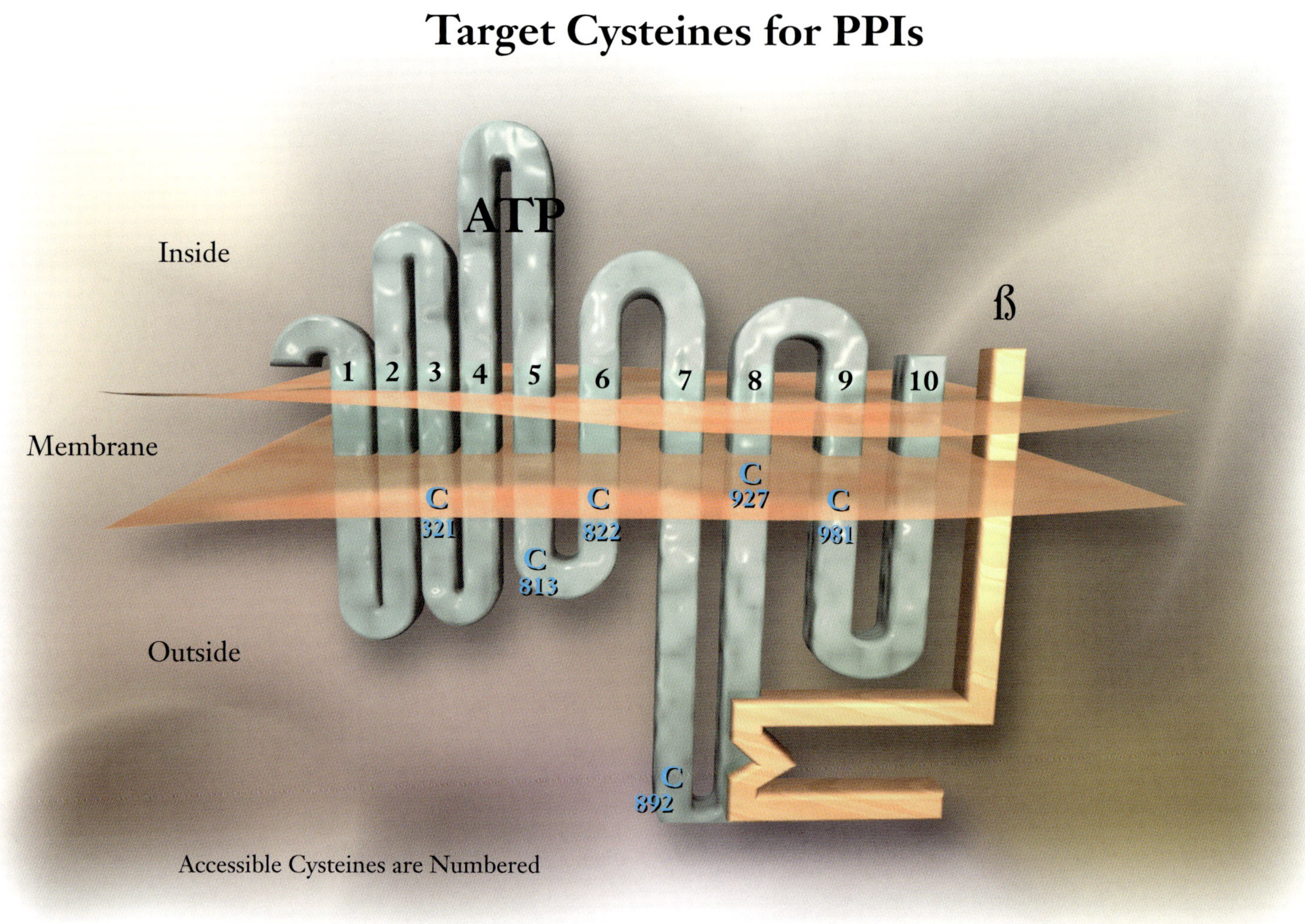

Figure 4. *— Experiments dedicated toward discovery of the cysteines that react productively with omeprazole were carried out in two ways. Radioactive omeprazole was used and the labeled peptides isolated after reaction with the enzyme under acid-transporting conditions, and reaction correlated with inhibition. From this, it was clear that reaction with the cysteines in the loop between M5 and M6 correlated with inhibition of the ATPase and with inhibition of acid production. Then the amino acids possibly involved are mutated to find those essential for inhibition. From these two approaches, it appeared that although the cysteine at position 813 was the site that was covalently labeled, it was still important to retain a structure that was like cysteine at position 822 for omeprazole to access cysteine 813. It seems that omeprazole and the other PPIs bind in the region of cysteine 822 and then react with other cysteines.*

Acid-Catalyzed Activation

In the acid space itself there are no SH groups for the compound to react with, and in the membrane, the major protein is the gastric H^+,K^+ ATPase. From the sequence of the catalytic and beta subunits of the pump, the cysteines exposed on the beta subunit are all disulfide linked. These might react with the omeprazole sulfenamide but would reform immediately, thus being irrelevant to pump inhibition. In the catalytic subunit, from analysis of membrane structure, there are six cysteines sufficiently exposed on the outer surface of the pump, in positions 321, 813, 822, and 892 as well as perhaps 927 and 981, to react with activated omeprazole.

Therefore, the basis of covalent inhibition of the pump is formation of a disulfide with cys 813 of the gastric ATPase, directly within the loop connecting the 5th and 6th transmembrane segment. Studies in animals with radioactive omeprazole in which the animal was examined for distribution of radioactivity thoroughly confirmed the specific targeting of these PPIs to the stomach, the parietal cell, and the stimulated secretory canaliculus. A series of studies in the test tube using a gastric gland model of acid secretion also directly showed that omeprazole is targeted only to active pumps in stimulated parietal cells.

Principles of Omeprazole Therapy

Therefore, the cell mechanism of omeprazole inhibition depends on the acid secretory status of the stomach. Usually, once-a-day therapy before eating is used, as the covalent inhibition provides long-lasting acid secretory inhibition. When omeprazole is taken, the active pumps are inhibited, but the cell returns to its resting

Inhibition of Gastric ATPase

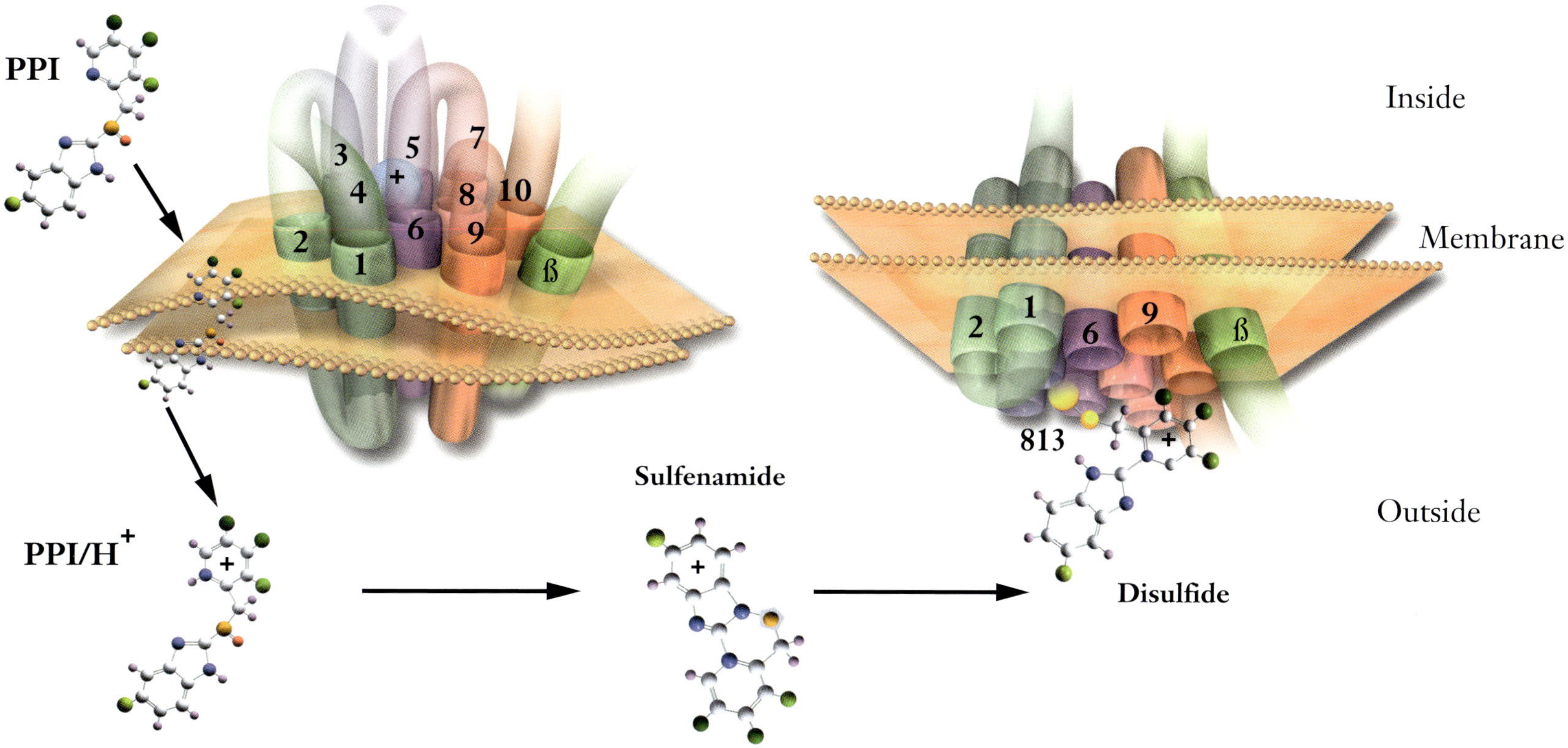

Figure 5. — A conceptual illustration of the acid gradient driven accumulation of PPIs followed by acid-catalyzed conversion to the sulfenamide and then reaction to form disulfides with cysteines in the loop between the 5th and 6th transmembrane segments. A view is shown from above and from below the membrane inserted acid pump, illustrating the transmembrane segments, the connecting loops on the cytoplasmic face (left), and on the outside surface (right).

state when the stimulus (ie, food) has left the stomach. In contrast, H2-receptor antagonists tend to return the cell to its resting state if only histamine is being used by the stomach to stimulate acid secretion.

Omeprazole and the other PPIs are acid unstable; therefore, they have to be protected against the acidity of the stomach. Various formulations have been tried. In the case of omeprazole, it is provided as enteric-coated granules in a soluble capsule, with the coating dissolving and liberating the drug when the pH rises to 6.1 or above. The covalent inhibition, the biosynthesis or turnover of the pump, and perhaps some degree of reversal of the disulfide linkage set the scene for the onset of action of the PPIs and the time it takes to reach steady-state inhibition, which was found to be about 70% of maximal acid output on once-a-day dosage.

The half-life of omeprazole in plasma is about 30 to 60 minutes in healthy subjects; therefore, effective acid inhibition can only occur while the drug is above threshold concentration, which is about 1μM. The time that the drug is above that concentration is about 2 hours. So any of the pumps that are present in the canalicular membrane over that period of time will be inhibited. Any pumps that were not active and any pumps synthesized over the next 24 hours will contribute to acid secretory capacity before the next daily dose of the drug. The half-life of the pump is about 50 hours. Thus, in theory, about 25% of the original pumps will be replaced each day. It is also probable that not all pumps are active during the 2 hours while the drug is present in above-threshold levels in the blood; perhaps about 75% are active. These will be inhibited covalently, leaving, after the first dose, about 50% of the secretory capacity (25% old plus 25% new pumps) intact at the time when the second dose is given. Here again, 75% of the pumps are inhibited, leaving 12.5% of the original secretory capacity, and during the next 24 hours, 12.5% of the pumps are replaced, resulting in about 25% of secretory capacity remaining when the third dose is given.

Therefore, with omeprazole, there will be inhibition of acid secretion on the first day after dosage. However, steady-state, and therefore optimal pH for healing active duodenal and benign gastric ulcers, will not usually occur until after the fourth day of treatment, given a single daily dose, as demonstrated in studies with normal volunteers.

The Selectivity of Omeprazole

The rationale for the specific targeting of omeprazole to the active acid pump has been discussed. It is worth, however, reemphasizing the basis for this extraordinary selectivity. The highly acidic space of the canaliculus of the parietal cell is about 1000 times more acidic than any other acid space in the body. With a pH of 1.0, this gives a therapeutic index of 1000 to the benefit of the PPI. The acid catalyzed conversion adds weight to this therapeutic index, as at these acidic pH levels, the conversion occurs in fractions of seconds further increasing the concentrating ability of this space for the PPI. The other family members of the gastric ATPase, such as the Na^+,K^+, colonic H^+,K^+ and Ca^{2+} ATPases, lack the cysteines that are the target of the PPIs. Finally, although there is a small amount of the gastric H^+,K^+ ATPase expressed in the medullary collecting duct of the kidney, the acidity is never high enough to concentrate omeprazole, and the contribution of this pump to renal physiology appears minimal.

The Effects of Inhibition of Acid Secretion

Although acid secretion into the stomach is a characteristic of fish, amphibia, and mammals, its absence appears to have few deleterious effects in humans. For example, the stomach is achlorhydric in pernicious anemia, and if the anemia is treated, there is no influence on longevity. With the beginning of anti-secretory drug therapy for acid-related diseases, fears have been expressed as to the potential consequences of acid suppression, beginning with cimetidine but not ending there, and continuing today.

Cellular Pharmacology of PPIs

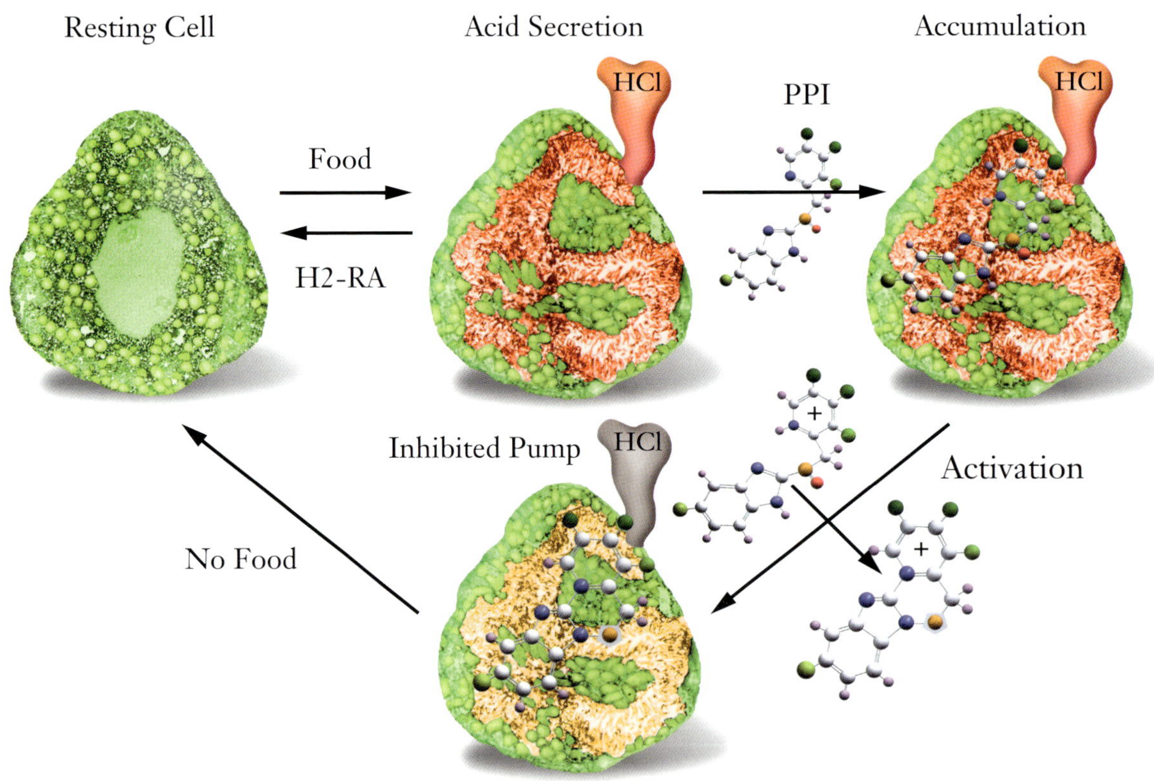

Figure 6. — This illustrates the parietal cell contribution to the biologic principles of PPI therapy. The parietal cell is stimulated, for example, by the administration of food, such as breakfast. After the PPI is given, it accumulates in the acid space of the parietal cell. In this space, the prodrug is activated by acid and binds the pump covalently. This results in inhibition of acid secretion. When food leaves the stomach, the cell returns to its resting state. H2-receptor antagonists also return the cell to the resting state, provided histamine stimulation is a component of activation of acid secretion. PPIs inhibit acid secretion irrespective of the nature of the stimulatory pathway.

After the development of cimetidine, several companies realized the advantage of producing a longer-acting H2-receptor antagonist, and several were in development. However, these drugs produced gastric tumors in rats, which precluded their introduction as medications. It was not considered that these tumors were carcinoids, resulting from the hypergastrinemia produced by inhibition of gastric acid secretion in the face of food stimulation of the G cell.

During development of omeprazole, in the required long-term carcinogenicity studies in rats, at very high doses it was found that rats developed hyperplasia and then carcinoid tumors of the ECL cells after 2 years' treatment. This resulted in the development of omeprazole being halted until this phenomenon could be explained. In a series of experiments, it was shown that this ECL cell phenomenon was entirely the result of the large increase in serum gastrin found following administration. The important experiments in rats were that with antrectomy (removal of the G cell), there was no change in the ECL cell population and that long-term administration of other PPIs or high doses of H2-receptor antagonists, or fundectomy, also produced the ECL cell carcinoids. Hence, the effect observed was due to the removal of acid feedback inhibition of gastrin release from the G cell. The development of omeprazole continued, and it was first launched in 1988. In long-term clinical trials involving more than 3000 patients, gastric biopsy specimens have not revealed gastric carcinoid induction in people. These careful surveys of the gastric mucosa after long-term treatment with omeprazole have revealed ECL hyperplasia but have been regarded as indicating the safety of this medication because no case of ECL carcinoids, dysplasia, or neoplasia has been found in these patients.

The Rise of Omeprazole

That the target of omeprazole and other PPIs is the gastric acid pump contributes significantly to their improved antisecretory effects. The formation of a relatively stable inhibitory disulfide bond with the pump differs from the displaceable binding of the H2-receptor antagonists. In several studies, the greater effectiveness of omeprazole was shown in rates of healing of active duodenal ulcer, active benign gastric ulcer, and erosive esophagitis compared to ranitidine.

In addition to concerns about ECL carcinoids, there were other obstacles to have general acceptance of omeprazole as a first-line therapy for appropriate acid-related disorders. At first, it was thought that omeprazole caused achlorhydria. It was obvious, however, that this was rare and that full acid inhibition could be desirable. Then it was claimed that omeprazole caused unscheduled DNA synthesis (UDS) in gastric cells; that is, omeprazole was thought to be carcinogenic. However, UDS was not demonstrated, and, moreover, high doses of omeprazole were not conclusively shown to be mutagenic in *x* assays.

Undoubtedly, these and similar concerns delayed the acceptance of omeprazole, but now it has become not only the first-line treatment for acid reflux disease but a leading prescription drug in the world. Omeprazole is an effective medicine for appropriate patients with a variety of acid-related disorders and has a well-established adverse events profile (see attached prescribing information for discussion of approved indications for omeprazole in the United States).

The Effectiveness of Antisecretories

How good is omeprazole, and is there any future development in the area of acid control that might provide alternative therapy? The most frequent means of analyzing effects of acid inhibitory drugs is intragastric pH metry. A typical experiment in human volunteers shows a gradual onset of elevation of intragastric pH reaching a steady state after 4 days of treatment.

In a series of meta-analyses — studies done on data after the clinical trial had taken place — various conclusions could be drawn. In the case of duodenal ulceration, in order to achieve optimal healing, it appeared sufficient to elevate intragastric pH to a level greater than 3.0 for about 16 to 18 hours per day. The average diurnal pH in healthy people is about 1.4. As pH is on a logarithmic scale, inhibition of about 90% of secretion would appear adequate for optimal healing of duodenal ulcer. In the case of GERD, a greater elevation of intragastric pH appeared to be required: that is, elevation of intragastric pH to > 4.0 for optimal healing of the lesion. In other studies, it appeared that perhaps elevation to pH of 5.0 was required for eradication of *H. pylori* in combination with antibiotics.

Onset of Inhibition of Acid-Secretory Capacity (Theoretic) Once-a-Day Dosing

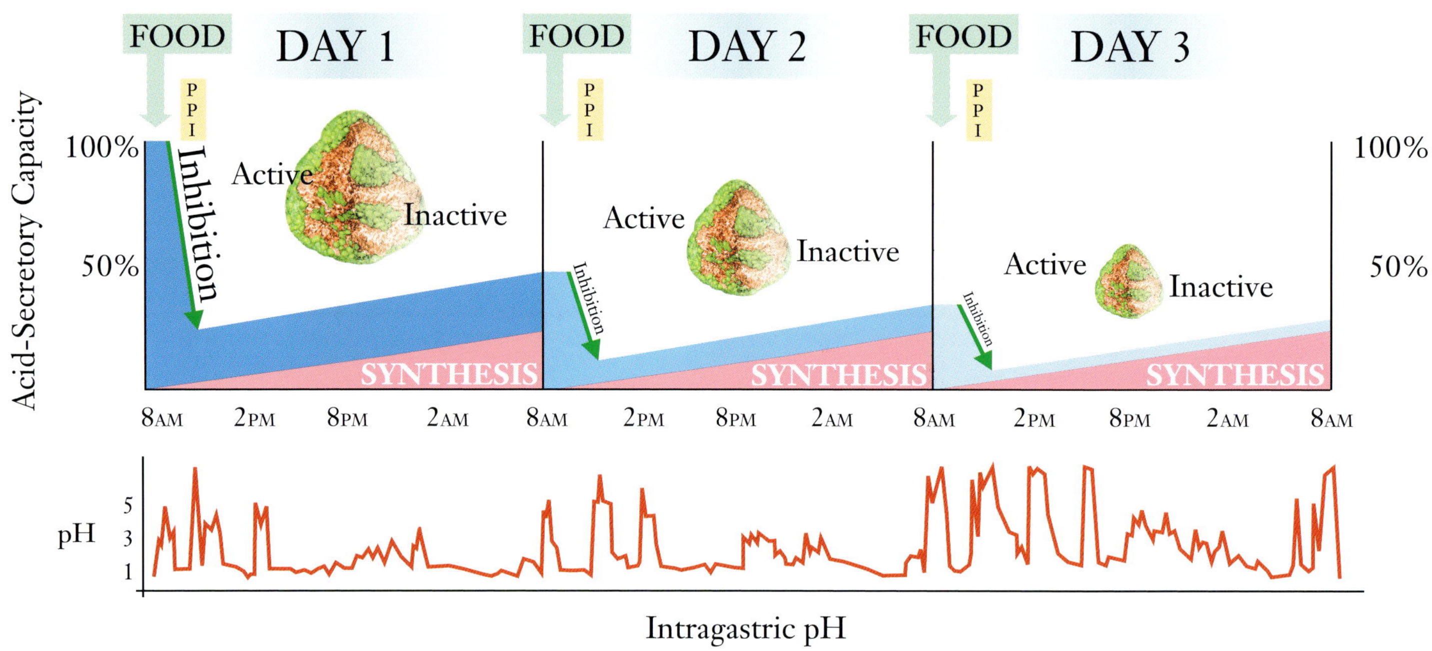

Figure 7. — Illustration of the onset of steady-state inhibition achieved, in theory, with once-a-day dosing of a PPI with covalent inhibition of the pump and a steady rate of synthesis of the pump with a half-life of about 50 hours. It is assumed that 75% of acid pumps are activated with breakfast. A typical pH profile over 3 days of treatment is shown, corresponding to the theoretical analysis above the pH metric curves. The calculations assume that 75% of total pumps are active during plasma presentation of the PPI and that the half-life of the pump in humans determines recovery and is 50 hours, as found in rats. Steady state inhibition of acid secretion will not occur until the fourth day of treatment, given a single daily dose, as demonstrated in studies with normal volunteers.

It is difficult to use omeprazole or similar compounds to achieve absolute inhibition of acid secretion at any given time. Therefore, if abolition of acid secretion is desirable, another approach should be taken: for example, a drug that fully inhibits the acid pump irrespective of its status. Some companies are therefore developing a different type of inhibitor of the gastric acid pump, the acid pump antagonists (APAs), which have immediate onset of action. These can also readily be formulated in a time-release fashion to give essentially continuous full inhibition of acid secretion.

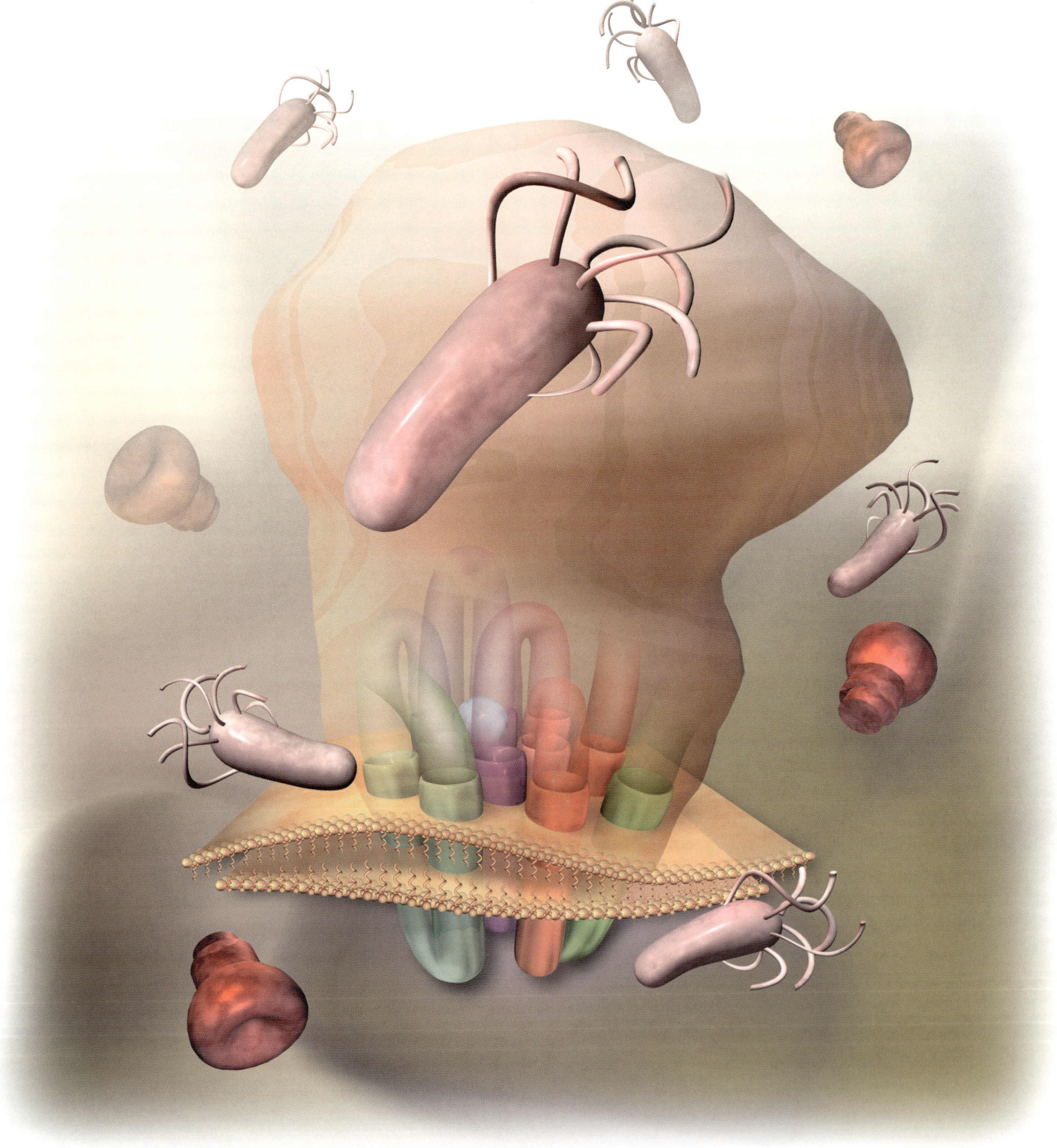

Chapter VI

HELICOBACTER PYLORI

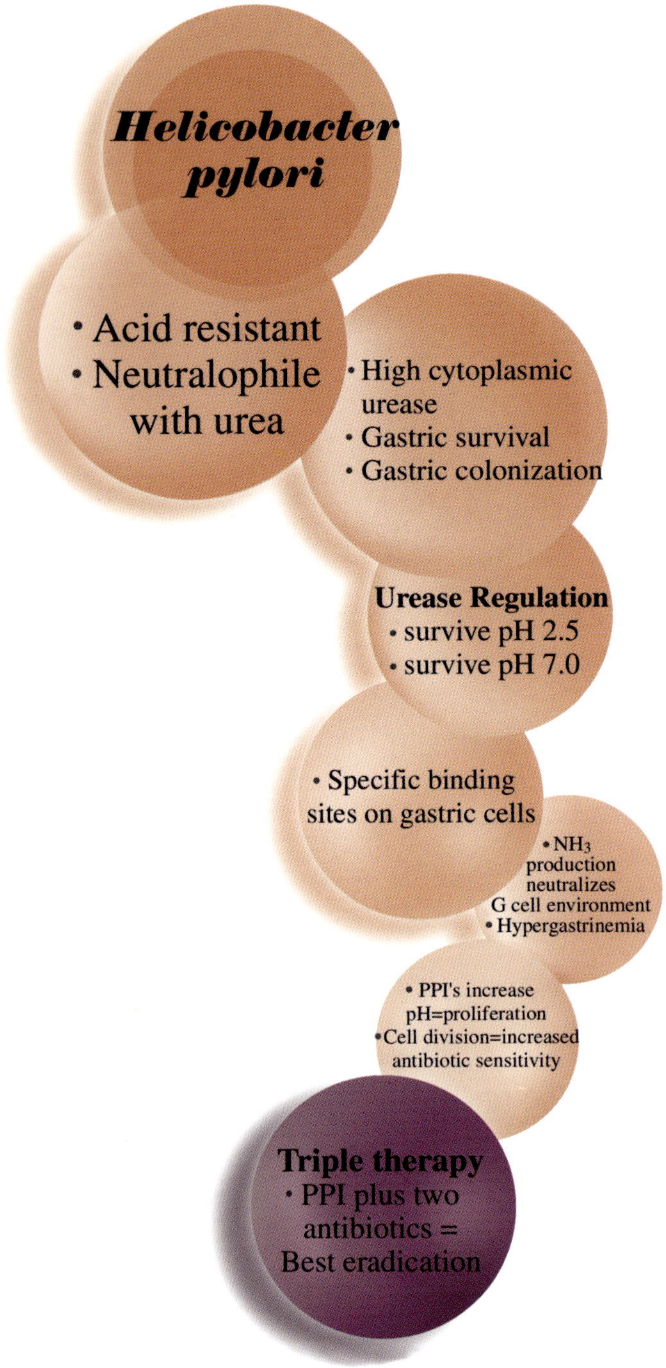
Helicobacter pylori
• Acid resistant
• Neutralophile with urea
• High cytoplasmic urease
• Gastric survival
• Gastric colonization
Urease Regulation
• survive pH 2.5
• survive pH 7.0
• Specific binding sites on gastric cells
• NH_3 production neutralizes G cell environment
• Hypergastrinemia
• PPI's increase pH=proliferation
• Cell division=increased antibiotic sensitivity
Triple therapy
• PPI plus two antibiotics = Best eradication

Helicobacter pylori

The arguments about the etiology of duodenal and gastric ulcer had continued unabated since the beginning of the description of the diseases. By the 20th century, it was generally accepted that acid was necessary for the appearance of the disease, but why only a few people suffered from peptic ulcers was not known. Considerable research went into attempts to correlate levels of acid secretion and the presence of disease. Even the number of parietal cells was counted and correlated with disease. The gist of all the data was that if there was a correlation between levels of acid secretion and disease, people with duodenal ulcer as a group had somewhat higher acid secretion and a larger number of parietal cells than normal, but no correlation was found between levels of acidity and gastric ulcer disease. It was recognized, however, that ingestion of several drugs, often anti-inflammatory agents such as aspirin, were related to some gastric ulcers and bleeding.

Eventually, when it became possible to control secretion of acid in a reproducible manner by the administration of daily doses of H2-receptor antagonists, it was found that reduction of acidity enabled healing of peptic ulcers, but to prevent such ulcers, maintenance on these drugs was essential.

This resulted in a spate of speculations about genotypic variation in the population to account for the recurrence of ulcers in patients who already had ulcers. This extended previous speculations about genotype and ulcer disease. Another rather remarkable finding was that ulcers tended to recur in the same location, as if the healing was imperfect or as if the driving force for ulceration was still present.

Perhaps stronger inhibition of acid secretion would result in better healing and eliminate ulcers. With the advent of omeprazole, it became possible to test this hypothesis. As with H2-receptor antagonists, although healing was faster, the rate of recurrence was identical. Nevertheless, by the time these data became available, the mysterious force had been identified. Many physicians, however, refused to acknowledge the significance of the observations published by two physicians in Perth, Western Australia.

One, a pathologist, Robin Warren, had taken advantage of the improvement in quality of biopsies taken under fiber optical endoscopes. He observed a bacterial association with areas of gastric ulceration but was not taken very seriously by physicians in the local hospital at the time of his discovery in 1979, coincidentally the year in which omeprazole was patented. However, a young GI fellow, Barry Marshall, took his observations more seriously, and together they attempted to culture bacteria from ulcer patients. Over a long weekend, they achieved success and named the bacterium *Campylobacter pylori*. In an heroic experiment, Marshall ingested the bacteria and developed symptoms and acute gastritis, which he later eliminated with high levels of antibiotics. A letter appeared in *The Lancet*, describing the organism and its association with disease. Rapidly thereafter, its association with recurrence of ulcer was demonstrated. In the succeeding few years, first infection by *C. pylori* became accepted as the cause of ulcer recurrence and then of ulcer disease when acid secretion was present. As various gene sequences became available toward the end of the 1980s it was recognized that the organism belonged to the *Helicobacter* species and was renamed *Helicobacter pylori*. Today it is known that there are animal species such as *H. felis* and *H. mustela* that live in the cat and ferret stomach, respectively. It has also been found that there are *Helicobacter* that do not dwell in the stomach. What is the difference between gastric and nongastric *Helicobacter*?

It was then, of course, up to the pharmaceutical industry to provide the physician with the means to eradicate this organism from the stomach. The path to eradication was perhaps slow, as, after all, the organism, although living within the cavity of the stomach, is outside the body and effects of antibiotics are not enhanced by cells such as macrophages.

The Organism

H. pylori is a spiral, motile, gram-negative organism. Gram-negative suggests a relatively dye impermeant outer shell. *In vitro,* it grows best at neutral pH and has the same pH range for growth as does *E. coli.* From this, it can be classified as a neutralophile, which is an organism that avoids extremes of pH. However, as it is able to infect the stomach, it must at least survive gastric acidity before colonization. It may also have to survive gastric acidity during its growth. If it is a neutralophile, then it must also be acid tolerant.

The whole gene sequence of the organism is now known. Two different strains have been sequenced. One had minimal subculture; the other had been passaged several times. There is some measure of disagreement as to the total number of predicted genes. The bacterium sequenced from the multiple passage was suggested to have 1590 open reading frames, the clinical isolate 1495. Therefore, there are fewer genes predicted to be present in the more naive organism — 95, to be exact — than those predicted to be present in the subcultured organism. Within any given strain of bacteria, dependent on its history, genetic variation can occur by, for example, deletion of genes not required during culture or for survival in a particular host. Of the genes, about 875 can be classified functionally, about 300 are conserved between different species, and about 345 are *H. pylori* specific. These similarities between the genes of *H. pylori* and those of other organisms allow identification of the function of about 60% of the genome. Within the genome there are about 300 membrane proteins, some of which have identifiable function, some of which do not. Often a membrane protein is a better drug target than cytoplasmic proteins in mammalian cells. However, in bacteria, targets for antibiotics can also be cytoplasmic, such as the 23S RNA that is the target for clarithromycin, or the DNA that is the target for the ketoconazoles.

Variations between the two strains also extend to variation in the last codon of the triplet, but this results in general conservation of amino acid sequence but probably an over estimate of the variability of gene expression by different organisms when using restriction enzymes. Some variation also exists in the location of the genes on the chromosome: 85% having identical neighbors. This low level of gene shuffling and conservation of gene strings suggests little evolutionary divergence, which has been a point of speculation before these two published sequences. There were 206 strain-specific genes, of which 125 were specific to *H. pylori* compared to other sequences in the gene bank. It is difficult to say at this time whether genes other than those in the pathogenicity island will relate to clinical consequence.

It would be nice to be able to survey all these genes and define those that are essential and absent from the host or other bacteria. This would enable the identification of target gene products that, if inhibited, would eradicate the organism. Here we would look for genes not known to be targets for normal antibiotics so that treatment of the infection would not result in more pathogenic bacteria becoming antibiotic resistant. Efforts are under way to systematically define which of the ~ 1500 genes are essential for survival either at neutral or acidic pH.

Appearance of *Helicobacter pylori*

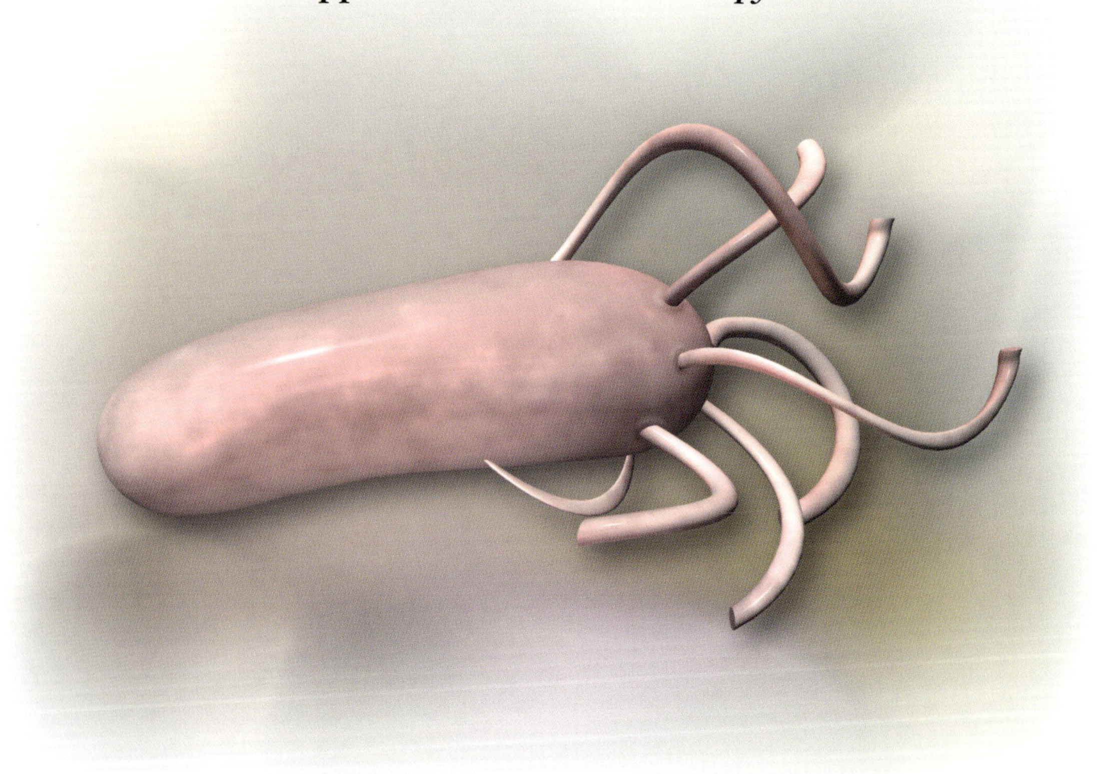

Figure 1. *— The general appearance of* H. pylori, *a spiral-shaped gram-negative organism with multiple flagellae placed at one pole of the organism.*

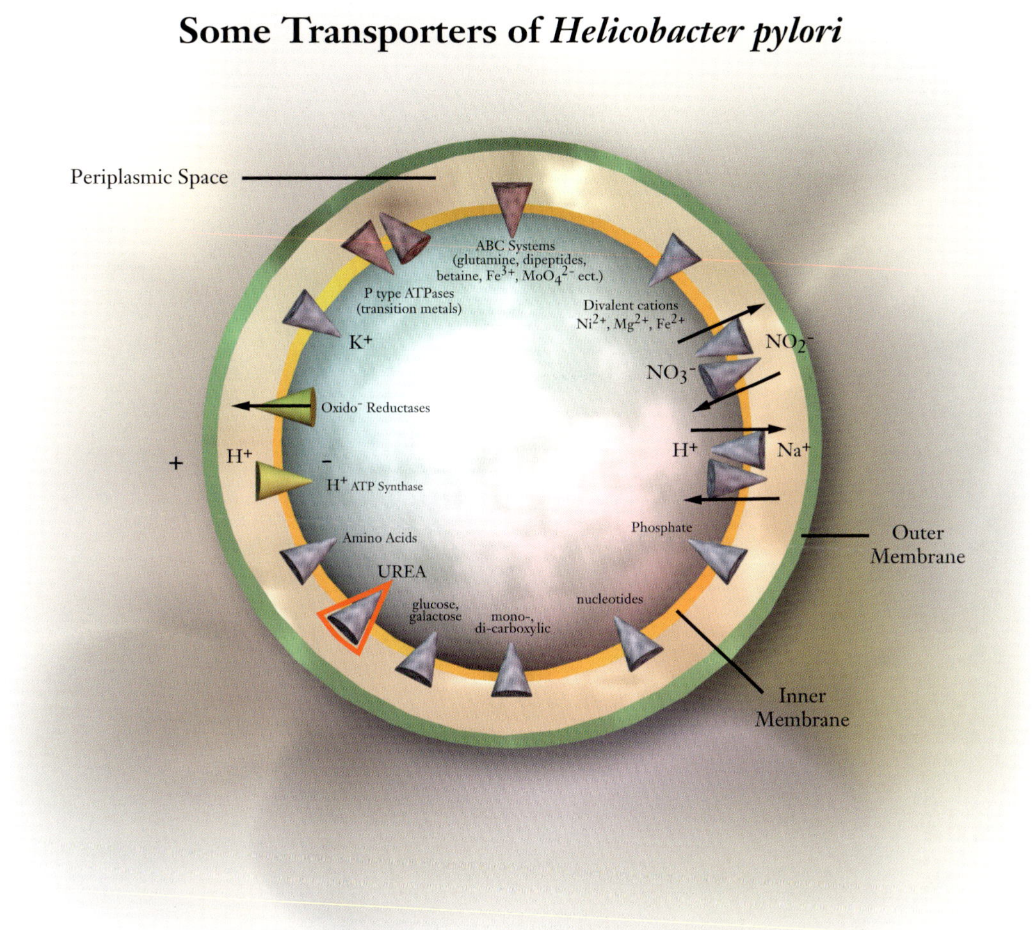

Figure 2. *— The various transport processes identified by gene homology in the genome of* H. pylori. *Some of these are ATP-driven transporters, some are H^+ symporters, and some are exchangers. There are probably others as yet unidentified. The urea channel responsible for acid resistance is highlighted.*

Bacteria have various sets of genes or gene clusters that are dedicated to orchestrating different sets of responses to variations in their environment. For example, in the absence of nutrients, cell division takes an enormous toll on viable organisms. Therefore, genes have evolved to produce what is known as a *stringency response*, in which cell wall biosynthesis and cell division are impeded. Other sets of genes interact to alter the metabolism of the organism as well as cell wall constituents so that a new form of the organism—a spherical coccoid form—becomes the major constituent of bacterial cultures, especially if the cultures are allowed to age. Paramount to *H. pylori* is survival and success in an acidic environment.

Acid and *H. pylori*

One means of gastric success is avoidance of acidity, which may be very difficult in the human stomach. However, different regions of the stomach are likely to have different acidity. The fundus, where acid is secreted, is more acidic at its surface than the antrum, where acid is absorbed rather than secreted. Hence, the motility of the organism is important, at least for avoidance of the more acid regions of the stomach. Consistent with this, organisms in which motility genes have been deleted are not able to infect animal models.

Another means of gastric success is toleration of acidity. Strategies developed by different strains of bacteria are different, depending on whether the organism is acidophile, neutralophile, or alkalophile. What is important for bacteria, as for mitochondria in animal cells (often thought of as symbiotic bacteria), is the maintenance of enough of an energy gradient across their inner membrane in order to enable synthesis of ATP, the energy currency of bacteria, as for animal cells. It is also of course important to maintain a constant cytoplasmic pH to enable normal bacterial cell function. Neutralophiles, such as *E. coli* or *B. subtilis*, tolerate pH down to about 4.0 and at pH values lower than that, die. The same is true of *H. pylori* in normal growth media *in vitro*. Death also occurs at pH values greater than 8.2.

The energy gradient vital to the life of bacteria is simply the electrochemical gradient of protons: that is, the transmembrane pH gradient added to the transmembrane potential driving hydrogen ions into the bacterium. Therefore, if the bacterium is an acidophile, the pH gradient across the membrane is large and the membrane potential is small or even positive inside to keep the driving force for ATP synthesis constant at about -200 mV or 3.5 pH units inward. The opposite holds for alkalophiles; as the pH gradient is small, the membrane potential is large. How about a neutralophile such as *E. coli* or *H. pylori*?

Here the organism can live between pH 4.0 and 8.5. At pH 8.5, the membrane potential is the sole driving force for ATP synthesis. At pH 4.0, it is the pH gradient that takes over, and in between these two external pH values, the sum of the two stays constant. This does not mean that everything else stays the same. For example, in bacteria, correct folding of membrane proteins depends on an adequate interior negative membrane potential in order to position clusters of positively charged amino acids, such as arginine and lysine, on the cytoplasmic side of the membrane. So, as the membrane potential falls, such insertion slows and even stops, accounting in part at least for the optimal growth of these neutralophile organisms at around neutral pH.

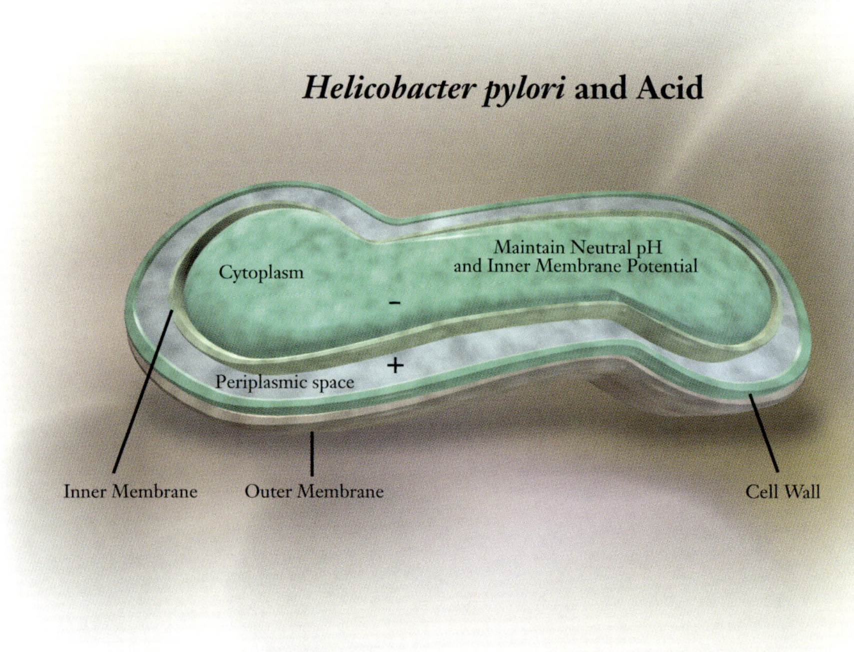

Figure 3. *— General structure of bacteria showing the outer membrane, the cell wall, and the periplasmic space external to the energizing membrane (the inner membrane), separating the space from the cytoplasm. An interior negative potential is maintained to allow the organism to survive by enabling synthesis of ATP and membrane protein synthesis.*

For growth in the stomach, acid-tolerance mechanisms must be added to allow maintenance of the membrane potential for growth at the acidic pH of the stomach. This means that the pH of the periplasmic space be maintained within the limits required for effective membrane potential generation at around -100 mV, as measured by a potential sensitive dye in cultured *H. pylori.*

The Periplasm

Bacteria have an outer membrane, a cell wall, a periplasmic space, an inner membrane, and a cytoplasm. In contrast to eukaryotic cells, the cytoplasm is devoid of membranous structures. The energizer system is present in the cytoplasmic membrane, and the outer membrane is relatively permeable to quite large molecules due to the presence of outer membrane proteins or porins. The outer membrane is composed of glycolipids and the cell wall of complex carbohydrates. The inner membrane is ion tight, as are most biologic membranes, and is composed of a phospholipid bilayer interrupted by integral membrane proteins. In terms of maintaining energy supply and membrane protein synthesis, it is the gradient across the inner membrane that counts, and, for growth in acidic media and survival in strong acid, neutralophiles have to guard the pH in the periplasmic space quite jealously.

Urease

The major means whereby *H. pylori* achieves acid tolerance to the variations in the pH of its gastric environment is the use of urease. This enzyme hydrolyzes the available urea that diffuses from the blood into the stomach and hydrolyzes it producing CO_2 and NH_3:

$$NH_2\text{-}\overset{\overset{\displaystyle O}{||}}{C}\text{-}NH_2 + H_2O \longrightarrow 2NH_3 + CO_2$$

The NH_3 protonates, absorbing acid to form NH_4^+. This enables neutralization of gastric acid until theoretically the pKa of the NH_4^+/NH_3 couple is reached at about pH 9.0.

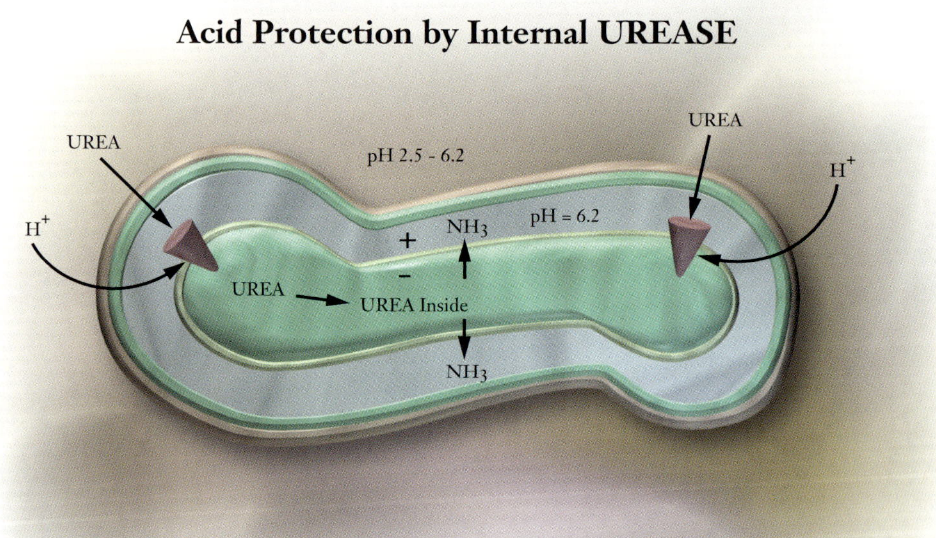

Figure 4. *— An illustration of the guarding of the pH of the periplasmic space by acid activation of urea access to internal urease. At pH 6.2 and below, urea gains access to the interior of the organism, permitting internal urease to generate* NH_3*. This diffuses into the periplasmic space alkalinizing this space until pH 6.2 is achieved, when urea permeability decreases preventing further alkalinization by internal urease. The membrane potential at a periplasmic pH of 6.2 is found to be -101 mV.*

Regulator of UREASE Activation

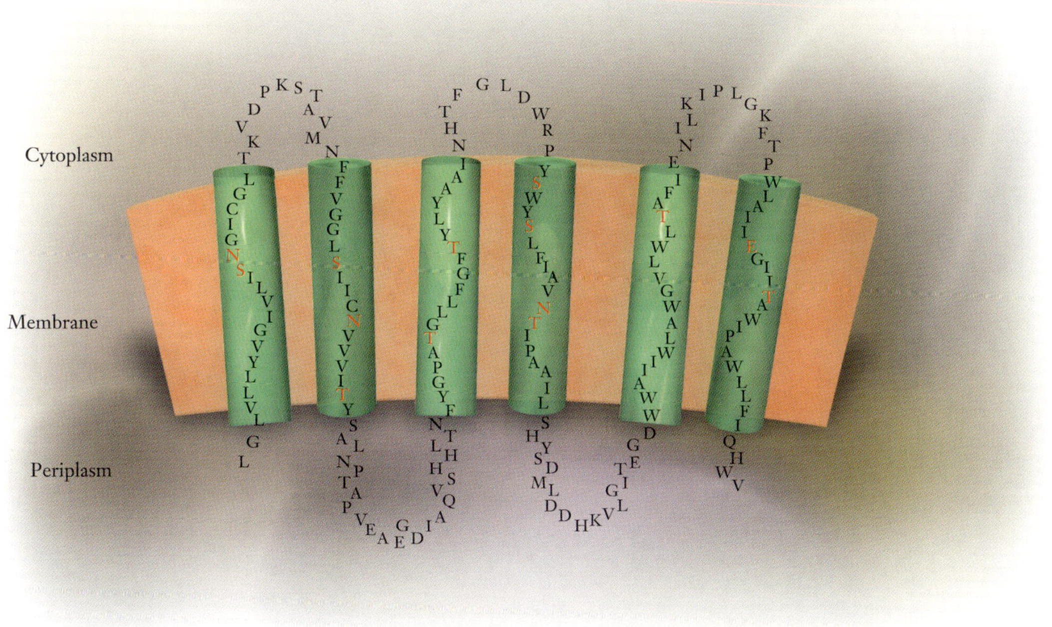

Figure 5. — The two-dimensional structure of ureI, the urea transporter responsible for acid activation of intrabactorial urease. There are 5-6 histidines in the periplasmic doman and 1 histidine in the cytoplasmic domain. Mutation of any of the histidines in the first periplasmic loop do not affect acid gating whereas mutations of any of the last 3 histidines inactivates the protein. The hydrophilic amino acids in the membrane region are colored red and may be implicated in its urea transport activity. This molecule may function on its own or be complexed with other proteins in H. pylori. This molecule acts as a proton-gated urea channel and is the link between bacterical urease and gastric colonization.

There are two urease compartments: urease that is bound to the surface of the organism and urease that is in the cytoplasmic compartment. The pH optimum of the urease that is bound to the surface is between pH 7.5 and 8.5, depending on how the measurements are made. All agree that there is virtually no activity of the urease at pH 4.5 or less. There is even irreversible activation of the surface urease at that pH. Therefore, either this surface urease has little to do with gastric survival of *H. pylori* or *H. pylori* never experiences a pH as low as that. Some would argue that the surface of the stomach is close to neutrality. This is based on measuring surface pH using open-tipped microelectrodes. These workers do agree that when the pH of the bathing solution drops to pH 2.0, surface pH becomes identical to bulk pH. Using fluorescent dyes and confocal microscopy, one worker claims that there is no pH gradient at the gastric surface, in opposition to the microelectrode army. Given that the bulk pH of the gastric lumen often falls to 1.0 or even less, it would seem reasonable to suppose that the organisms are often exposed to acidic pH values less than 4.0, at which they die in the absence of a specific acid tolerant response, and that that response cannot depend on the activity of the surface urease. Again, although some believe that this urease is secreted by the bacteria, direct experimental evidence argues that it results from lysis and adhesion to the bacterial surface. Some have called it altruistic lysis, but little in nature is altruistic, especially in primitive organisms.

Their secret, closely guarded for millions of years, is to use their internal urease wisely. Untrammeled function of this urease would often result in large alkalinization of the cytoplasm with resultant death. The urease comprises about 15% of cellular protein, the largest quantity of urease known in bacteria. In young organisms, less than 10% of total urease is found outside, 90% inside. It is inactive at neutral pH, but as the pH falls below 6, urease activity switches on, reaching a maximum at about pH 5.0; it stays constant down to a pH of 3.0 and then dwindles as the pH falls further. When urea is added to intact bacteria at pH levels below 6.0, there is a rapid restoration of membrane potential due to elevation of periplasmic pH to 6.2. This potential is reached irrespective of the starting pH and appears to be a set point for the acid tolerant response of these organisms.

The Urea Channel

The urease gene cluster consists of two regions. The first encodes the two subunits, urease A and urease B. This is followed by a promoter region, and then five further genes: *ureI*, *ureE*, *ureF*, *ureG* and *ureH*. The function of the latter four genes is thought to be in urease assembly, as this enzyme requires Ni^{2+} to be inserted into its active site after synthesis. The enzyme is also assembled into its mature hexameric heterodimeric form. The function of *ureI* is not known.

However, removal of *ureI* from the genome results in an inability for survival at acidic pH and inability to infect mice or gerbils. Furthermore, there is no further acid activation of urease and no restoration of membrane potential in the absence of the *ureI* gene product. It seems therefore that in some way this protein regulates the acid activation of internal urease. Not surprisingly, *Helicobacter* species that live in the stomach all express the *ureI* gene product. Those *Helicobacter* that do not inhabit the stomach do not have the *ureI* gene. Searching in the data base for genes like *ureI* finds two genes with some similarity that seem to be part of the amidase gene cluster, tentatively thought of as amide transporters. Urea is also an amide. So what is the structure of the *ureI* protein?

Chapter VI

Evidence for Urea Channel in *H. pylori*

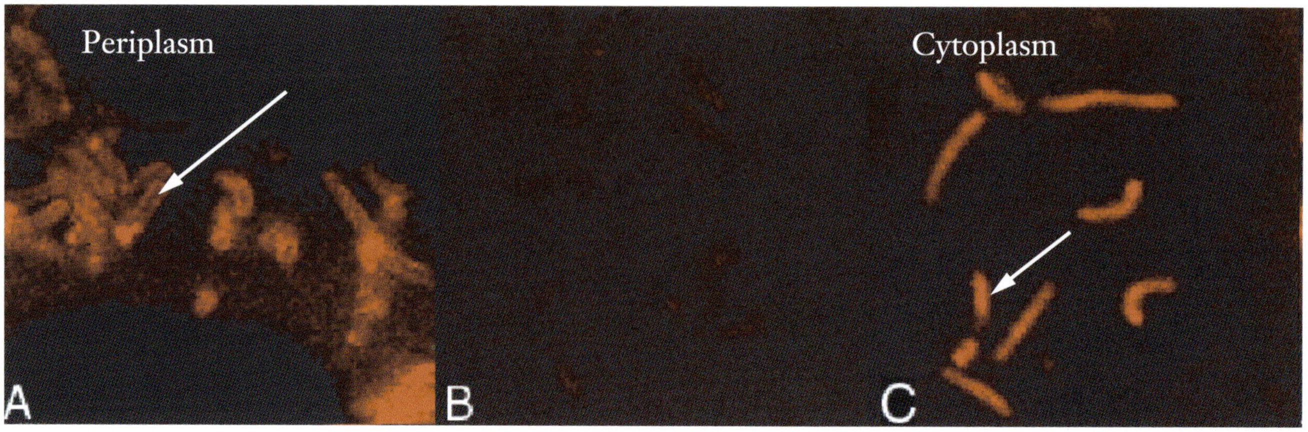

H. pylori + urea pH 5.5 | *H. pylori ureI-* + urea pH 5.5 | *H. pylori ureI-* + urea pH 5.5 + Nonidet

BCECF Acid as pH probe

Figure 6. *— Illustration of the role of ureI as regulator of pH of periplasmic space. On the left, urea is added at pH 5.5 to normal bacteria. The flourescent pH probe, BCECF, immediately increases its fluorescence in the periplasmic space due to activation of internal urease and early elevation of the periplasmic pH. The same organisms but with* ureI *removed show no response of BCECF with the addition of urea at pH 5.5. However, urease is still active, because with the addition of a mild nonionic detergent (0.01% $C_{12}E_9$), there is a rapid elevation of pH in the cytoplasm due to access of urea to the cytoplasmic urease.*

From the amino acid sequence, this protein is a cytoplasmic membrane protein with six membrane-inserted helices, oriented so that the N and C terminals face the periplasmic space. In the second periplasmic loop, there are three histidines. Histidine is an amino acid with a pK_a of around 6.0, admirably poised to respond to external pH of around 6.2. This protein can therefore sense and respond to acidification of the periplasmic space. Its function can be to allow urea entry into the cytoplasm, acting as an amide transporter and therefore a urea permease. Alternatively, this protein could respond to pH by transmitting a signal to the cytoplasmic urease, enabling its activation. However, this would mean that urea has free access to an inactive cytoplasmic urease. Homogenization of the bacteria does not produce an inactive urease, perhaps denying the possibility that UreI protein acts as a sensor for removal of inhibition of internal urease. The most likely hypothesis is that at pH less than 6.2 this protein functions as an amidoporin.

Habitat

The gastric mucosa has a varied menu for those bacteria that choose to become its denizens. There are many different cell types in the gastric epithelium such as surface cells, neck cells, parietal cells, and peptic cells. The geography is variable: narrow acid- and pepsin-secreting fundic glands, larger shorter antral glands secreting pepsinogen and HCO_3^-, and reabsorbing acid and acid secretion sites in the fundus but not the antrum. Within given cells, there is also structural variations in the plasma membrane above the tight junction exposed to the bacteria. There are the tight junction proteins themselves, the molecules, such as e-cadherin, immediately above the tight junction, and a panoply of proteins present on the apical rather than basal surface of the epithelium.

The organism itself has specialized surface structures adapted to adhere to cells; in particular, it adheres to the cells of the gastric mucosa. Some of these appear to mimic human surface proteins or carbohydrates or at least structures that usually bind to these. In a culture system in which bacteria and a human cell line are mixed to see where the bacteria end up, it appears that the organisms prefer to bind to regions just above the regions of contact, perhaps recognizing the extracellular domain organized by the presence of e-cadherin.

In vitro data have clearly shown that *H. pylori* can survive between pH 4.0 and 8.2 in the absence of added urea. In the presence of urea, they can survive down to a pH of 2.5, based on the acid-tolerant mechanisms discussed here. Their location in the stomach immediately after infection is not known. It appears that, after acute infection, there is inhibition of gastric acid secretion that then returns as they begin to colonize the stomach. Their site of colonization is either the fundus or the antrum, especially within antral glands. They are found in the mucus and at the apex of the surface epithelial cells. In general, antral colonization is more frequent than fundic colonization, presumably because in many persons, the pH at the fundic surface is too low for habitation. It

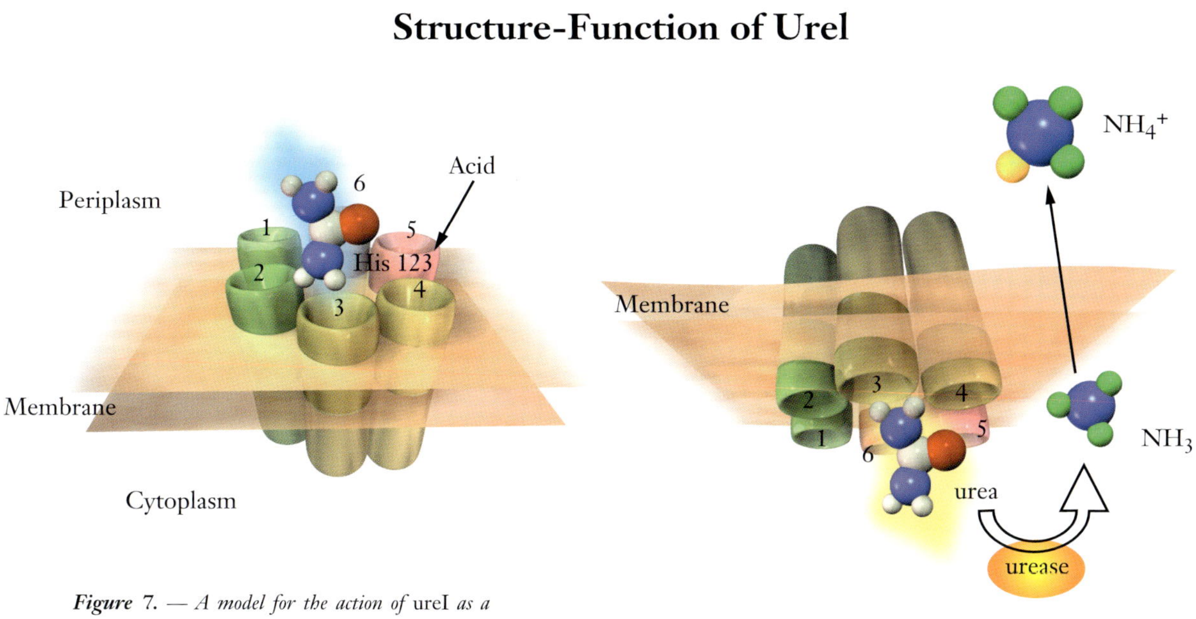

Figure 7. — *A model for the action of* ureI *as a proton-gated urea channel shown by expression in Xenopus oocytes. With acidification of the periplasm, and prtonation of histidine at position 123 in the amino acid sequence, the urea channel opens allowing very rapid entry of urea for hydrolysis by intrabacterial urease. The NH_3 produced diffuses across the inner membrane of the organism and by forming NH_4^+ in the periplasm, protects* H. pylori *against gastric acidity.*

is found that, during treatment with proton pump inhibitors, there is migration of the organism toward the fundus, as if inhibition of acid secretion makes the fundic environment more amenable. There is, however, also a decrease of the organism in the antrum, as if the pH elevation in that region is uncomfortable. This is perhaps because the surface urease is able to elevate the pH too much for the health of *H. pylori*, exceeding the pH 8.5 at which they can survive. Thus, *in vitro* data are easily able to rationalize the sites at which the organism is found in the stomach.

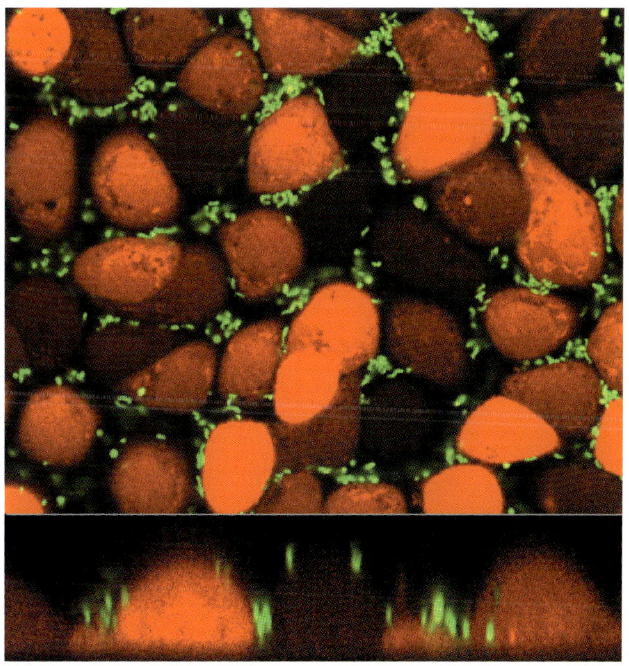

Figure 8. — H. pylori *expressing green fluorescent protein cocultured with human gastric AGS cells stained with Snarf-AM. The cells are stained red; the bacteria are green. It can be seen that the bacteria are distributed on the periphery of the cells, and a section in the z-axis shows that they are located just above the regions of adhesion between the cells.*

Duodenal ulcer is also a possible sequel to *H. pylori* infection of the stomach. Here, one finds regions of gastric metaplasia, thought possibly to be due to excessive exposure of this part of the duodenum to acid. On these cells, it is claimed, one finds *H. pylori*. It is clear however that infestation of the duodenal ulcer with *H. pylori* is a rarer observation than finding the organism in the antrum. Antral infestation is a risk factor for duodenal ulceration.

Pathogenicity

Infection by *H. pylori* has a variety of possible consequences for the host. Everyone who is infected gets gastritis: that is, an inflammatory response in the wall of the gastric mucosa. The locale of this inflammation depends on where the major component of the infection resides: antrum or fundus. About 20% of infected persons may get either duodenal or gastric peptic ulcer disease. Why these particular individuals? One line of investigation, for which there is reasonable evidence, suggests that the bacterial genotype plays an important role. The pathogenicity island, a set of genes that are similar to other pathogenic factors in other bacteria, may be an important determinant. The presence of genes such as *CagA* and *VacA*, or genes elsewhere in the organism, such as *ICE*, appear to predict a tendency toward ulcer disease. However, the presence of these particular proteins is not a fully accurate predictor of pathogenic as compared to commensal strains. For example, *CagA* is expressed in bacteria inhabiting the Chinese population, but the frequency of peptic ulcer disease in this population is similar to that of other nations. *VacA* is often present in the absence of disease or is absent in the presence of disease.

Infected patients generate antibodies against a large number of the bacterial proteins, with no one particular protein antigen being overrepresented in the infected population. It seems as if almost all bacterial proteins are present to the host immune system, whether they are cytoplasmic or peripheral.

H. pylori is a lysogenic type of organism, which means that they lyse readily and express genes that enable lysis. Evidently, if they lyse, all bacterial proteins are potentially antigenic and those with equal antigenicity generate equal levels of antibodies. The presence of antibodies has been used by several manufacturers to provide kits for diagnosis of infection.

Lysis may also be the means whereby surface urease appears in *H. pylori* cultures. From labeling of the organisms and determining exterior and interior proteins, it does not appear the urease is selectively found, relative to other bacterial proteins, on the outside of the bacteria. This suggests that lysis, rather than secretion, is responsible for the presence of surface urease.

A molecule present in all infections is NH_3. This is a weak base, and just as it is able to be protonated and neutralize the periplasmic space, it can also penetrate mammalian cells and generate interior alkalinity. It could be that this alone is sufficient to begin the inflammatory cascade, and there are some data suggesting that administration of NH_3 in the form of NH_4Cl does result in gastric damage in rats. Perhaps this is the cause of the beginning of the inflammation; however, it is not the cause of peptic ulcer disease per se.

The ability of NH_3 to neutralize the environment of the organism may also account for the hypergastrinemia seen in infected persons. The antral gastrin (G) cell is stimulated by luminal amino acids, by transmitters released by gastric nerves — for example, gastrin-releasing peptide and acetylcholine — and is inhibited by somatostatin released from antral D cells. However, at a gastric luminal pH of 3.0 or below, gastrin release from the G cell is inhibited, either because of a direct effect of pH on this cell, or an effect of pH on the D cell. This is a feedback regulatory mechanism for acid secretion; after digestion of food and loss of buffering capacity, the fall of pH results in the shut down of acid secretion.

As NH_3 production accompanies acidification of the organism, if there are bacteria in the vicinity of antral glands or within antral glands, a level of hypergastrinemia is expected and indeed is found. With hypergastrinemia, an increase of parietal cell and ECL cell mass would be expected, as is found in patients with duodenal ulcer disease. Hence, such patients would tend to have higher acid output capacity than uninfected people. In addition, several large studies suggest that patients with duodenal ulcers have higher acidity than normal.

Effect of *Helicobacter pylori* Urease on Gastrin Release

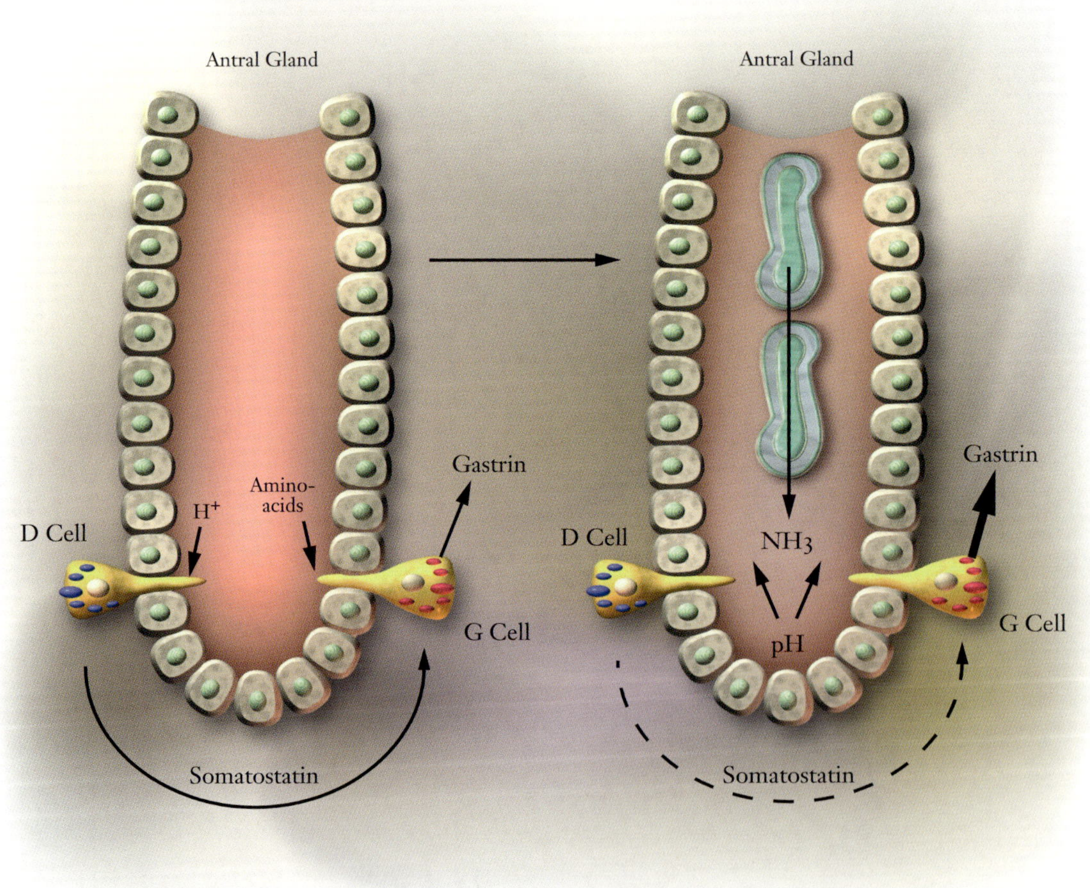

Figure 9. *— A model explaining the increase of serum gastrin seen in patients infected with* H. pylori. *To the left is a normal gland in which the G cell is stimulated by amino acids and is inhibited by acidification of the antral gland lumen. To the right is shown* H. pylori *producing* NH_3*, which tends to neutralize the gland lumen and results therefore in inappropriately high levels of gastrin by interfering with the physiologic feedback of high acidity.*

The effect of *H. pylori* on the fundic epithelium seems to have more important consequences than on the antral epithelium. Here, after some time, the fundic gastritis can result in a degree of fundic gland atrophy and even intestinal metaplasia. The latter is considered to be a precancerous condition, and this has resulted in the organism being classified as a class 1 carcinogen. Epidemiologic studies have shown a correlation between infection and gastric cancer.

H. pylori as a Commensal

Although the role of *H. pylori* in generation of peptic ulcer disease, gastritis, and gastric cancer would appear to suggest all *H. pylori* should be eradicated, there appear to be consequences of eradication that are not entirely positive. After eradication, it appears that intragastric pH control by proton pump inhibitors is not as good as before eradication in the same patients. It also is suggested that symptoms of gastroesophageal reflux disease (GERD) may be worsened and that Barrett's esophagus may be exacerbated. If this view is correct, in those cases in which *H. pylori* infection has no gastric or duodenal consequence other than inflammation, the organism may be regarded as a commensal organism, rather than as a pathogen. If this view comes to be accepted, it is important to be able to predict which organism is pathogenic and which is commensal. With the availability of all the gene sequences of the organisms, a new technology may become available: the use of chip arrays to determine the level of expression of all the genes of *H. pylori*. With this tool, direct correlation may be made between gene expression and disease, enabling informed analysis of the basis for pathogenicity or commensality.

Effects of Medium pH on Protein Synthesis

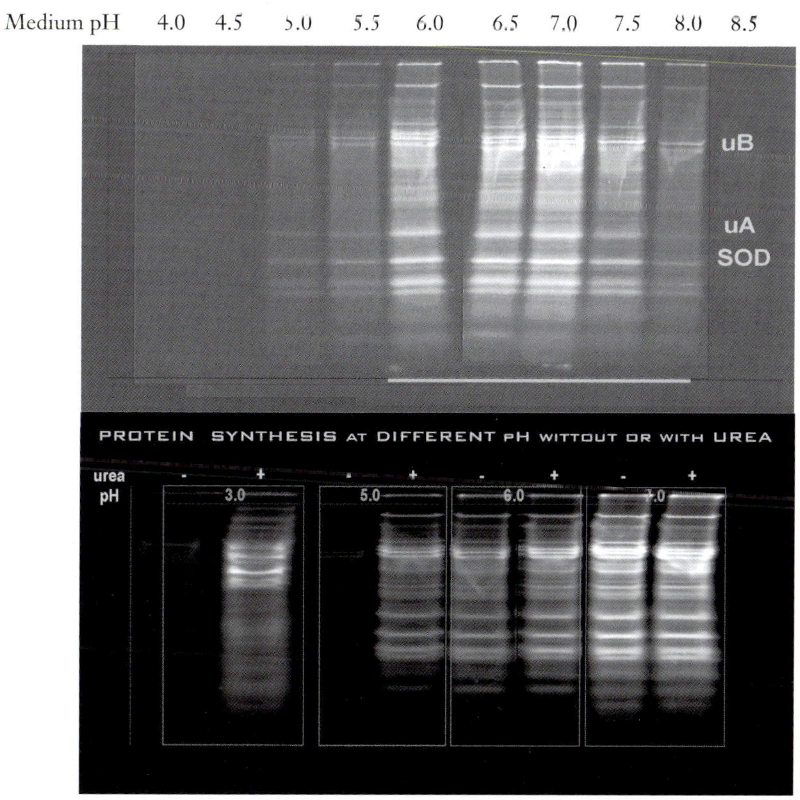

Figure 10. — The effect of acidification of a test meal (EnsureTM) on the results of a 13C urea breath test for diagnosis of H. pylori *infection. This shows that acid activation of UreI to allow activity of intra-bacterial urease is important when diagnosing some patients on PPI therapy (courtesy Pantoflickova, Dorta and Blum).*

Growth

Although survival of the organism in the presence of urea extends from a gastric environment of pH 2.5 to 8.2, this is not true of growth. Urease activity at 2.5 mM urea can elevate periplasmic pH to 6.2 over that pH range, and this is within the growth curve of the organism. This can be seen when we measure protein synthesis at different fixed medium pH and look at the effect of the presence of urea. Thus, with this level of urea, the organism is able to grow in the regions of the stomach where it is able to elevate the pH to 6.2. Of course, the urea level in the stomach is not always 2.5 mM, and it is possible that there is just enough urea available to elevate periplasmic pH to levels compatible with survival but not growth.

From this *in vitro* approach, one is left with the suspicion that *H. pylori* will tend to occupy a fairly selective niche in the wall of the stomach, where its growth would be dependent on a balance between the prevailing pH, the local concentration of urea, and perhaps the state of binding to epithelial cells. Unfortunately, we do not know what the actual pH is in the environment of an infection nor do we know the concentration of urea. It seems that the cells comprising the epithelial cells of the mucosa do not have a urea transporter with homology to renal or red cell urea transporters; hence, urea accesses the gastric lumen by diffusion, presumably mostly through tight junctions. If urease inside the organism is activated by acid, the cytoplasm will constitute a sink for uptake of urea. The urea concentration at which the organism is able to elevate the periplasmic pH to 6.2 is not known. However, in those regions in which the organism is multiplying, periplasmic pH is between pH 6.0 and 8.0. This may be due to a locally high pH or effective action of the organism's urease. Almost surely, such an environment is not going to be identical in the universe of the gastric epithelium and may even vary with the state of the disease. Therefore, at any given time, some organisms will be in active growth, while others will be in a nondividing state, but still surviving a pH lethal in the absence of urea and urease activity. This has important implications for antibiotic therapy from which the antibiotics require protein synthesis or cell wall biosynthesis for their bacteriostatic or bactericidal effects.

Eradication

Given that infected patients with duodenal ulcer disease should have the organisms removed, eradication is an important consideration. Over the years, several protocols have been tried, but only recently has a degree of consensus been achieved as to how to reach this goal. Perhaps the first such substance used that may have had benefit because of its effect on the bacteria was bismuth. This divalent cation appears to be toxic to the organism and also to be retained in the stomach for a long time. However, bismuth must be administered in combination with other drugs, such as metronidazole, plus tetracycline, and a histamine-2 receptor antagonist to give effective eradication.

The use of antibiotics became obvious once the presence of infection was realized. Soon thereafter, it was found that antibiotics *in vitro* were potent bactericidal or bacteriostatic agents with appropriate MIC values, especially antibiotics such as amoxicillin, clarithromycin, and metronidazole. However, they did not work *in vivo*. Several reasons could be given for this. Perhaps they were not stable in gastric acid. Perhaps they did not get to the organism that was hiding from them. Perhaps when they got to the organism, its state (ie, dividing or nondividing) was insensitive. For example, a nondividing organism will not respond to the penicillin class of antibiotic. An organism that does not require protein synthesis will not respond to clarithromycin.

Based on this idea, various acid secretion inhibitors were tried in combination with antibiotics. At first, it was thought that a combination of a single antibiotic with omeprazole would be effective in eradication.

Now triple therapy has become the standard approach in which a proton pump inhibitor, such as omeprazole, is given twice daily along with two antibiotics: clarithromycin and amoxicillin. Clarithromycin binds to the 23S RNA and inhibits protein synthesis. Amoxicillin binds to penicillin binding proteins and inhibits the transpeptidase reactions necessary for cell-wall biosynthesis, resulting in a bactericidal effect on the organisms. So what is the role of the proton pump inhibitor such as omeprazole?

At one time, it was thought that omeprazole and its congeners had a direct effect on the organism, but further experimentation showed that this was an *in vitro* artifact. Now it is thought that the effect of proton pump inhibitors taken in combination with amoxicillin and clarithromycin can be accounted for by pH elevation. This either makes the antibiotics more available to the organism or makes the organism more sensitive to the antibiotics. The latter seems more likely, when the growth characteristics of *H. pylori* are considered.

In the normal gastric mucosa, given the variation in pH that is expected, some regions will contain growing organisms, but some will contain nondividing organisms. If a proton pump inhibitor is given, the pH will rise and more organisms will be growing and fewer will be nondividing. This results in an increased susceptibility to antibiotics. Metronidazole, which targets DNA and not just dividing bacteria, shows no synergism with proton pump inhibitors.

Current eradication rates with appropriate protocols with omeprazole reach from the 77th to 90th percentile (per protocol analysis) and from the 69th to 83rd percentiles (intent-to-treat analysis) in clinical trials. Perhaps in the field, this eradication rate is not achieved because of compliance with a rather complicated regimen requiring the taking of three pills twice a day for 10 days in the absence of inducements to compliance such as pain.

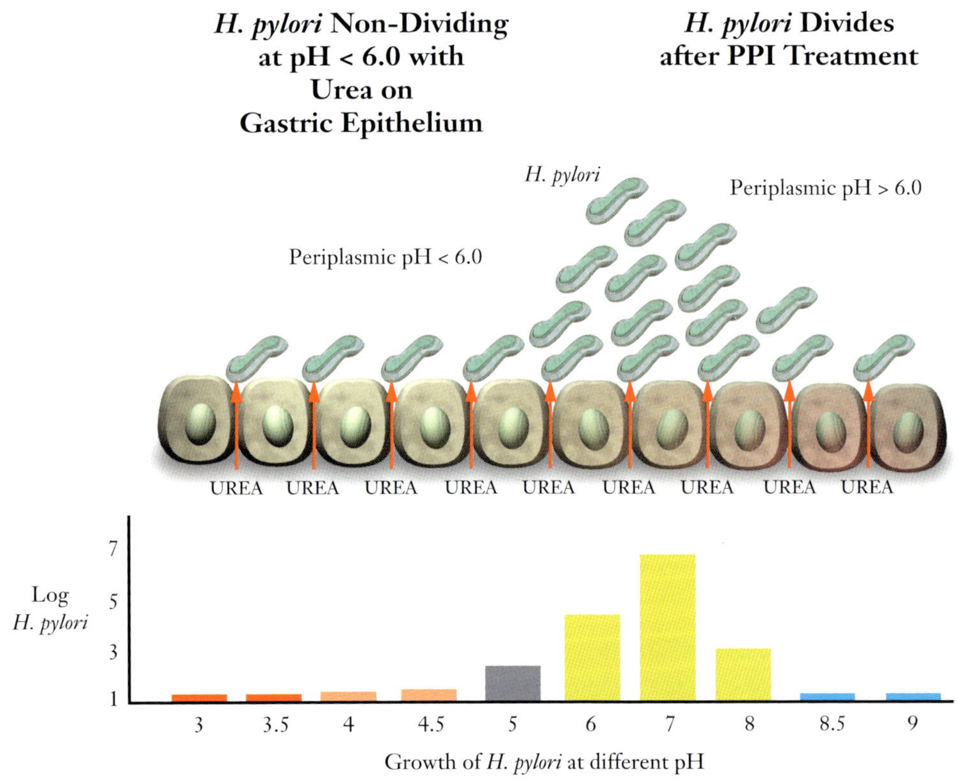

Figure 11. *— An illustration of the mechanism of synergism of proton pump inhibition with growth-dependent antibiotics. On the left are illustrated regions of the stomach in which urea concentrations are insufficient to raise the periplasmic pH to 6.2 but sufficient to enable survival of* H. pylori. *When proton pump inhibitors are given, the pH of this region elevates to the point at which urease activity raises the pH to levels that cell division can occur, resulting in antibiotic sensitivity.*

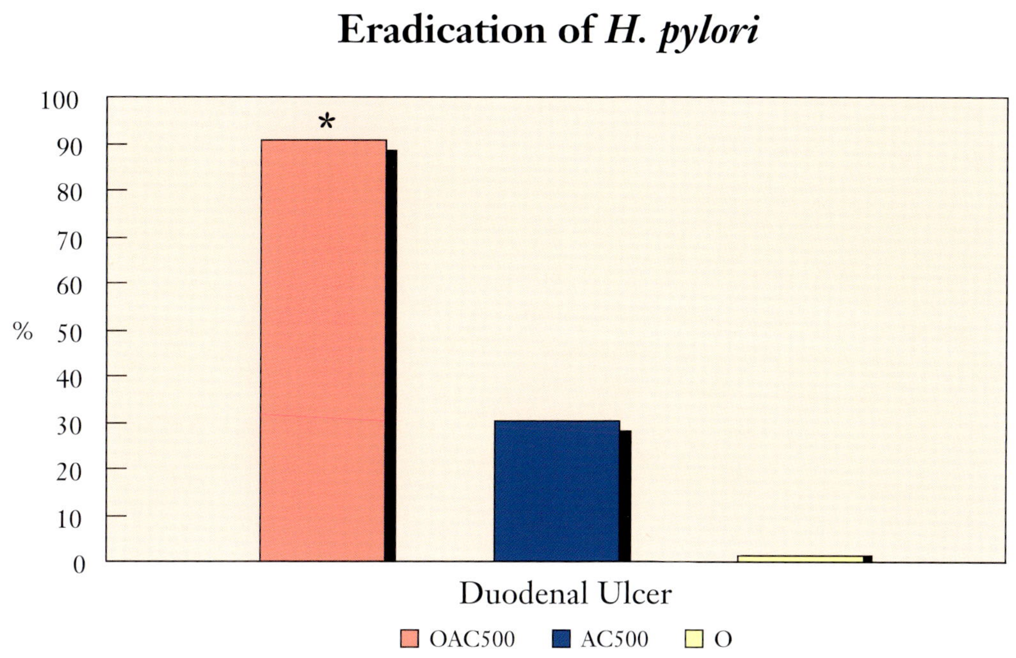

Figure 12. — The results of studies in which various eradication protocols were compared, with single drug (omeprazole (O), 40 mg once daily), two antibiotics (amoxicillin (A), 1g and clarithromycin (C), 500 mg, both taken twice daily), or triple therapy (omeprazole, 20 mg, amoxicillin, 1g, and clarithromycin, C, 500 mg, twice daily). Clearly, triple therapy was the most effective combination.

In view of the results of eradication therapy and because of the presence of metronidazole resistance, a combination of proton pump inhibitor in combination with amoxicillin and clarithromycin is an approved therapeutic regimen. However, in the event of clarithromycin resistance, alternative microbial therapy should be used (See attached prescribing information and the Note to Prescriber in the back of the book for additional prescribing considerations for clarithromycin and amoxicillin).

Noninvasive Diagnosis of Infection and Eradication

It is important to know if a patient is infected and, if treatment is undertaken, to determine whether eradication has been successful. The most reliable noninvasive technique appears to be the urea breath test, whereby the breakdown of ingested ^{13}C or ^{14}C urea is measured as a diagnostic and evaluation tool. Here it is important to ensure acidity at the time of urea administration to enable activation of internal urease. This can be done by administering urea in citric acid buffer at pH 3.0. This should prevent some of the false negatives seen in patients taking proton pump inhibitors.

Alternatively, a stool antigen test has been suggested or a serologic method wherein 3 or 4 low MWt antigens are tested. These require careful evaluation.

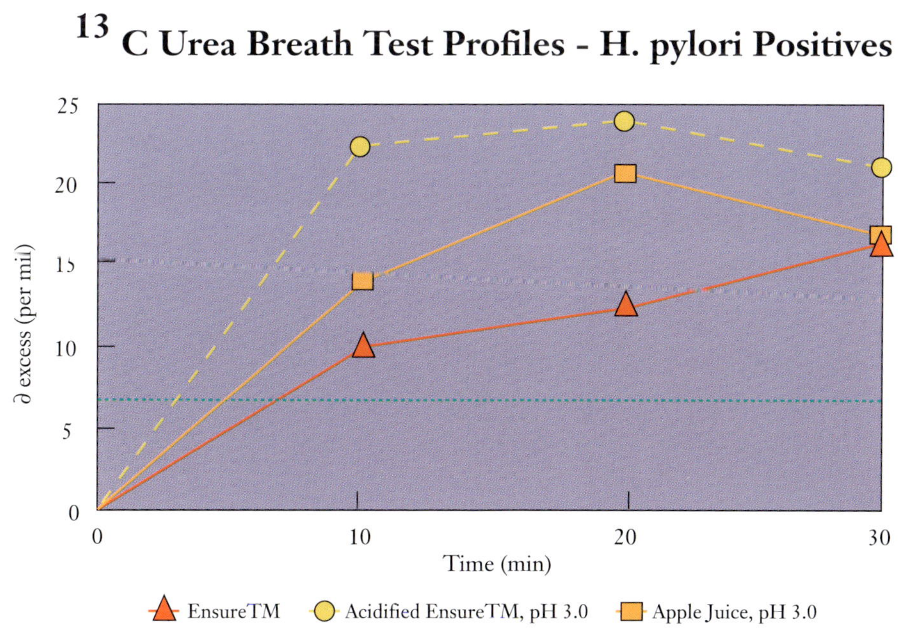

Figure 13. — The effect of acidification of a test meal (Ensure™) on the results of a ^{13}C urea breath test for diagnosis of H. **pylori** *infection. This shows that acid activation of UreI to allow activity of intrabacterial urease is important when diagnosing some patients on PPI therapy (courtesy Pantoflickova, Dorta, and Blum).*

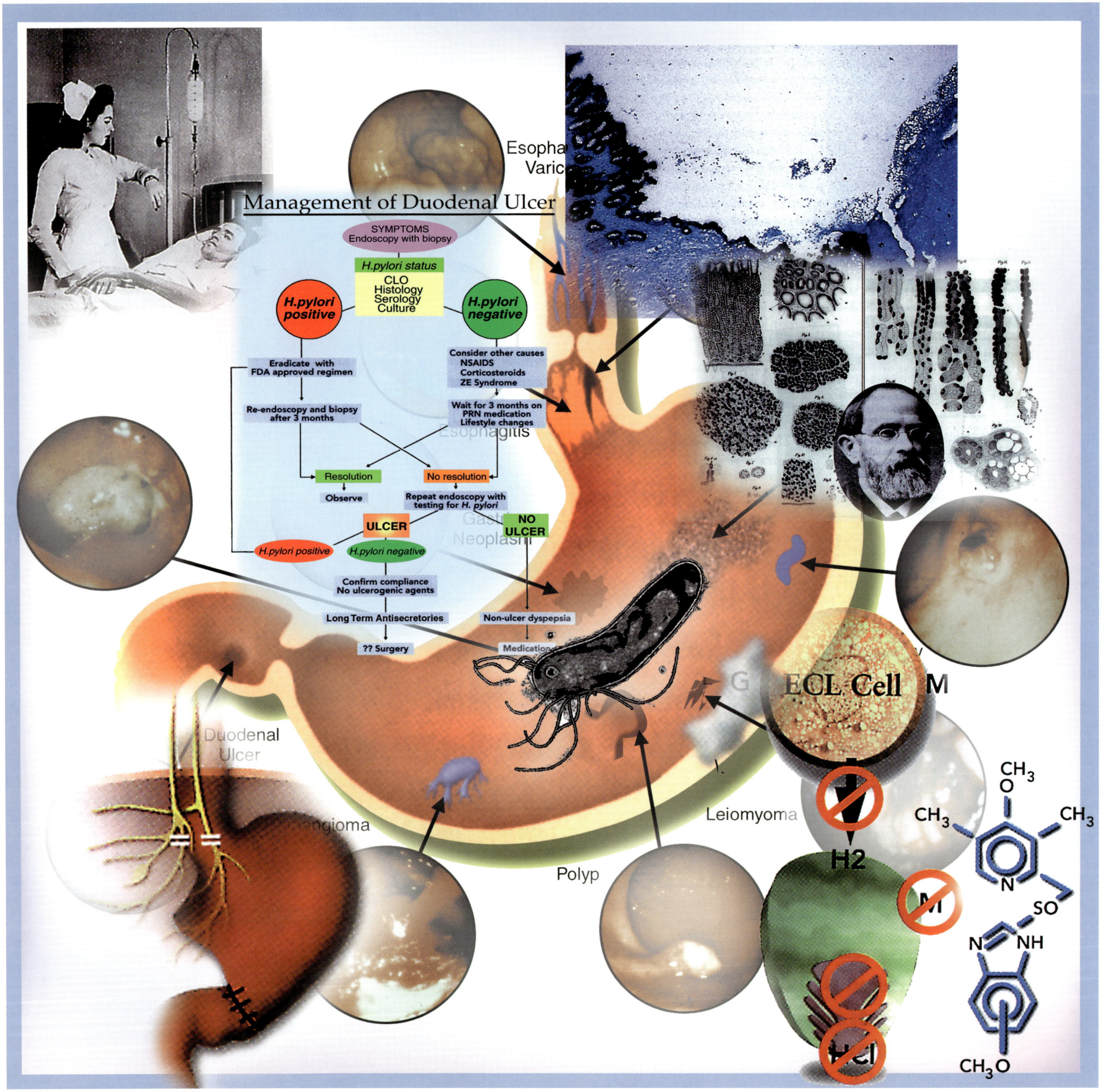
Management of Duodenal Ulcer
SYMPTOMS
Endoscopy with biopsy
H.pylori status
CLO
Histology
Serology
Culture
H.pylori positive
H.pylori negative
Eradicate with
FDA approved regimen
Consider other causes
NSAIDS
Corticosteroids
ZE Syndrome
Re-endoscopy and biopsy
after 3 months
Wait for 3 months on
PRN medication
Lifestyle changes
Resolution
No resolution
Observe
Repeat endoscopy with
testing for H. pylori
ULCER
NO ULCER
H.pylori positive
H.pylori negative
Confirm compliance
No ulcerogenic agents
Long Term Antisecretories
Non-ulcer dyspepsia
?? Surgery
Medication
Esophagitis
Duodenal
Ulcer
Leiomyoma
Polyp
ECL Cell
G
M
H2
HCl
CH3
O
CH3
CH3
N
SO
N
NH
CH3O

Chapter VII

Gastric Ulcer and Duodenal Ulcer Disease

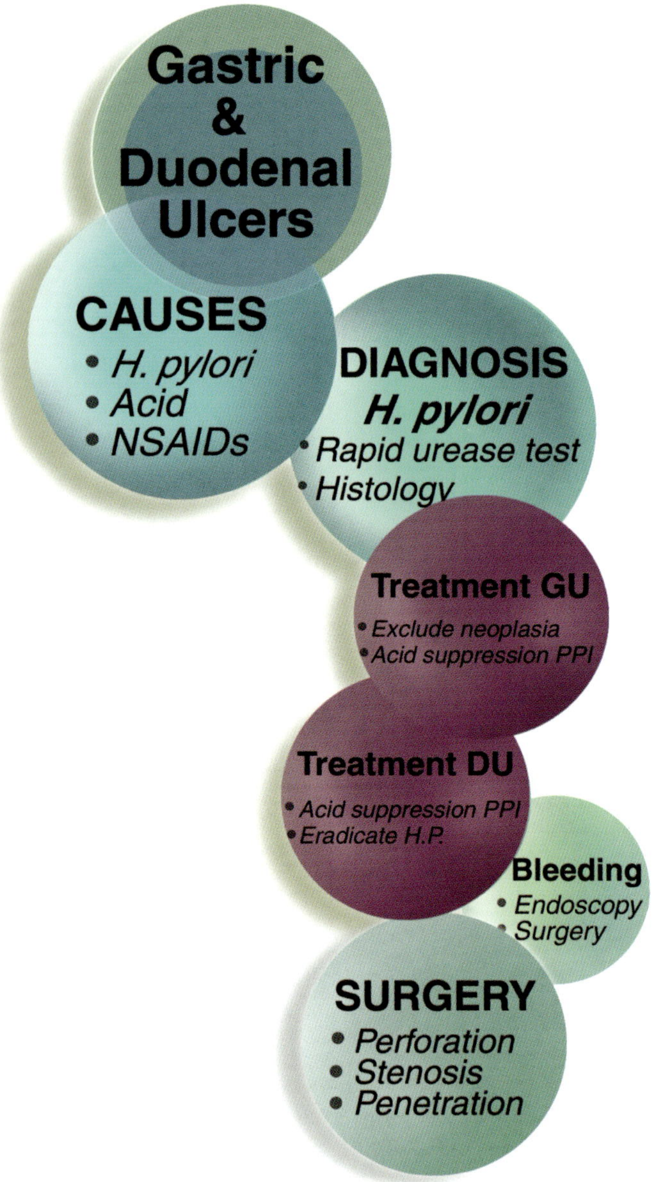
Gastric & Duodenal Ulcers
CAUSES
• H. pylori
• Acid
• NSAIDs
DIAGNOSIS
H. pylori
• Rapid urease test
• Histology
Treatment GU
• Exclude neoplasia
• Acid suppression PPI
Treatment DU
• Acid suppression PPI
• Eradicate H.P.
Bleeding
• Endoscopy
• Surgery
SURGERY
• Perforation
• Stenosis
• Penetration

Gastric Ulcer and Duodenal Ulcer Disease

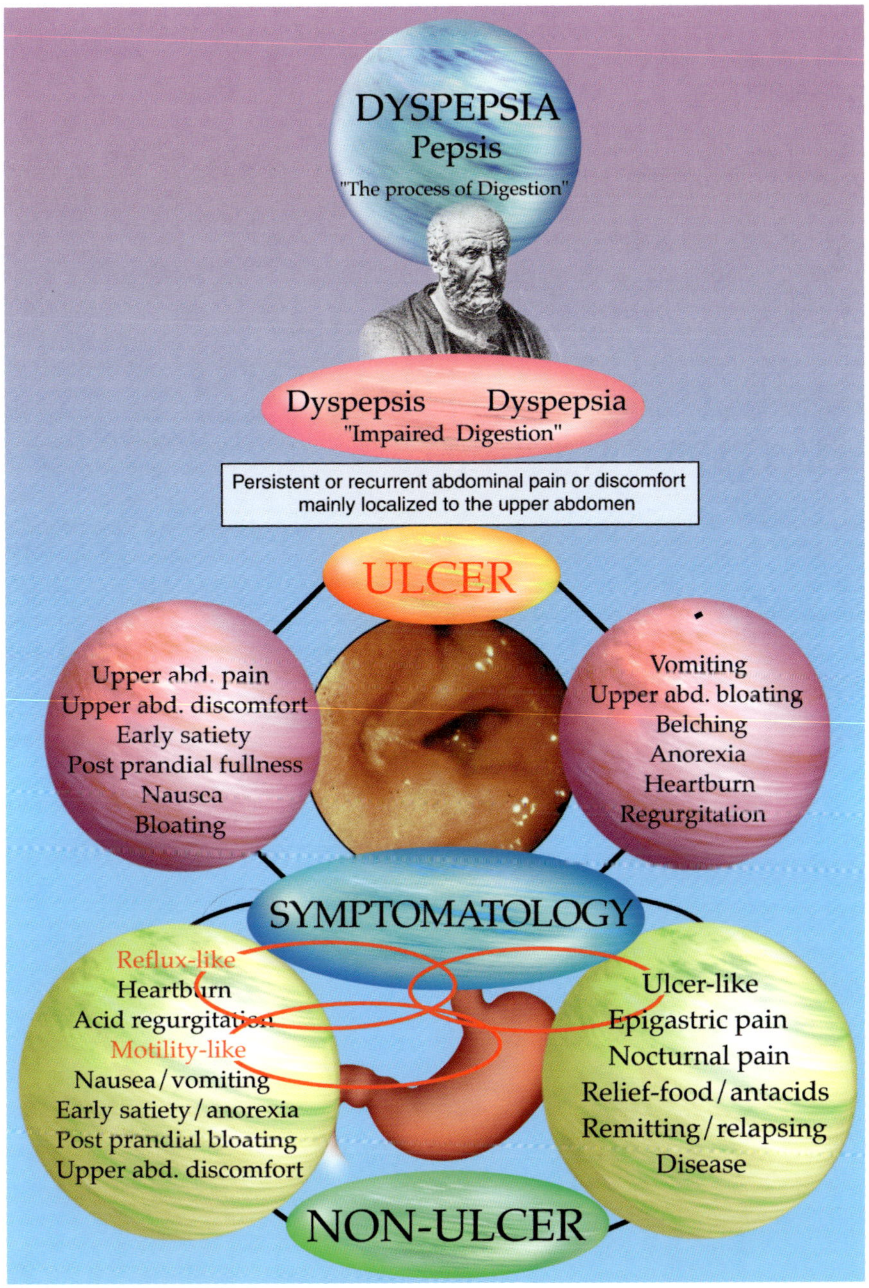

Figure 1. — *The archaic Hippocratic assessment of abdominal discomfort under the broad heading of dyspepsia has remained in common use for more than two millennia. However, the semiotics of symptomatology fail to adequately delineate the pathologic cause of the "disordered digestion"* (dys-pepsis). *Patients and physicians must regularly confront the difficulty of relating subjective evaluation of visceral affect to mucosal damage, particularly if it is not apparent through endoscopy.*

Introduction

Duodenal Ulcer

Although the incidence of duodenal ulcer disease has steadily declined in the United States since the turn of the century, approximately 500,000 new cases and 4 million recurrences annually are reported. Contrary to previous thought, duodenal ulcer disease does not "burn out," and without treatment, symptoms not only persist but exhibit a progressive increase in severity with time. As the duration of the untreated disease is often in excess of 30 to 40 years, the loss of health-related well being, costs to society, and the likelihood of complications are significant. The lifetime risk of duodenal ulcer in the developed world is about 10%, and the point prevalence is between 1% and 2%. Duodenal ulcer is the major lesion in Western populations, whereas gastric ulcers are more frequent in Asian countries, particularly Japan. Geographic incidences appear to a large part to inversely reflect the prevalence of *H. pylori*, which increase as the level of economic development decreases in a particular area or country. The prevalence of *H. pylori* in the United States has been as high as about 45% and higher in blacks than whites (70% versus 34%). In children in developed countries, the prevalence is low, with an acquisition rate of 0.3% to 1% per year that remains constant until about the fifth decade of life, whereafter a substantial increase occurs. This "cohort effect" in persons older than 45 years of age is believed to reflect the higher rate of acquisition among children born before 1950 and is regarded as reflective of improved social conditions.

It is now generally accepted that *H. pylori* is the major etiologic factor in duodenal ulcer disease, although the precise mechanism by which infection leads to ulceration is unclear and controversial. The significant reduction in the rate of duodenal ulcer recurrence following eradication of *H. pylori* further supports its role as a major etiologic factor, although recurrence of ulcer disease in the presence of eradication is still unexplained except in cases of covert use of nonsteroidal anti-inflammatory drugs (NSAIDs). The advent of H2-receptor antagonists in the treatment of duodenal ulcer disease resulted in a significant reduction in hospital admissions, but such issues as tolerance and the persistent high rate of relapse of GERD remained a difficulty.

The introduction of PPIs changed the approach to treatment of duodenal ulcer disease. Furthermore, the combination of a PPI with antibiotics to eradicate *H. pylori* has resulted in a dramatic decrease of the rates of recurrence and relapse of duodenal ulcer with the odds of developing a recurrent ulcer being approximately five times greater if *H. pylori* is not eradicated.

Meta-analysis for predicting the degree of acid inhibition necessary to provide an optimal healing for duodenal ulcer showed this to be a mean intragastric pH of 3.0 for 18 hours per day, indicating that the duodenum was able to handle a significant pH load because of its ability to secrete HCO_3^-. This fact, as well as the presence of mural-related acid in the gastric wall itself and the common site of the ulcer at the unstable junctional zone of the antrofundic mucosa, have rendered gastric ulcer a more difficult treatment problem.

Gastric Ulcer

Although less prevalent (0.1% of the population in developed countries) than duodenal ulcer, gastric ulcer is associated with a higher mortality and a greater morbidity (hemorrhage, perforation, and obstruction). The relationship between gastric ulcer and *H. pylori* is less clear than for duodenal ulcer, with positivity apparent in 58% to 94% of patients. A large amount of the variability in the association reflects the use of NSAIDs, as exclusion of this variable results in prevalence rates closely comparable to those for duodenal ulcer. It seems unlikely that NSAIDs and *H. pylori* are related in the genesis of gastric ulcer, as the histology of the two lesions is different, and there is no evidence that NSAIDs increase susceptibility to *H. pylori* infection.

Frequent recurrence is common with gastric ulcer following therapy; ulcers recur in 35% to 80% of the patients within 6 to 12 months of healing. If recurrence of gastric ulceration occurs, rigorous endoscopic reassessment by biopsy for the presence of neoplasia should be undertaken. In those patients who experience complications, such as hemorrhage, perforation, or obstruction, appropriate surgical intervention is necessary. Although bleeding gastric ulcers may be endoscopically managed, a rebleed may warrant surgical intervention. Simple suture may suffice, but more often than not they are better managed by appropriately tailored surgical resection. In some circumstances, anatomic considerations may mandate resection, particularly in ulcers close to the gastroesophageal junction on the lesser curve. Chronic gastric obstruction usually in the juxtapyloric region usually mandates gastric resection with establishment of a Billroth II anastomosis. Overall, however, the picture of gastric ulcer disease as a difficult problem with a high level of complications, often necessitating surgical intervention, has declined significantly and has begun to resemble duodenal ulcer as a pathologic process amenable to conservative medical therapy except in complicated circumstances. Results of meta-analyses to predict healing of gastric ulcers as a function of pH have not been published. Still, current PPI therapy may require longer administration for healing of gastric compared with duodenal ulcers, presumably because there is still acidity within the gastric wall itself, impeding healing.

Relationship of Gastroduodenal Disease to H. pylori

The introduction of PPI therapy and the advent of *H. pylori* eradication have, in recent times, considerably improved therapeutic outcome for patients with duodenal ulcer. The failure of a gastric ulcer to heal in the face of compliance with a curative regimen (PPI therapy and/or withdrawal of NSAIDs) should be regarded as an alarm symptom or sign suggestive of gastric neoplasia. There are, however, data to suggest that recurrence of duodenal ulcer in patients who do not use NSAIDs and who are *H. pylori* negative, may be greater than previously estimated.

A number of epidemiologic studies have concluded that *H. pylori* infection is a major cause of gastric cancer worldwide. The matched odds ratio for this association ranges from 2.2 (95% confidence interval [CI] 1.0–8.0) to 6.0 (95% CI 2.1–17.3). The infection increases the risk of gastric adenocarcinoma by three to six times, possibly by promoting the development of chronic atrophic gastritis. In addition, *H. pylori* increases the likelihood of the development of the primary non-Hodgkin's MALT lymphoma by approximately sixfold.

Figure 2. — *Although the organism* H. pylori *accounts for the vast majority (85% to 95%) of duodenal ulcers, the precise mechanism by which it engenders mucosal ulceration has yet to be defined. Mastocytosis and gastrinoma are neoplastic diseases that cause ulceration by provoking excessive acid secretion by production of histamine and gastrin, respectively. Hypercalcemia, as a consequence of hyperparathyroidism, also increases acid secretion through a number of different mechanisms including increased release of gastrin. The mechanisms of burn and acute stress-related ulceration are controversial and may include microcirculatory disturbances, mucosal hypoxia, and centrally mediated neural events. Crohn's ulceration reflects a local manifestation of the ill-understood inflammatory disorder that may be of polyvalent pathogenesis. Posterior fossa lesions are associated with centrally mediated medullary alterations in acid secretion as well as dysregulation of local mucosal microcirculatory homeostasis. NSAID-related ulceration represents locally induced mucosal damage, resulting from at least drug-related alterations in prostaglandin biosynthesis.*

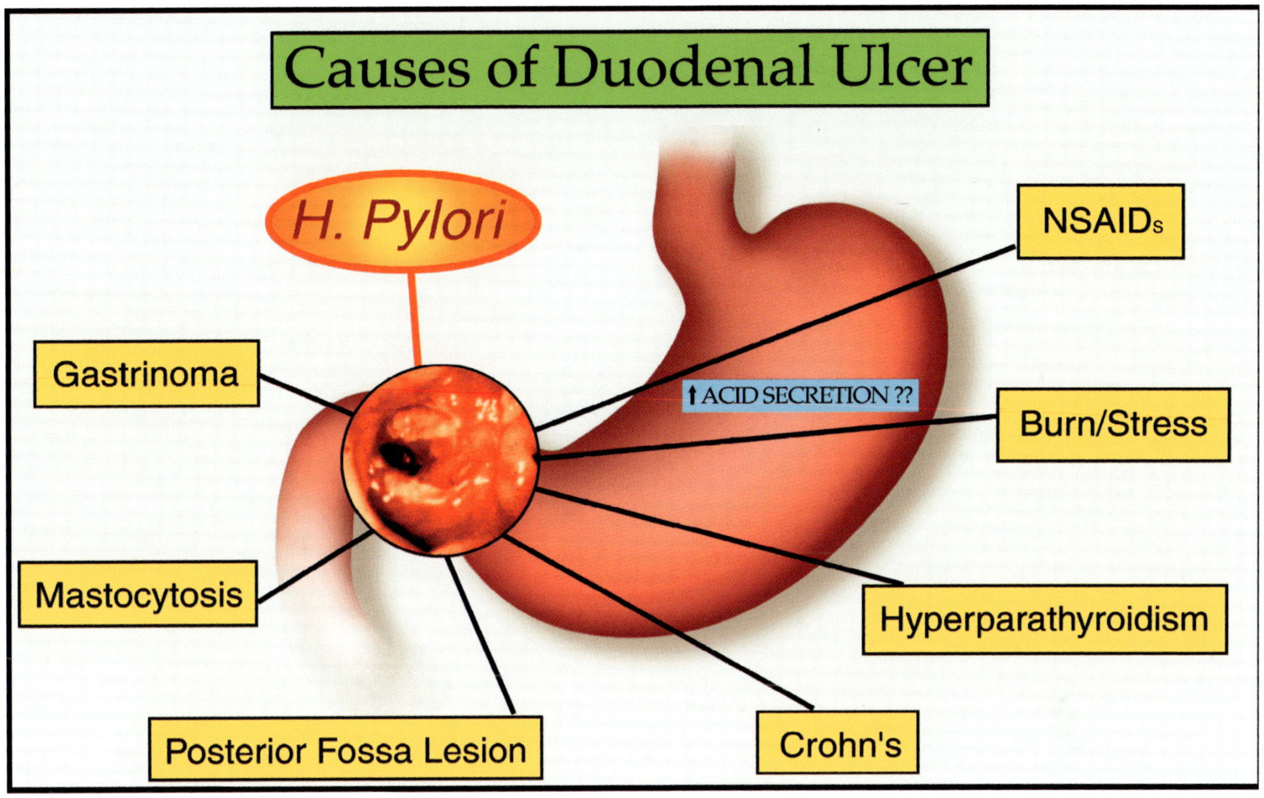

Impact on Health-Related Resource Allocation

The cost of peptic ulcer disease to society reflects both indirect expenses related to decrease in health-related well being and loss of productivity as well as expenditure associated with management of the disease itself. In 1990, it was estimated that the annual direct costs related to diagnosis and treatment of peptic ulcer disease in the United States was between $3 and $4 billion compared with the $2.5 million estimated in 1975. Data from 1997 indicate that the total direct and indirect costs had risen to $5.65 billion and that peptic ulcer disease accounted for about 37% of direct medical expenditures for acid-related disorders. Patients with ulcers were calculated to generate excess yearly costs of $1183 per person compared with matched controls.

Pathogenesis

The pathogenesis of duodenal ulcer may best be viewed as representing a complex scenario involving an imbalance between defensive and aggressive factors of which the most notable now appears to be *H. pylori*. Ulceration has been broadly conceived of as a process by which the mucosa is unable to sustain itself against extrinsic aggressive factors. Previously, considerable attention had been directed to the role of acid and bile in the generation of mucosal damage. The entropic term cytoprotection was proposed as a generic entity, embracing the concept of gastric mucosal defensive mechanisms. In broad terms, these were regarded as preepithelial, epithelial, and subepithelial. Healing represents mucosal restitution and the reestablishment of epithelial cell continuity independent of cell proliferation and is linked to the expression of growth factors and the maintenance of mucosal integrity.

NSAIDs compromise these mucosal defenses through both direct local toxic effects and systemic effects: specifically, the inhibition of cyclooxygenase type 1 and type 2 (COX1 and COX2, respectively), the enzymes responsible for the biosynthesis of prostaglandins. The subsequent depletion of endogenous prostaglandins results in a decreased production of mucus and bicarbonate by the epithelium and a reduction in gastric mucosal blood flow. The disruption of prostaglandin-mediated defenses contributes to a breakdown of the mucosal barrier, leading to the formation of ulcers in the gastric or duodenal wall. Researchers also suggest that an inhibition of prostaglandin synthesis may

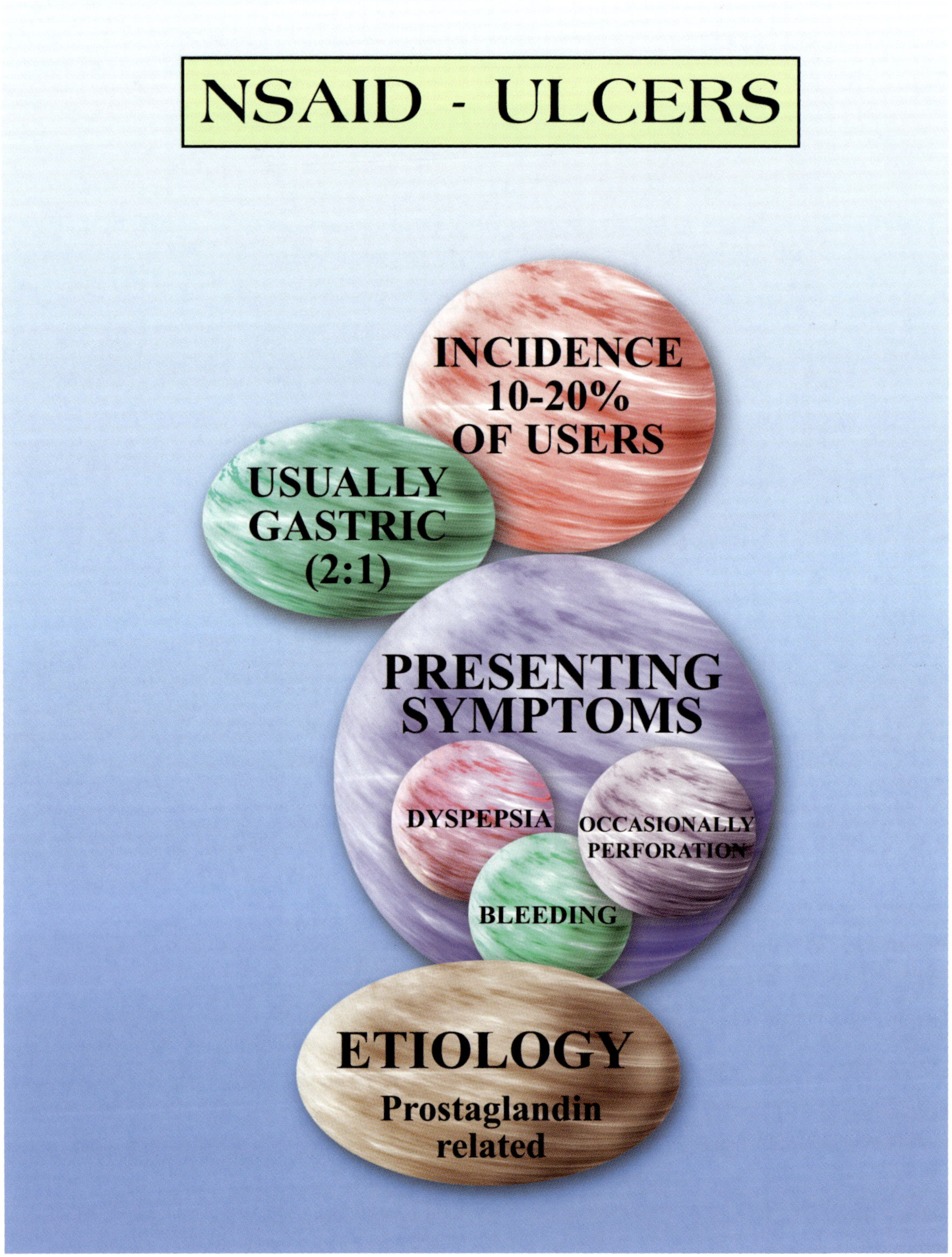

Figure 3. — *The widespread use of NSAIDs for a variety of different ailments has resulted in their significant contribution to the disease spectrum associated with gastroduodenal ulceration. The clinical impact is particularly evident in the elderly population group that commonly uses such medications for the amelioration of osteoarthritic or rheumatoid-type diseases.*

cause a diversion of arachidonic acid through the lipoxygenase pathway, thereby increasing leukotriene synthesis. As leukotrienes are inflammatory mediators, this mechanism may also play a role in NSAID-induced gastrointestinal injury.

The "mucosal barrier" was conceived and variously considered to embrace the mucous bicarbonate barrier, specialized apical ion transport systems, and tight junctions that provided an anatomic barrier for diffusion of acid and pepsin. Innumerable studies have correlated levels of secretion of acid with ulceration, and although pepsin is well accepted as a cofactor in ulceration, its precise role in the pathogenesis has been ignored in favor of a preoccupation with neutralizing or inhibiting acid secretion. Confounding variables such as cigarette smoking, alcohol ingestion, "stress," and spicy foods have been identified, but their precise involvement in the genesis of mucosal damage is ill defined.

The subject of *H. pylori* was dealt with separately but is worthy of brief comment in the context of noxious agents affecting the gastric mucosa. There is a critical association between gastric metaplasia in the duodenal cap and *H. pylori*, which appears to confer a predisposition to duodenal ulcer disease. Similarly, there is an association between the eradication of *H. pylori* infection and reduction of the risk of recurrence of duodenal ulcer. The identification of *H. pylori* in 90% to 95% of patients with duodenal ulcer and 60% to 80% of patients with gastric ulcer, compared with 25% to 30% incidences in symptomatic control subjects, confirms its relevance in the genesis of mucosal ulceration of the duodenum in particular. Although the prevalence of infection increases with age and is more common in those with deprived socioeconomic circumstances, it is apparent that, in some countries, infection is not always involved with peptic ulceration. Such observations have raised the issue as to whether all types of *H. pylori* are of equal pathogenicity. Nevertheless, given that lifetime prevalence for duodenal ulcer is approximately 10% for men and 5% for women, the importance of *H. pylori* as a component of the disease process is substantial.

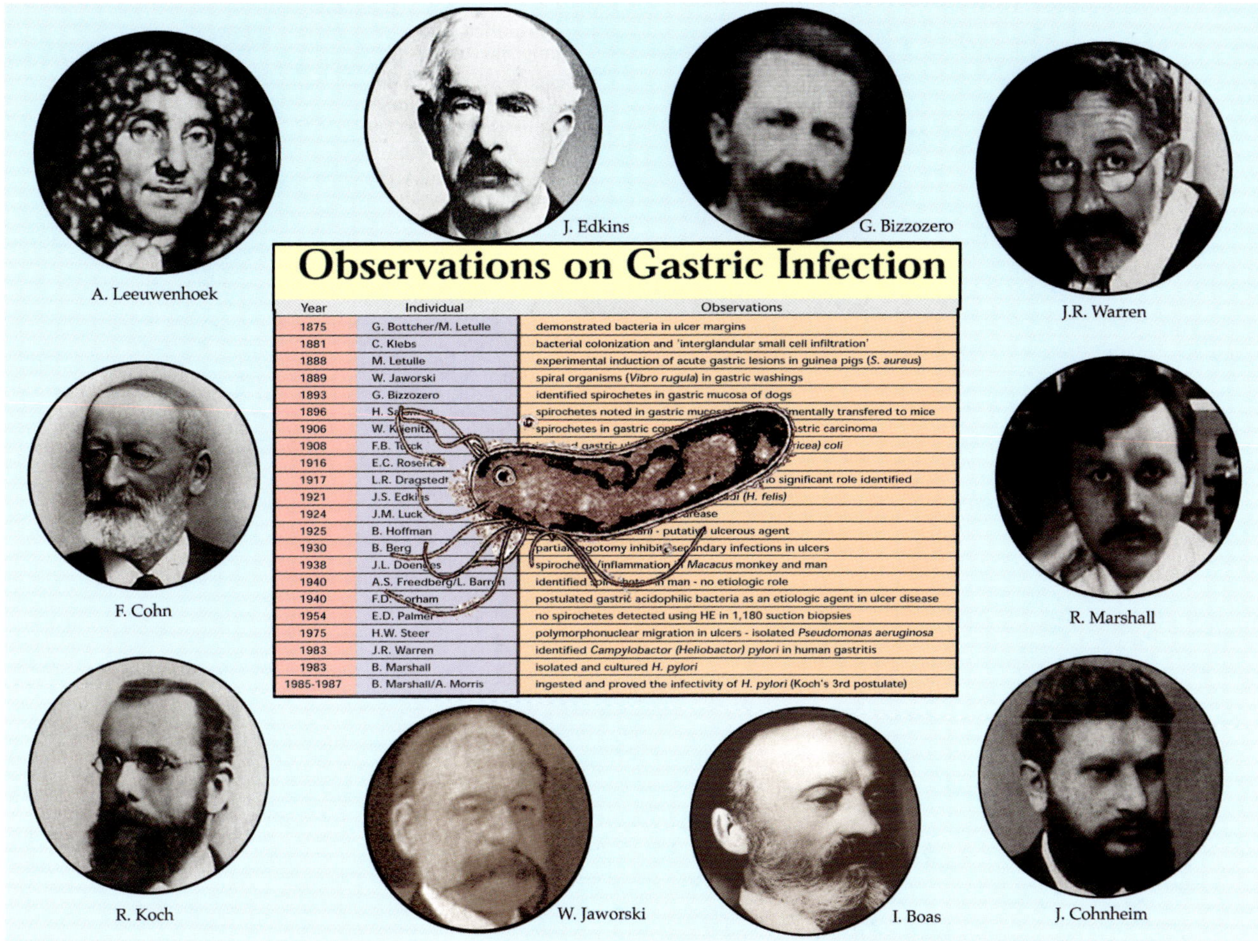

Figure 4. — *The presence of bacteria in the stomach has been noted for more than a century. Leeuwenhoek (1632–1723) was the first to identify organisms in the mouth and colon but did little more than note their presence. Cohn (1828–1898) provided a morphologic classification, and his protégé Koch (1843–1910) thereafter developed the concept of species-specific infectious diseases. Bizzozero, in 1883, noted the presence of spiral organisms in the gastric mucosa but did not pursue this observation in deference to his discovery of blood platelets. In 1889, Jaworski proposed that a gastric spiral organism* (Vibrio rugula) *was pathogenic, but Boas, who regarded the work as a technical artifact, disputed this observation. Boas believed the Oppler-Boas bacterium to be the entity responsible for gastric cancer and refuted Jaworski's results as the chemical effect of hydrochloric acid on mucus. In 1921, Edkins described* Spirella regaudi *in the gastric juice of cats and investigated whether its presence interfered with digestive function. Other notable proponents of the pathogenicity of gastric organisms included Salomon (1896) and Cohnheim (1839–1884). Almost a century would elapse before the conundrum of peptic ulceration and infection was resolved. In 1983, Warren and Marshall defined the role of* H. pylori *as a gastric pathogen and implicated it in the genesis of mucosal ulceration of the stomach and duodenum.*

Diagnosis

The recognition of symptomatology involving epigastric discomfort related to the ingestion of food is broadly grouped under the nomenclature of dyspepsia. The establishment of dyspepsia as a cardinal presenting symptom rapidly leads to upper gastrointestinal endoscopy. The confirmation of the diagnosis of ulcer disease requires not only the identification of the site of the lesion but also the determination of the presence of *H. pylori*. This can be undertaken by histologic staining or identification of urease in the biopsy material, but serology and breath testing are other possibilities. The sensitivity and specificity of such tests are important criteria, although costs will probably become the ultimate determinant in the decision. Of particular relevance in the history should be the determination of alarm symptoms or signs such as weight loss, vomiting, the development of back pain, or failure to relieve symptomatology with antacids. In general, such features suggest the development of either a complication (bleeding, penetration, perforation, stenosis) or that the ulcer may be neoplastic or due to other causes. Apart from noncompliance with therapy, ulcers recalcitrant to treatment or those that recur are usually due to aspirin, intake of NSAIDs, or, rarely, a gastrinoma.

Detection of H. pylori

The diagnosis of *H. pylori* can be undertaken by the use of noninvasive or invasive tests. Invasive methodology involves endoscopy with gastric mucosal biopsy and either histology, culture, or rapid urease testing. The rapid urease test is probably the most useful in routine practice, as, in addition to being highly sensitive (85% to 95%) and specific (98%), it is easy to perform, relatively inexpensive, and provides a rapid result. Although the histologic demonstration of the organism has a high sensitivity (85% to 90%) and specificity (93% to 100%), its routine use is limited by its high cost. Culture of the organism is probably the ideal diagnostic technique but is difficult and has a high rate of failure compared with other diagnostic strategies. Culture may be of use in checking bacterial sensitivity, particularly with patients for whom eradication has failed or macrolide antibiotics or nitro-imidazoles are under consideration as future therapy.

The noninvasive methodologies available for the diagnosis of *H. pylori* include radiolabeled urea breath tests and enzyme-linked immunosorbent serologic assays (ELISAs). The drawbacks of the serologic studies are related to the relative lack of sensitivity, although they are easy to perform and relatively inexpensive. Serologic tests are not useful in monitoring the success of eradication therapy, as immunoglobulin G (IgG) and immunoglobulin A (IgA) titers may only drop by 20% to 50% within the month of the cessation of therapy. The currently available labeled urea breath tests are the nonradioactive ^{13}C test and the radioactive 14C test. Current studies suggest that both are equally specific (99%) and sensitive (90% to 98%). The 14C test is less costly and has recently met with approval of the Food and Drug Administration (FDA). The ^{13}C test is expensive, and the equipment is expensive and not widely available.

In duodenal ulcer disease it is important to identify the presence of *H. pylori* before the institution of therapy. If upper endoscopy detects duodenal ulcer disease, a gastric biopsy should be used to test for *H. pylori*, preferably by means of the rapid urease test. It is important that at least two biopsy samples be evaluated (fundic and antral) because if antisecretory therapy has been initiated, the organism may be present only in small numbers and may have migrated (a consequence of acid-suppressive therapy and the alteration of its ideal pH milieu) from its original site. Eradication of the organism can be confirmed after 4 to 6 weeks after the end of treatment of duodenal ulcer disease by use of the noninvasive urea breath test. In those patients who exhibit relapse or recurrence of symptomatology, the presence of *H. pylori* should be meticulously assessed.

Medical Management

Ulcer Healing and Acid Suppression

There is a direct correlation between the healing rate of duodenal ulcers and the degree of suppression of 24-hour intragastric acidity associated with the use of antisecretory agents. PPIs produce healing in a greater proportion of duodenal ulcers than the H2-receptor antagonist ranitidine. As the primary determinant of

Figure 5. — *The majority of duodenal ulcer disease is related to the association of* H. pylori *infection and synchronous acid-induced damage. The failure of ulcer healing despite compliance with an appropriate regimen of acid suppression and* H. pylori *eradication should initiate consideration of either covert or less common causes of mucosal ulceration.*

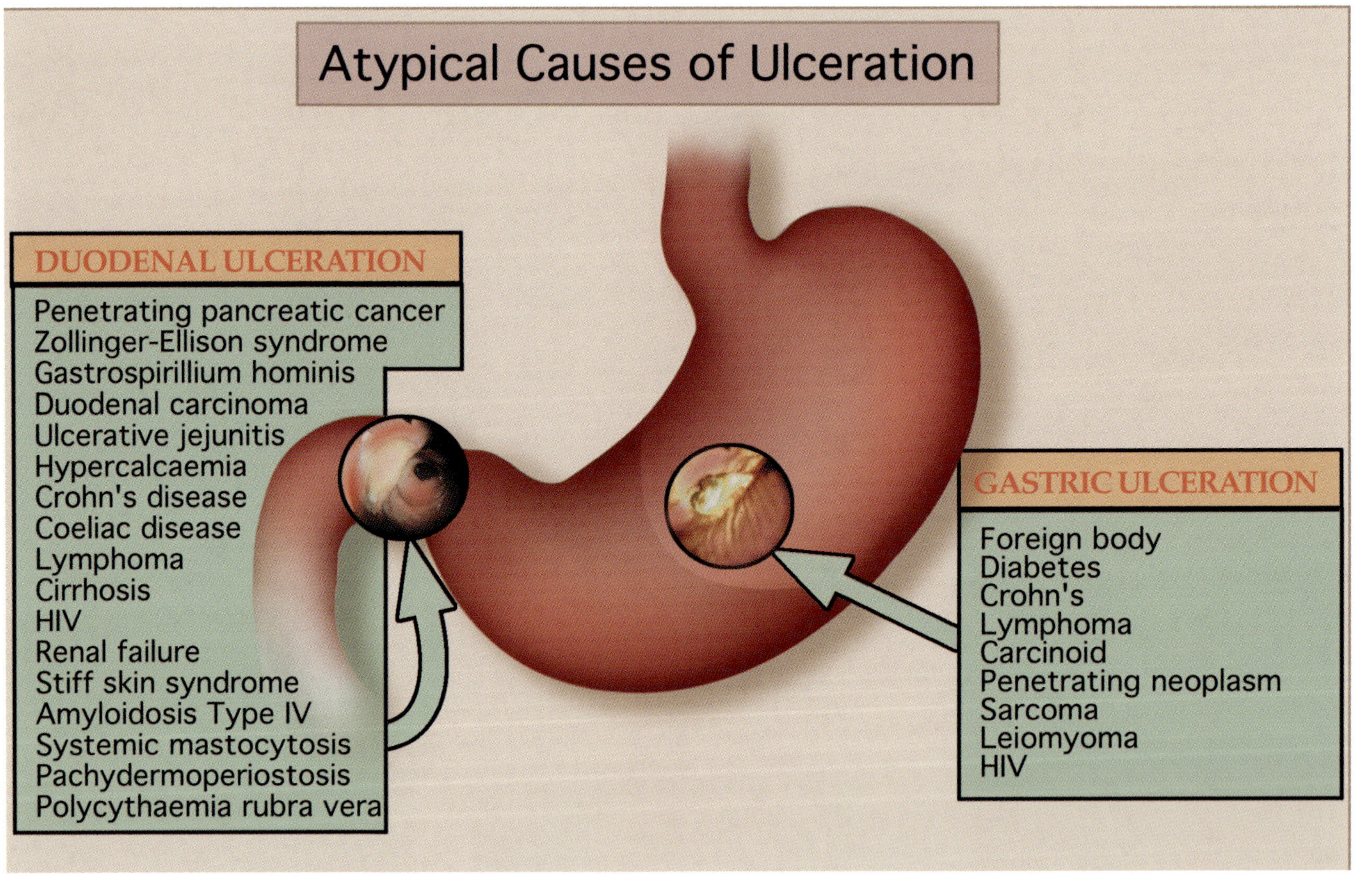

duodenal ulcer, healing is represented by the fraction of the day for which intragastric pH is maintained above 3.0 as well as the duration of treatment itself. Thus, duodenal ulcers can be healed within 4 weeks if intragastric pH is maintained above 3.0 for between 18 to 20 hours per day. In this respect, the PPI class of drugs are more effective, as they inactivate the H^+,K^+ ATPase enzyme and produce inhibition of both peripherally and centrally mediated gastric acid secretion. The H2-receptor antagonists act by competitive antagonism at the H2-receptor of the parietal cell to inhibit histamine-mediated acid secretion. Such agents are therefore somewhat less effective in controlling food-stimulated gastric acid secretion, as cholinergic mediated stimulation is not inhibited. Comparable observations are available demonstrating the utility of acid suppression in patients with gastric ulcers. Omeprazole (40 mg daily) produces consistently higher rates of healing than H2-receptor antagonists.

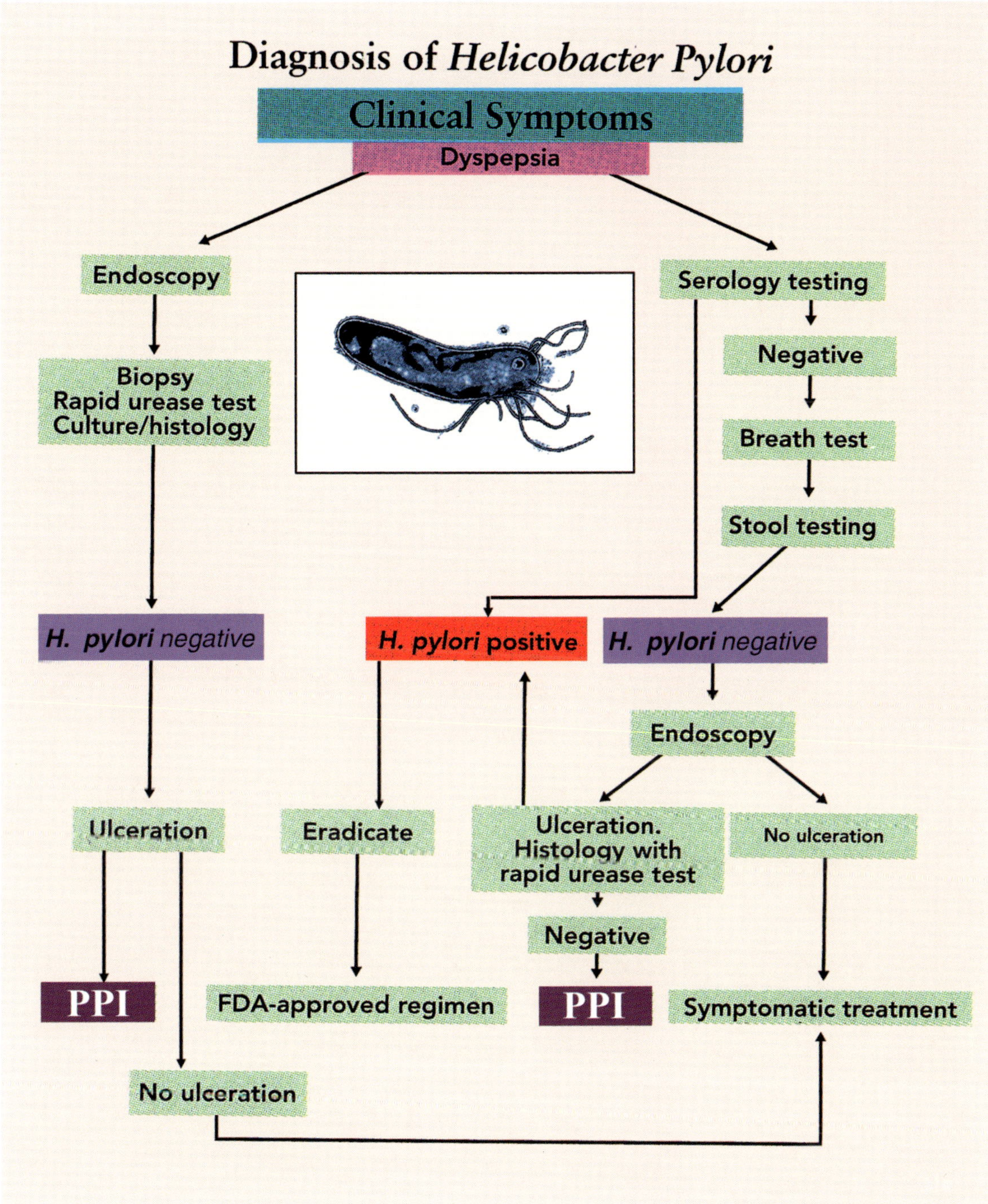

Figure 6. — *An outline of the general strategies available for the diagnosis and management of dyspepsia considered to be due to* H. pylori-*related mucosal disease.*

Duodenal Ulcer

There is considerable overlap between 24-hour intragastric pH measurements in normal persons and in patients with duodenal ulcer. Nevertheless, there appears to be greater gastric acid secretion in patients with duodenal ulcer than in normal subjects, particularly at night. Overall, however, the 24-hour pH profile is not predictive of the duodenal ulcer in an individual patient, and other factors, particularly duodenal bicarbonate secretion, have been proposed to be implicated in the genesis of duodenal ulceration. Pharmacodynamic studies of the acid-suppressive effects of antisecretory drugs and meta-analytic studies that evaluated duodenal ulcer healing indicate that healing rates for duodenal ulcer correlate with the suppression of gastric secretion. There are three critical determinants predictive of duodenal ulcer healing: the degree of acid suppression, the duration of acid suppression within a 24-hour period, and the length of treatment. The healing rates for duodenal ulcer correlate with the degree of acid suppression, and a daily intragastric pH of 3.0 for more than 18 to 20 hours achieves maximal healing rates for duodenal ulcers at 4 weeks. Although increasing acid suppression to an intragastric pH greater than 3.0 did not significantly improve healing, increasing the total duration of suppression of acid, by either lengthening treatment or during the individual 24-hour period itself, resulted in higher rates of healing. It was also evident that the therapeutic effect of H2-receptor antagonists reflected their ability to suppress nocturnal acidity better than daytime acidity.

Figure 7. — *This illustration shows a general outline of the diagnosis and management strategies available for duodenal ulcer disease.*

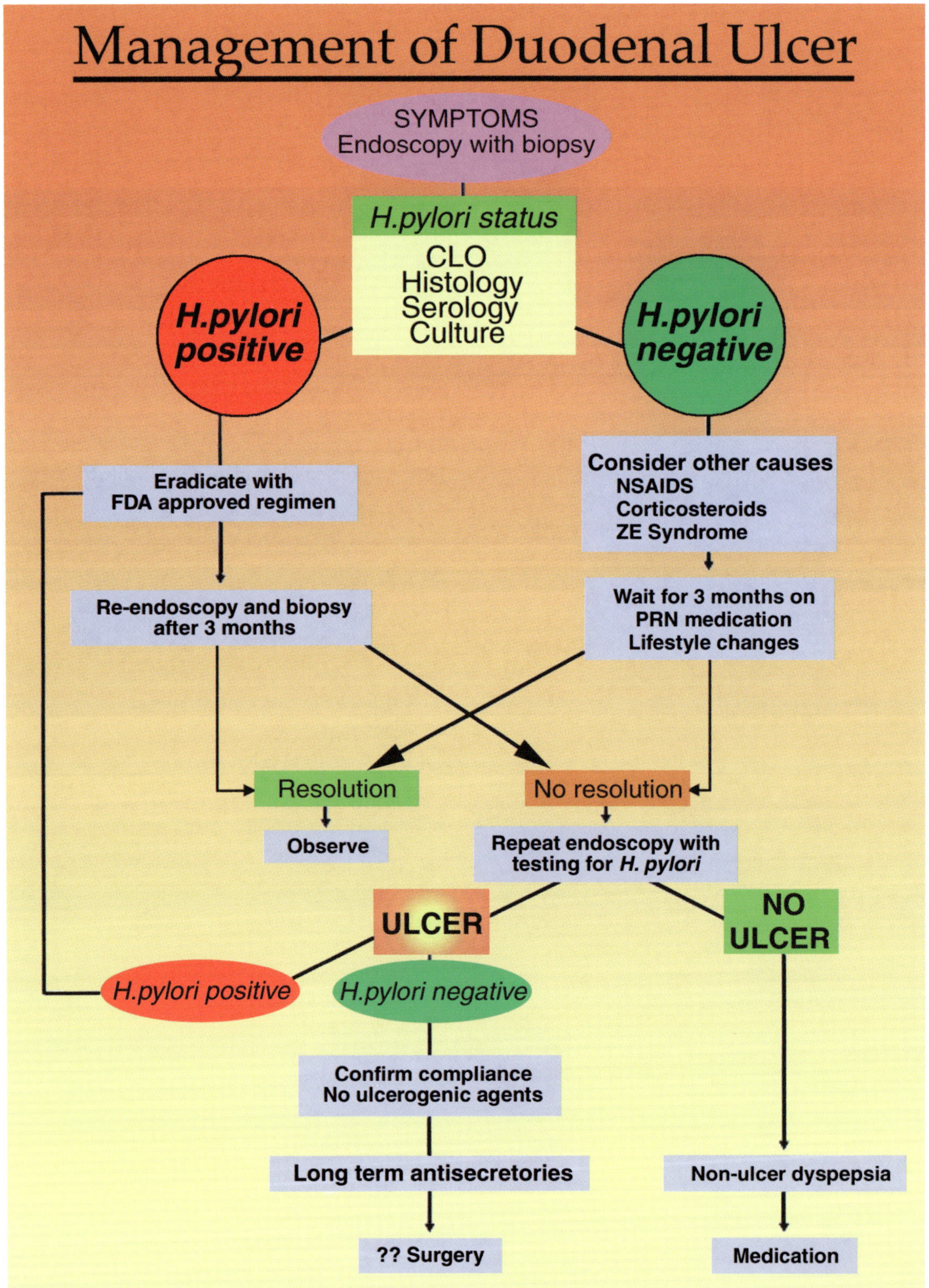

Synchronous eradication of *H. pylori*, if present, is mandatory to ensure successful treatment of duodenal ulceration. Acid-suppression therapy alone is associated with relatively high levels of recurrence. To ensure cure of ulcer and abrogate the likelihood of the development of complications, optimal treatment requires the combination of eradication of bacteria and the elevation of pH. The therapeutic regimens available for management of uncomplicated duodenal ulceration can be evaluated under the headings of acid-suppressive therapy and antimicrobial therapy and a combination of both entities. Surgery of uncomplicated duodenal and gastric ulceration may be regarded as unwarranted except in instances of perforation, failed conservative management of bleeding, gastric outlet obstruction, and the development of neoplasia. In the past, patients with gastrinoma usually required total gastrectomy, but PPI therapy has greatly reduced the need for acid-reduction surgery. Surgical intervention should be confined to a consideration of the removal of the neoplasm and/or its metastases, although this is rarely feasible.

Gastric Ulcer

The management of gastric ulcer has always been more difficult than duodenal ulcer. Patients with gastric ulcer are usually older, have defects in mucosal defense factor function, and may have other factors contributing to ulceration. Also, the intramural presence of acid and pepsin in higher quantities than in the duodenum may play a role. Although patients with gastric ulcer exhibit lower levels of gastric acid secretion than healthy controls, healing is reflective of similar critical determinants as identified in patients with duodenal ulcer. In gastric ulcer healing, however, the duration of treatment appeared to be the most important single determinant in predicting healing; all treatment modalities indicate an increase in healing rates from 4 to 8 weeks of treatment. Despite such observations, the degree of acid suppression is significant, as greater suppression of 24-hour intragastric acidity produces the highest healing rates. The suppression of 24-hour acidity appears to be more important than suppression of either night time or daytime acidity, and maintenance of gastric pH greater than 3.0 for 18 hours daily predicts healing in most gastric ulcers by 8 weeks.

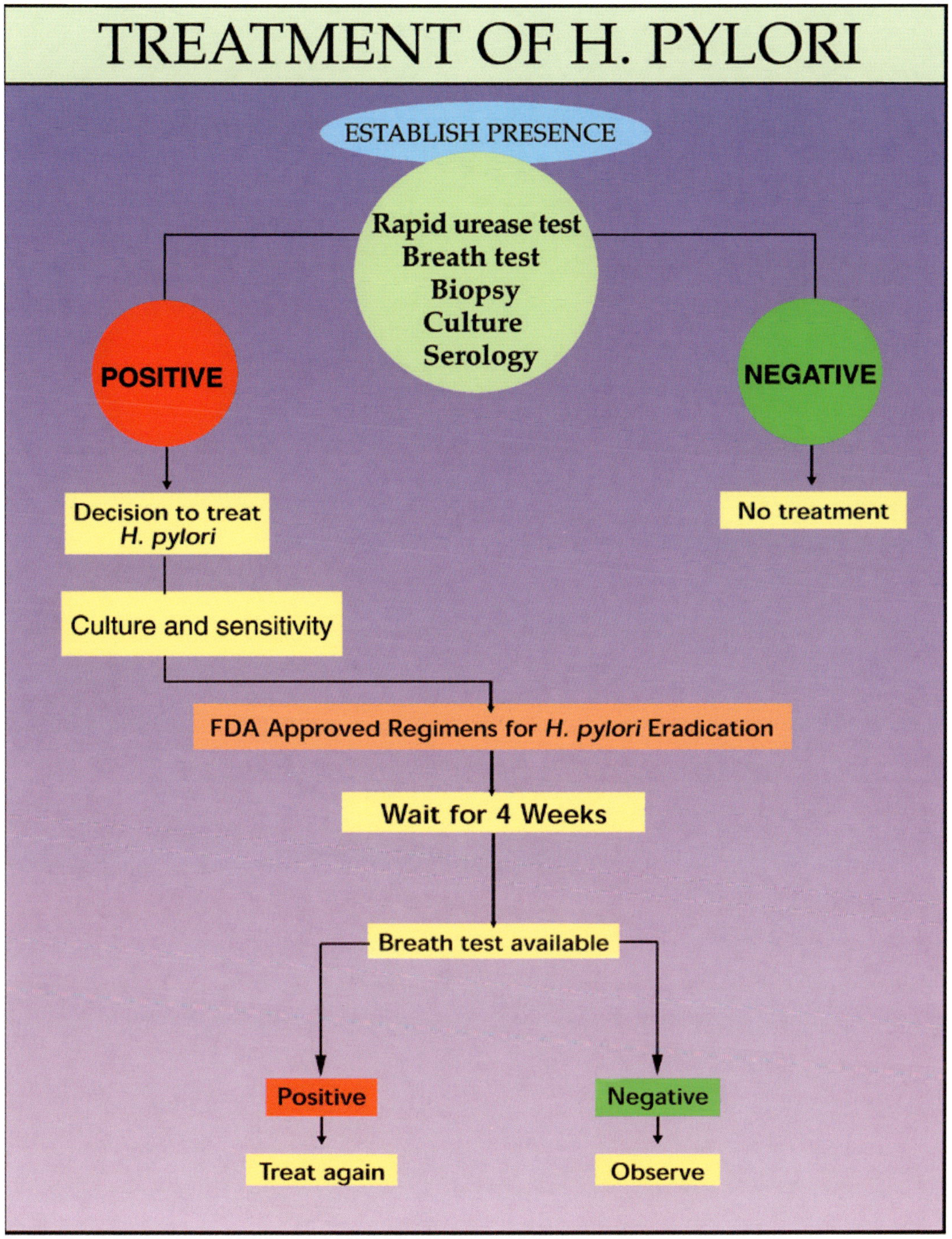

Figure 8. - *This figure shows a management strategy for* H. pylori *related duodenal ulcer disease.*

Eradication of *H. pylori*

Bismuth-Based Antimicrobial Therapy

H. pylori has been demonstrated to be sensitive in *in vitro* assays to a wide variety of antimicrobial agents including macrolides, beta-lactams, ketoconazoles, tetracyclines, gentamycin, rifampicin, nitrofuran, and some quinolones. Nevertheless, the use of any of these agents alone (monotherapy) has generally proved to render suboptimal results, with eradication rates of approximately 20%. Clarithromycin, a macrolide antibiotic, is more acid stable than its counterpart, erythromycin, and is well tolerated, more effective, and has an eradication rate alone of about 30%. It is however apparent that the use of more than one antibiotic has resulted in improved rates of cure. The most commonly administered combination is quadruple therapy, which includes the classic bismuth triple therapy of bismuth subsalicylate metronidazole and tetracycline in combination with a H2-receptor antagonist. A newer combination of ranitidine bismuth citrate with clarithromycin has been approved for eradication. It is claimed that this form of bismuth is more soluble and more available for bactericidal action.

Eradication and Acid-Suppressive Combination Therapy

Summated information indicates that an optimal management strategy for duodenal ulceration is the use of a PPI and two antibacterial agents. The treatment paradigm that is most frequently used is triple therapy with PPIs in combination with amoxicillin and clarithromycin. This is twice-daily treatment with omeprazole 20 mg with 1 g amoxicillin and 500 mg clarithromycin taken simultaneously (OAC), which, in trials, have given 69% to 90% eradication. With patients in whom previous eradication therapy has been unsuccessful or in patients who exhibit antimicrobial resistance to clarithromycin, alternative antimicrobial therapy should be instituted (See attached prescribing information and the Note to Prescriber in the back of the book for additional prescribing considerations for clarithromycin and amoxicillin).

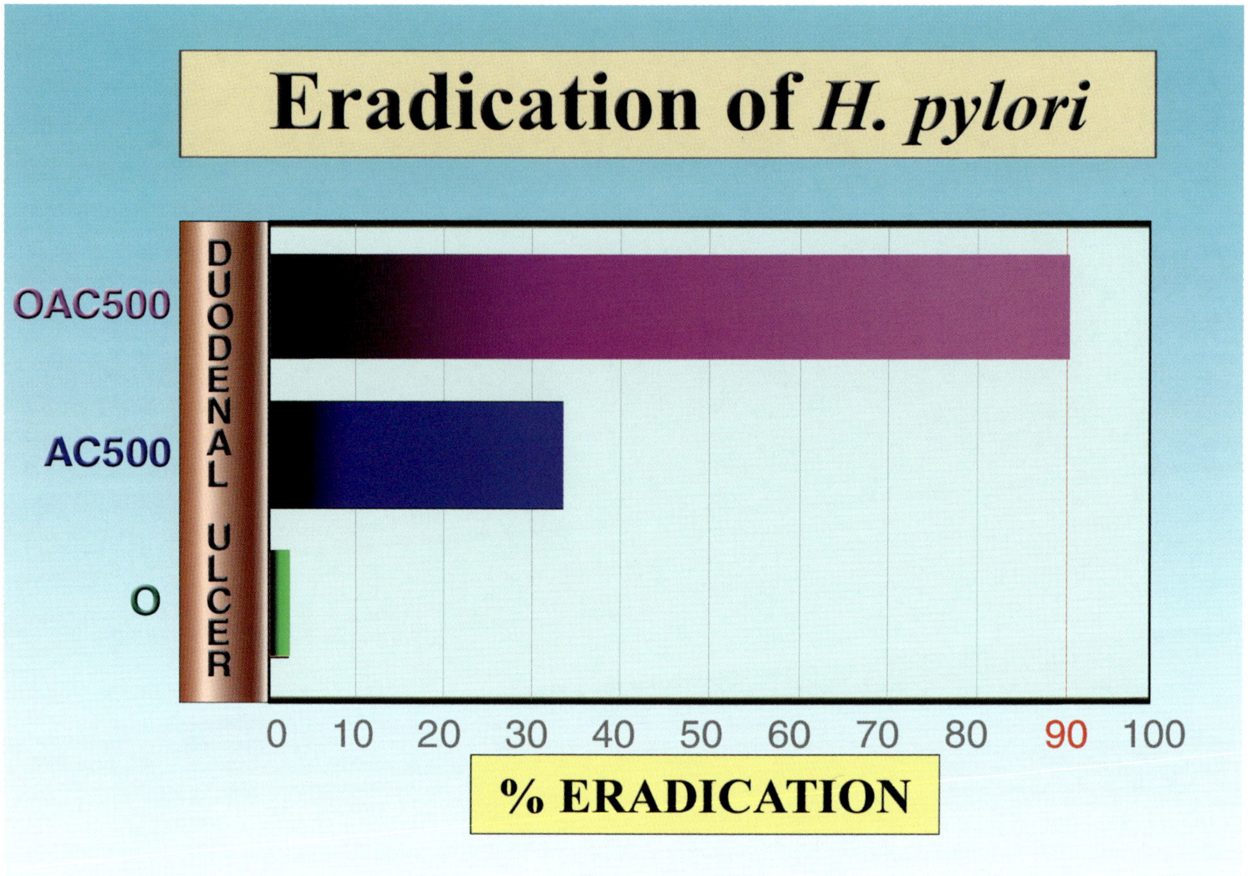

Figure 9. — *A table that summarizes the per protocol results of a study comparing twice-daily regimens; it is apparent that triple therapy is optimal to ensure good rates of eradication*

Treatment Failure of Duodenal Ulcer Disease

Although there are a number of reasons for a duodenal ulcer to recur, including NSAID use, failure of compliance, inadequate acid suppression, and gastrinoma, by far the most common is the failure to eradicate *H. pylori*. Thus, 68% of patients who remain *H. pylori* positive after eradication therapy develop recurrence of ulcer within 1 year compared with only 5% for those in whom the organism is eradicated. Use of a PPI with antibiotic regimens such as OAC produces *H. pylori* eradication rates of 69% to 90%, whereas monotherapy with a PPI fails to eradicate *H. pylori*. Although the failure to eradicate may actually represent reinfection, the true rate of reinfection in developed countries is probably less than 1% to 2% but may be higher in developing countries. Recurrence of *H. pylori* infection within 1 year probably represents recrudescence of an original infection that was suppressed rather than eradicated.

There is a group of patients in whom ulcers recur even after successful eradication of *H. pylori*. In such instances, once other causes of therapeutic failure (noncompliance, salicylate abuse, NSAIDs, gastrinoma) have been eliminated, approved maintenance therapy with antisecretories should be considered. Long-term antisecretory agents should thus be considered for patients in whom at least two attempts at *H. pylori* eradication have failed or those who have *H. pylori*-negative duodenal ulcer disease and possibly in patients with complicated ulcers, particularly those prone to recurrent bleeding.

Whereas surgery had previously been the mainstay of the management of chronic duodenal ulceration, and particularly its complications, the advent of H2-receptor antagonists — and, more recently, PPIs — has virtually abolished elective surgery in the consideration of the management of duodenal ulcer disease. Nevertheless, in a small group of patients with chronic or recurrent duodenal ulcer disease and complications, surgery may eventually become a consideration. Thus, apart from the issue of gastrinoma, surgery of duodenal ulcer disease may be considered primarily as a strategy only in the management of complications.

The Complications of Peptic Ulcer Disease

The complications of acid peptic disease occur most frequently in the setting of chronic ulceration, although such events may occur in an acute setting. In such circumstances, the acute presentation often represents exposure to drugs (NSAIDs, steroids, or alcohol) or the exposure to stressful events such as trauma, sepsis, burns, or major surgery. In the latter, bleeding and perforation are the most dramatic and the most common, whereas penetration and obstruction are less frequent and less acute and usually related to chronicity and recurrence of ulcer.

Bleeding

Bleeding is a relatively common complication of peptic ulcer disease, but in 70% to 80% of patients, once appropriate resuscitation has been instituted, spontaneous cessation occurs. A small group, however, exhibit severe persistent or recurrent bleeding, and, in such instances, a rate of mortality of between 6% and 10% may be predicted. Survival is adversely affected by factors that include active bleeding, the identification of a visible vessel at endoscopy, age over 65 years, rebleeding in hospital, and major intercurrent medical problems including cardiac and renal disease.

Early therapy can be instituted at diagnosis. At initial endoscopy, bipolar coagulation, laser sealing, or application of topical homeostatic agents or glue should be used, depending upon availability. The success of such methodology has led to a significant decline in the need for open surgical intervention. In circumstances in which surgery may be necessary but the patient's condition militates against open surgery, selective embolization may be an option, although this technique can result in severe sequelae including duodenal infarction or pancreatitis. In the event of endoscopic strategies failing to halt the bleeding, or the hemorrhage being too excessive to permit endoscopy, surgery should be rapidly undertaken and directed at identifying the bleeding vessels. These are then underrun and oversewn. In the past, ligation of the bleeding vessel was usually followed by a vagotomy and pyloroplasty or even a gastrectomy to decrease acid secretion and diminish the likelihood of a

Figure 10. — *The complications of duodenal ulcer disease are, to a certain degree, site dependent. They represent either failure to heal or the result of inappropriate or excessive healing. Anterior disease may result in free perforation into the peritoneal cavity. Posterior or posteromedial disease results may culminate in bleeding as the pancreaticoduodenal vessels are breached. If the process is more chronic and associated with thromboendarteritis obliterans, bleeding may not occur, but progressive ulceration results in penetration of the ulcer into the head or uncinate process of the pancreas. Repeated episodes of ulceration and healing result in excessive fibrosis and obstruction of the duodenal lumen, leading to gastric outflow obstruction. In the stomach, longstanding ulceration may very rarely be associated with neoplasia, although it is possible that such lesions may have been neoplastic ab initio.*

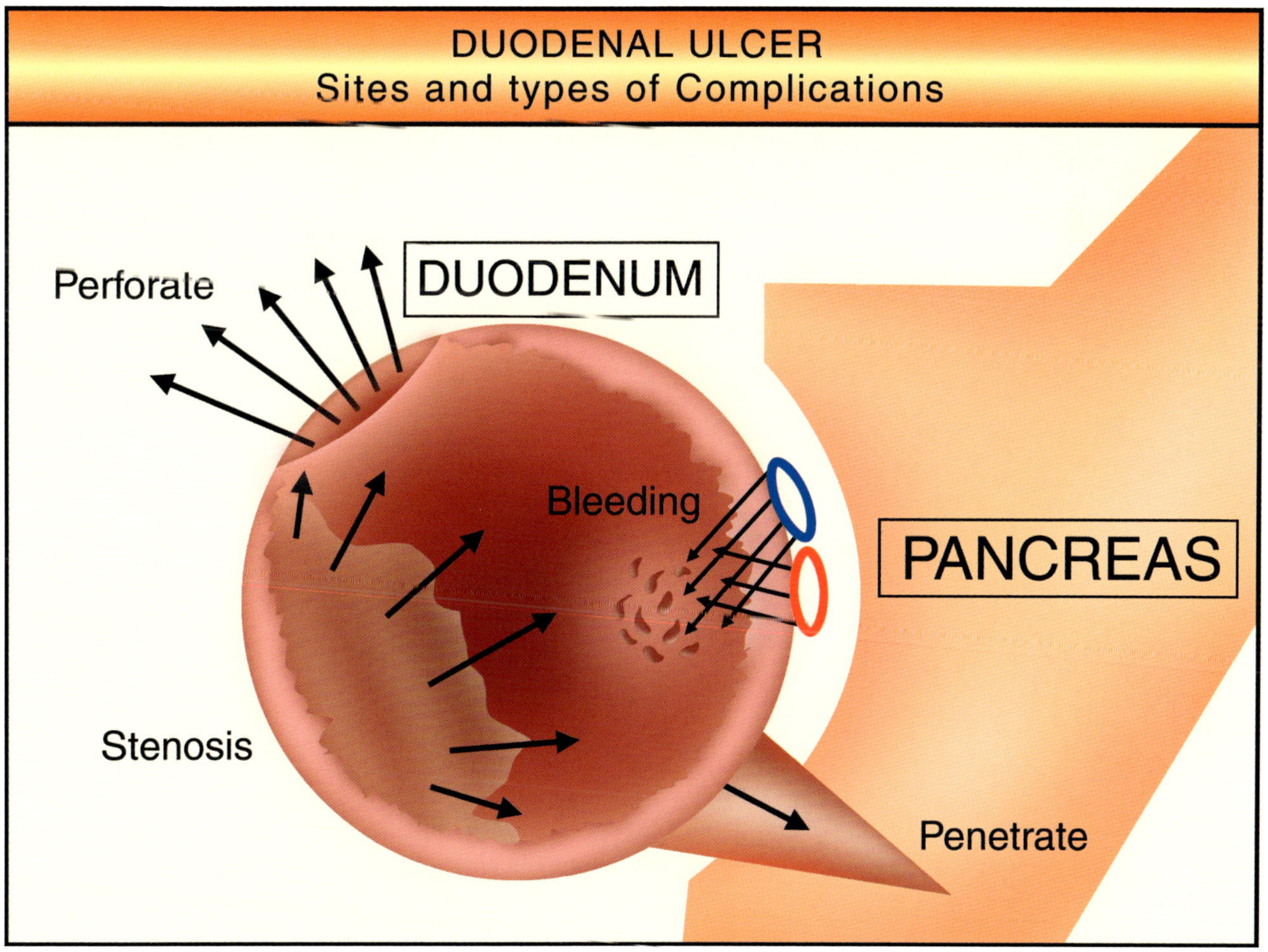

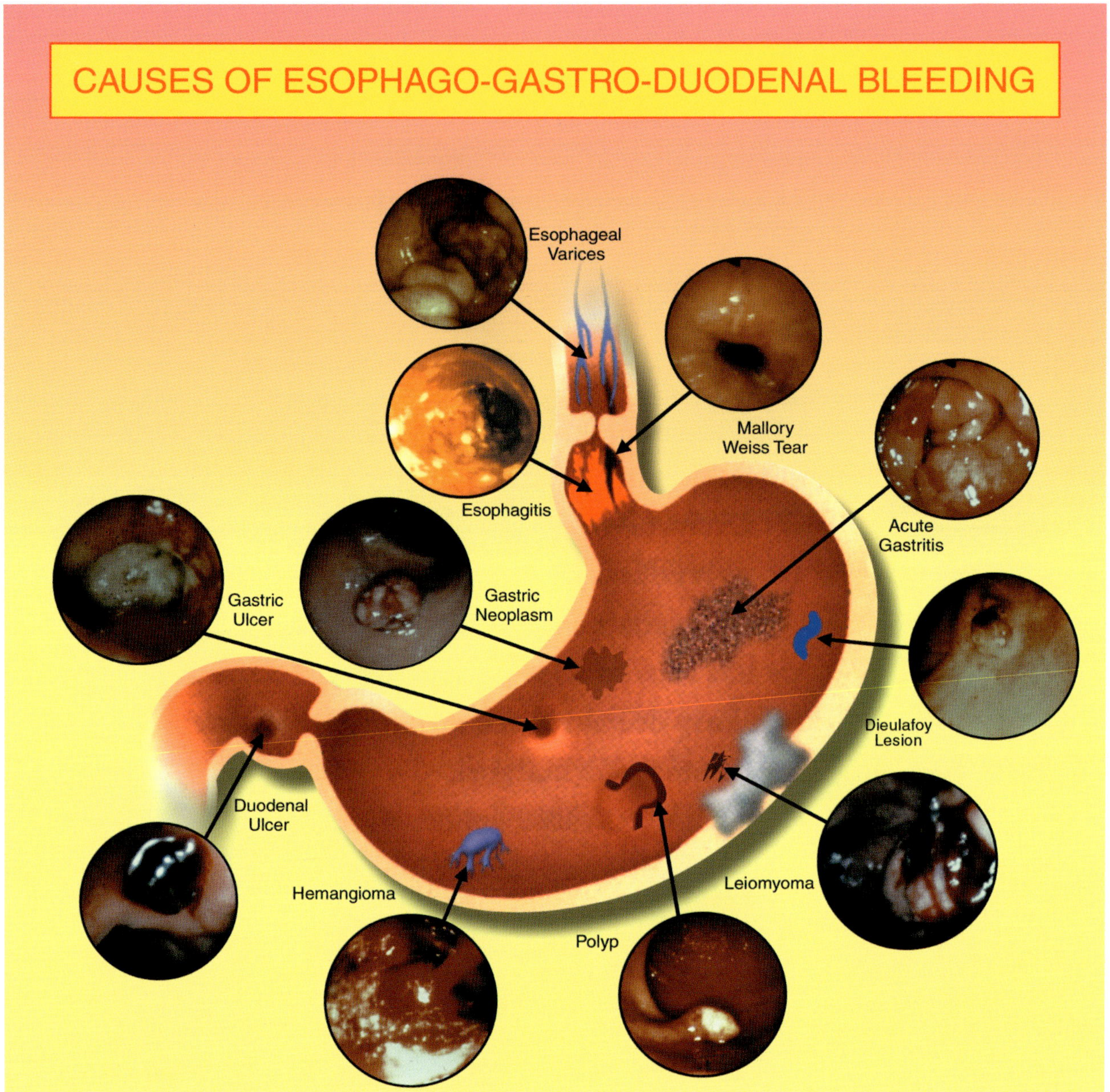

Figure 11. — *An illustration of the stomach with endoscopic inserts of the common causes of bleeding. There are a wide variety of causes associated with upper gastrointestinal bleeding, and the majority can be identified at endoscopy. Peptic ulcers account for the majority (50%–60%), gastric and esophageal varices (10%–15%), angiomas (3%–6%), Mallory Weiss tear (5%), erosions (5%), neoplasms (4%–6%), Dieulafoy's (1%) and others (10%–15%). These incidences can vary widely depending upon the socioeconomic milieu.*

rebleed. The availability and use of H2-receptor antagonists or PPI therapy for active duodenal ulcer and active benign gastric ulcer has to a large extent obviated the need for emergency gastrectomy and similarly decreased the incidence of recurrent bleeding from ulcer sites.

Perforation

Occasionally, the first indication of a peptic ulcer may be the perforation itself, whereas in some patients previous vague symptomatology may dramatically culminate in acute perforation with peritonitis. The pathogenesis of an indolent or even chronic disease transformed into an acute event is unclear but may represent a local vascular phenomenon whereby vessels supplying the ulcer base are acutely obliterated, and a local infarction occurs. In 1843, Edward Crisp, of London, reported 50 cases of perforated peptic ulcer and accurately summarized the dire clinical aspects of the condition at that time. He expressed considerable pessimism about the outcome, stating that "Once the perforation has occurred, the case must be considered hopeless. In surgery's present state, the idea of cutting open the abdomen and closing the opening is simply too quixotic to consider." In 1884, Mikulicz-Radecki, in Vienna, presciently noted that "Every doctor faced with a perforated

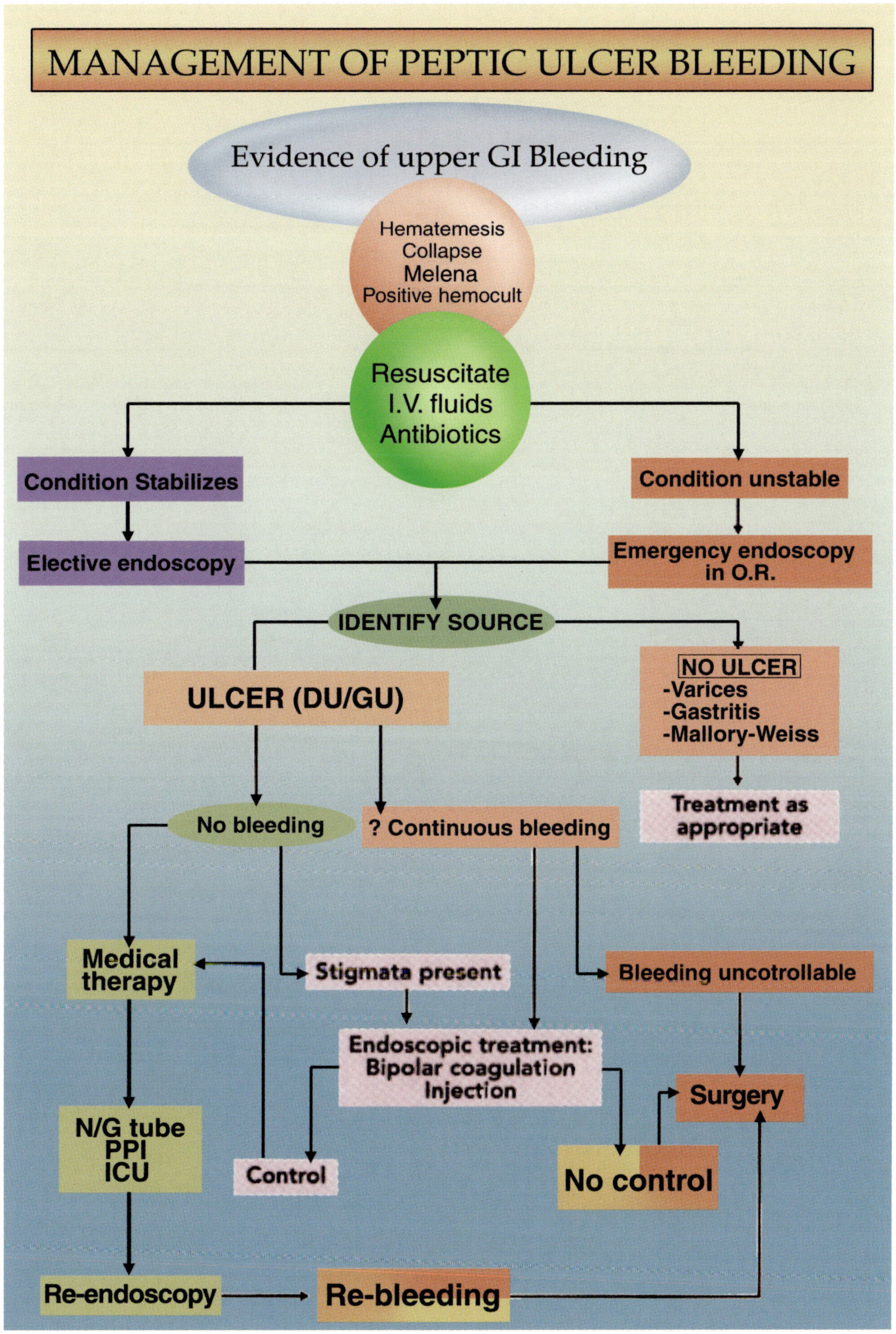

Figure 12. — *An outline of the general strategy necessary for the diagnosis and management of upper gastrointestinal bleeding. There are a number of independent clinical risk factors associated with a poor outcome from nonvariceal hemorrhage. These include age >60 years; serious comorbid medical or surgical issues; persistent hypotension or circulatory collapse; bright red blood per rectum, hematemesis, or blood in the nasogastric tube; initial transfusion requirements of >6 units; evidence of a coagulopathy; and a repeat bleed.*

ulcer of the stomach or intestine must consider opening the abdomen, sewing up the hole, and adverting a possible or actual inflammation by careful cleansing of the abdominal cavity." He did not undertake this procedure himself, and the first successful operation was performed on May 19, 1892, by Ludwig Heusner of Wuppertal, Germany.

At present, initial therapy for perforated duodenal ulcers includes laparotomy, peritoneal lavage, and omental patch repair, although developments in laparoscopic surgery have led to modifications of the acute management of the perforation itself. The laparoscope can be used to identify the perforation, lavage the abdomen, and suture or glue omental plugs into the defect. Large perforations can be managed by a combination of laparoscopic and endoscopic technique, whereby the laparoscopic introduction of the omentum into the duodenal lumen is followed by endoscopic suture or gluing of the omentum in place.

The need for concomitant or subsequent acid-reducing surgical procedures, such as vagotomy and gastrectomy, has been obviated by the introduction of medical therapy. Although mortality rates in the preantibiotic era for perforation were close to 25%, current mortality rates are less than 5% to 10%, with figures as low as 3%. Mortality reflects either delay in diagnosis or the presence of significant comorbid conditions consequent upon prolonged sepsis, advanced age, and cardiac or renal failure.

The advent of H2-receptor antagonists and PPIs for active duodenal ulcer and active benign gastric ulcer has, for the most part, precluded the need for consideration of subsequent definitive duodenal ulcer surgery for active duodenal ulcer and active benign gastric ulcer. In the era before PPIs, simple closure resulted in recurrence of ulcer in 52% of patients, of whom 28% would bleed, 15% would exhibit pyloric obstruction, and 9% would perforate. However, the clinical efficacy of suppression of acid secretion, combined with eradication of *H. pylori*, has led to the acceptance that simple duodenal ulcer closure and appropriate medical therapy thereafter is adequate.

The management of perforated gastric ulcers has similarly undergone an evolution in much the same fashion as perforated duodenal ulcers. Before the availability of H2-receptor antagonists and PPI therapy, the

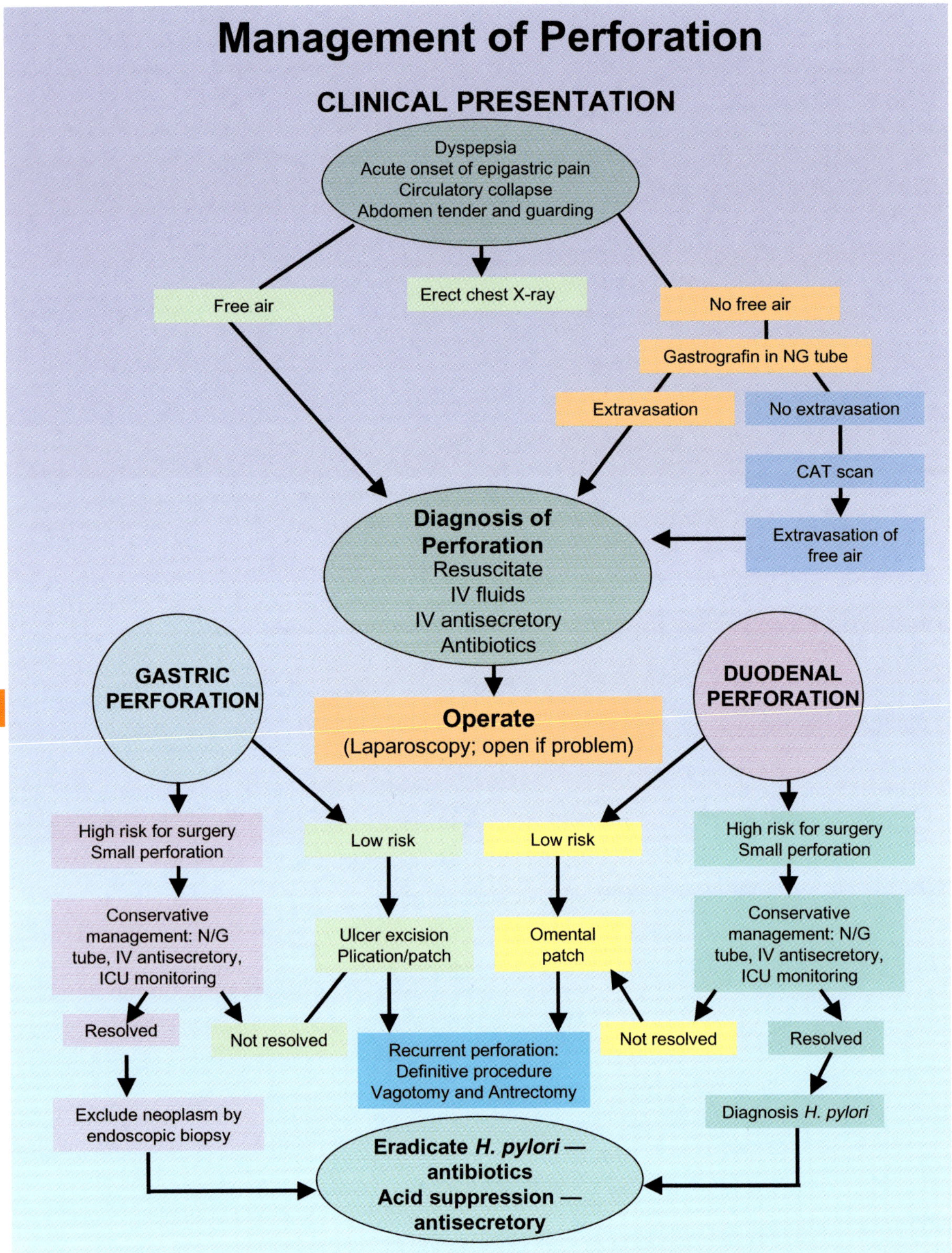

Figure 13. — *An overview of the diagnostic and therapeutic strategies available for the management of a perforated duodenal or gastric ulcer. In the majority of patients surgery is necessary, with conservative management reserved for those with either a substantial delay in diagnosis or considered too ill for open surgery and general anesthesia. As laparoscopic repair of a perforation is far less invasive and thus better tolerated by ill and elderly patients, this type of intervention may be considered the treatment of choice if available.*

majority of perforated gastric ulcers were managed by partial gastrectomy. However, with the availability of effective acid-suppressive medication, plication of the perforation and omental patch have become the standard of treatment. With perforated gastric ulcer, the need to confirm the absence of neoplasia is vital. Regardless of negative histology at the repair of the acute perforation, endoscopic reevaluation should be undertaken at 8 weeks with four-quadrant biopsies to confirm the absence of neoplasia.

Gastric Outlet Obstruction

This complication usually reflects prolonged untreated or inadequately treated duodenal ulceration and occurs as a result of bulbar cicatrisation. The gastric outlet gradually narrows, and function is impaired, and gastric emptying is initially slowed and then impeded. This process is accompanied by a sensation of early satiety and bloating, followed by a sensation of distention. Reflux symptoms may supervene as the stomach becomes overfilled, and disordered peristalsis drives food into the esophagus. This is associated with foul-smelling eructation and halitosis, consequent upon the bacterial colonization of stagnant gastric contents. In advanced gastric outlet obstruction, projectile vomiting of old undigested food occurs, and weight loss, as well as abdominal distention, and a succussion splash are apparent. Consideration should be given to the possibility of a prepyloric gastric cancer of the scirrhous variety, masquerading as a chronic duodenal ulcer, although this is rare.

In the majority of circumstances, surgery is required to manage gastric outlet obstruction due to progression of a chronic duodenal ulcer, although a trial of medical therapy may reverse obstruction due to an acute episode of ulceration. Endoscopic balloon dilatation has been used and in some circumstances may be of temporary benefit in allowing egress of gastric contents. It should be undertaken with caution, as perforation of the duodenal bulb may occur with accompanying morbidity or mortality. Usually restenosis occurs rapidly, and surgery is eventually required. Before surgery, passage of a large-diameter nasogastric tube with lavage and drainage of the gastric contents over a period of at least 5 days is necessary to empty the stomach and enable it to regain tone.

The use of oral nonabsorbable antibiotics and antifungal agents is of benefit in decreasing gastric bacterial colonization and obviating postoperative sepsis. The surgical procedure is directed at resection of the stenotic area of the duodenum and involves a partial gastrectomy with a Billroth-II gastrojejunal anastomosis. The resection of the strictured segment of the duodenum usually obviates the construction of a Billroth-I anastomosis, as inadequate duodenal length may result in excessive anastomotic tension. Vagotomy is ill advised, given its adverse effects; it is of little benefit in reducing acid secretion, provided an adequate antrectomy is undertaken. Safe closure of the duodenal stump is of critical importance, as leakage can cause catastrophic sequela.

Penetration

This complication is usually associated with a long history of untreated or inadequately treated peptic duodenal ulcer disease and was particularly common before the advent of acid-suppressive therapy. Clinically, it is presaged by alteration in symptomatology, and the classic picture of epigastric discomfort and nocturnal pain is no longer relieved by the ingestion of food or antacids. The site of the pain shifts from the epigastrium to the back and attains a constant, boring characteristic that is often worst at night and after meals. Under such circumstances, the consideration of pancreatic neoplasia may be raised, and even at endoscopy, the duodenal appearance can be suggestive of a neoplasm. The constant back pain often accentuated by food, and the failure of its relief with acid-suppressive medication usually mandates surgery. Under such circumstances, resection of the part of the duodenum containing the ulcer with a partial gastrectomy and Billroth-II anastomosis is the operation of choice. Surgery may be difficult, given the chronicity of the lesion, extensive fibrosis, and distortion of anatomy. Therefore, particular care should be exercised to avoid damage to the common bile duct and the head of the pancreas.

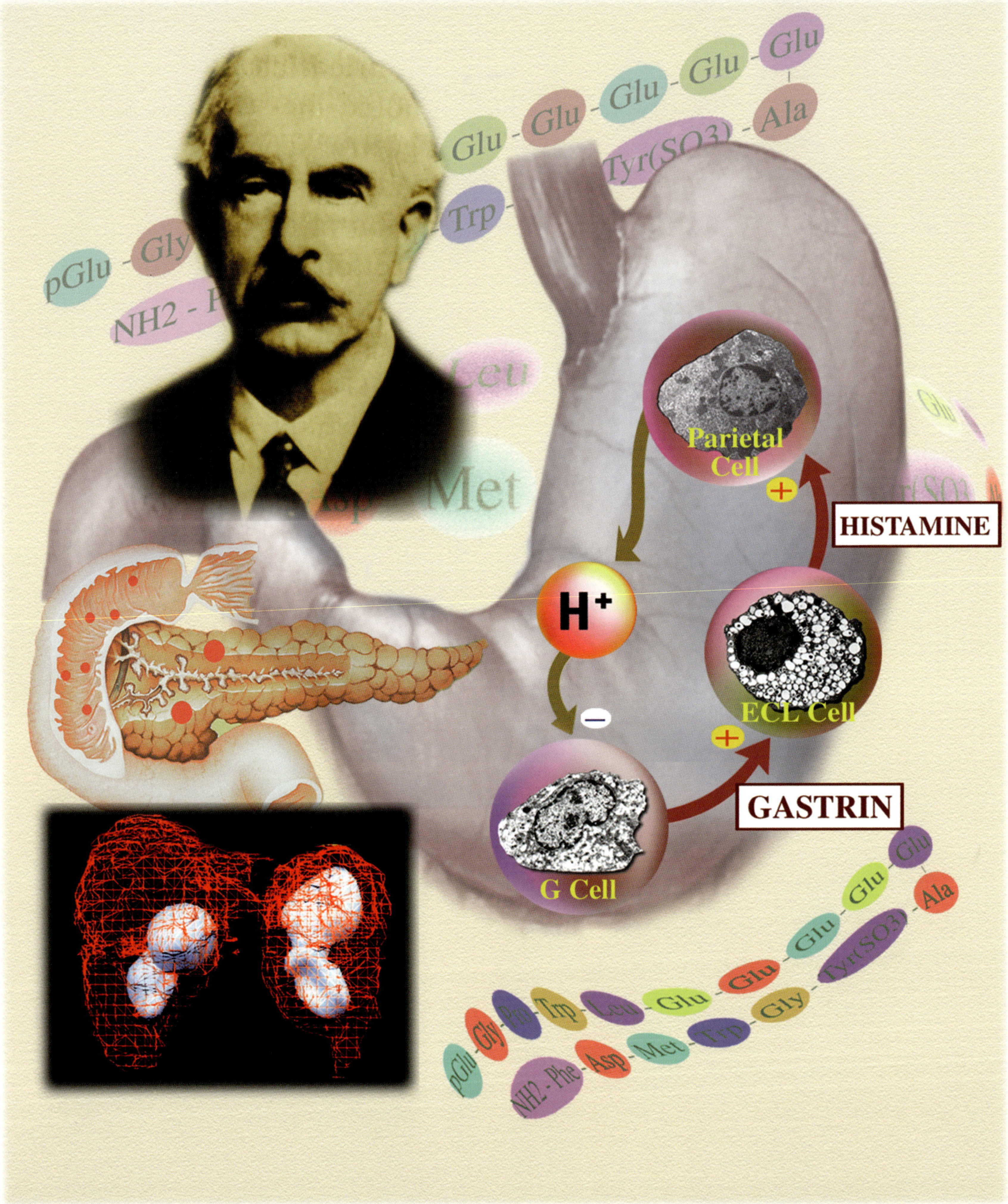

Parietal Cell
HISTAMINE
H^+
ECL Cell
G Cell
GASTRIN
pGlu - Gly - Pro - Trp - Leu - Glu - Glu - Glu - Glu - Glu - Ala - Tyr(SO3) - Gly - Trp - Met - Asp - Phe - NH2

Gastrin and Hypergastrinemia

Physiology

Hypergastrinemia

Gastrinoma

Treatment

Gastric Carcinoid

Background

Clinical Pathology

Classification

Prognosis

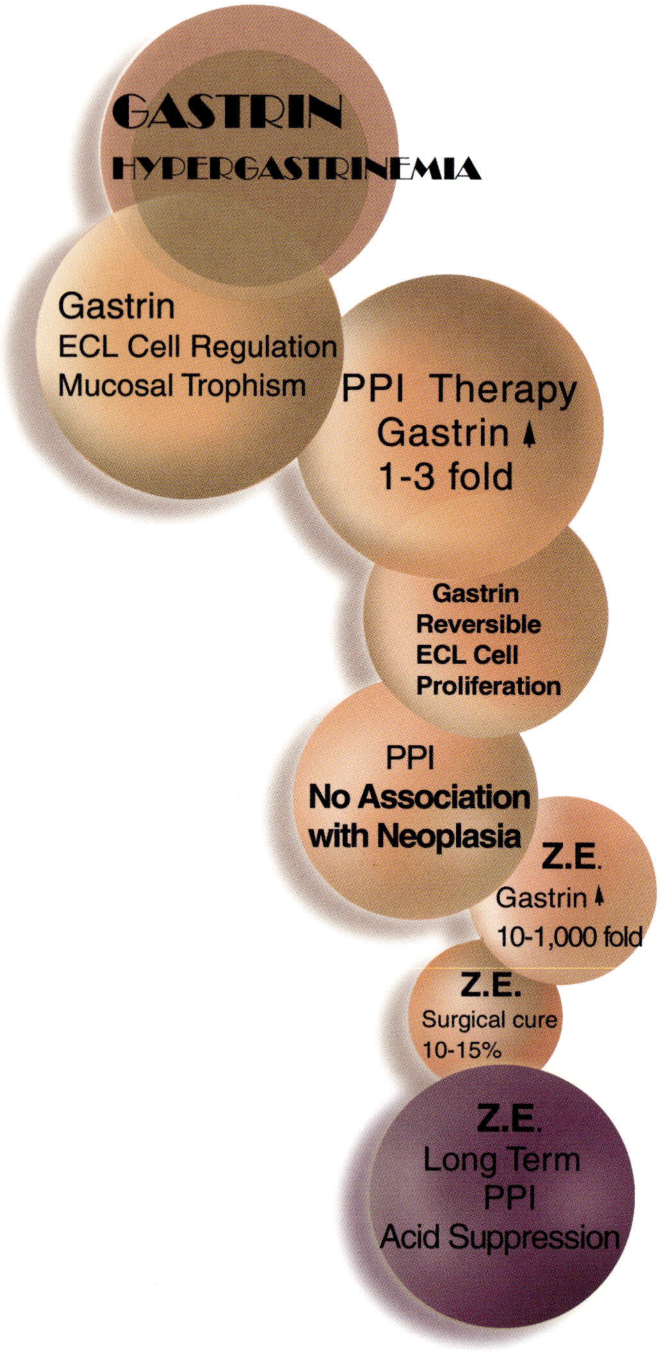
GASTRIN
HYPERGASTRINEMIA
Gastrin
ECL Cell Regulation
Mucosal Trophism
PPI Therapy
Gastrin ↑
1-3 fold
Gastrin
Reversible
ECL Cell
Proliferation
PPI
No Association
with Neoplasia
Z.E.
Gastrin ↑
10-1,000 fold
Z.E.
Surgical cure
10-15%
Z.E.
Long Term
PPI
Acid Suppression

Gastrin and Hypergastrinemia

Physiology

Gastrin is secreted by the G cells of the antrum in response to a number of stimuli including luminal pH and amino acids, gastric mechanical events, and neural input of both a central and peripheral nature. Although, in the adult, gastrin is synthesized mainly in the G cells of the gastric antrum and duodenum, small amounts have been identified in the pituitary and some vagal nerve fibers. In early life, the fetal and neonatal pancreas produce gastrin, which may be the source of neonatal hypergastrinemia. After birth, production of gastrin in the periphery is due to G cells in the antral mucosa. In the circulation, the predominant form of gastrin is a heptadecapeptide, G17, although both shorter and longer forms have been identified. Gastrin contains a COOH terminal amide resulting from post-translational amidation of a glycine-extended precursor. Gastrin shares an identical pentapeptide amide with CCK, which results in relatively similar binding to the CCK-B receptor. Cholecystokinin contains a tyrosine residue in the seventh position from the COOH terminal that is always sulfated, whereas gastrin has a tyrosine in the sixth position that may or may not be sulfated. The position and sulfation of the tyrosine residue appears to be critical for recognition by the CCK-A subtype receptor. Structural differences in the two peptides result in receptor subtype selectivity and thereby determine selective biologic activity.

Figure 1. — Gastrin plays a pivotal role in the regulation of acid secretion. In response to luminal stimulation (aromatic amino acids) and neural modulation (PACAP), the antral cell releases gastrin into the circulation. This activates CCK-B receptors on the fundic ECL cell, which releases histamine and engenders paracrine activation of histamine subtype 2 receptors on the parietal cell. In response to this stimulation, acid is secreted, which then provides a negative luminal feedback for gastrin release by the G cell.

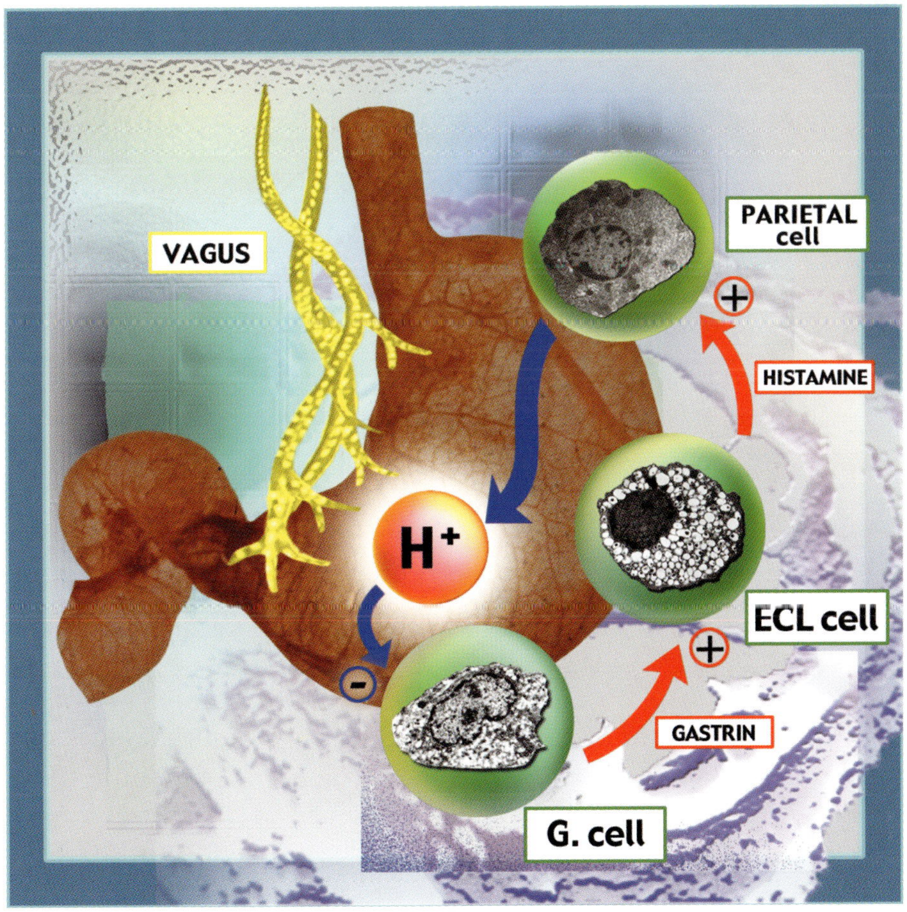

Meal-related increases in plasma gastrin reflect the summation of the effects of luminal amino acids, antral distention, and neural input of both a central and enteric type engendered by agents including PACAP and acetylcholine. The predominant negative regulatory mechanism for gastric secretion is provided by luminal pH, whereby a decrease of antral hydrogen ion concentration results in the activation of antral somatostatin cells that inhibit G-cell secretion of gastrin. Normal fasting gastrin levels are usually in the range of 50 pg/mL and may increase twofold to threefold after a standard meal.

As the G cells of the gastric antrum are of the "open" type with their apical surfaces reaching the glandular lumen, luminal contents (protons, amino acids) are able to directly modulate G-cell activity and the release of gastrin. Intracellular granules containing gastrin are abundant in the basal portion of the cells, and, upon stimulation, gastrin is released by an exocytotic process into the extracellular fluid whence it diffuses into the circulation and is conveyed to the gastric fundus. In this respect, gastrin meets the archetypal criteria of a true hormone originally proposed by Hardy in 1896.

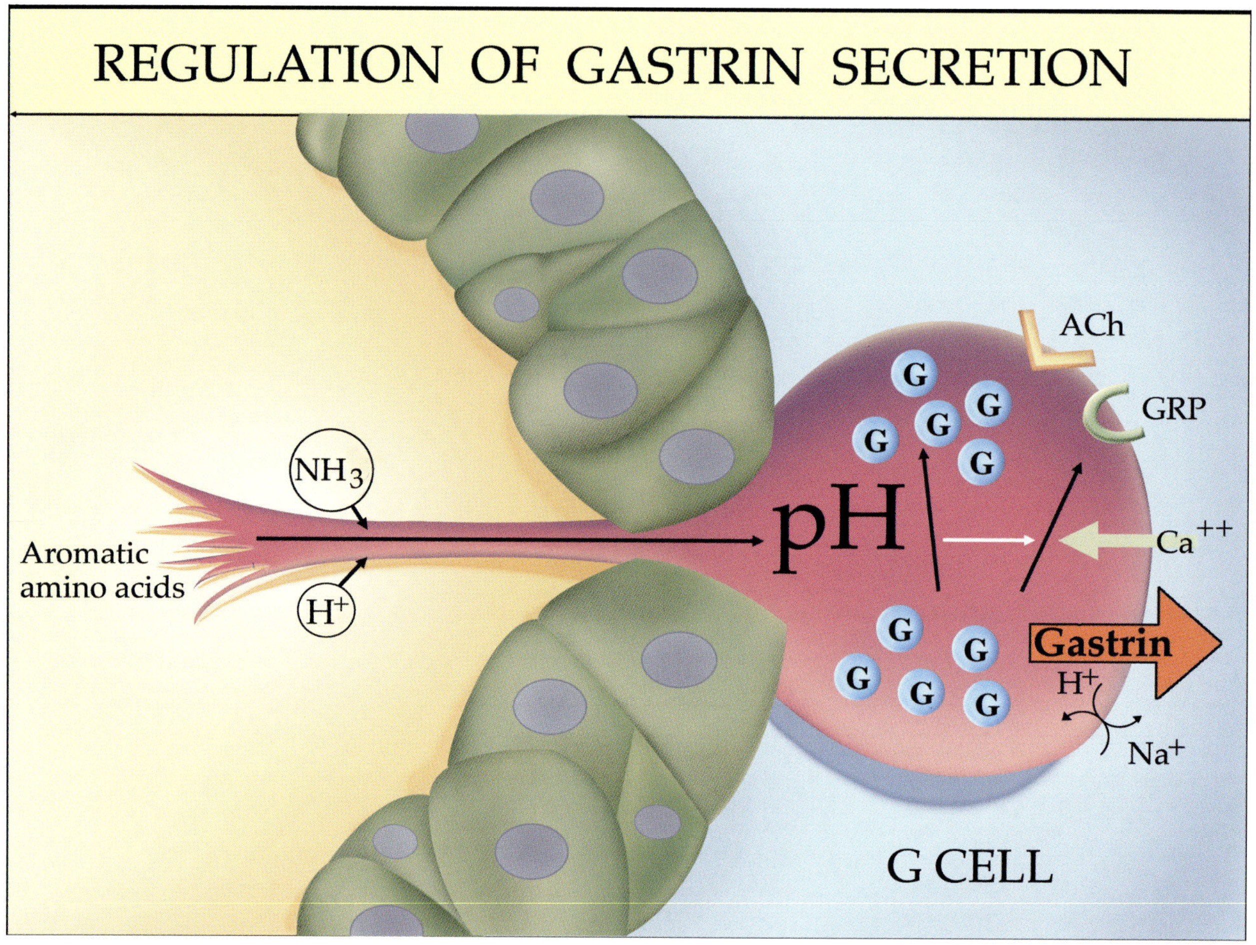

Figure 2. — A model of stimulation of gastrin release. The chief regulators are aromatic amino acids and pH in the antral lumen, and acetylcholine and gastrin-releasing peptide (GRP) acting through receptors located on the basolateral cell surface. The apical surface has been illustrated in such a way as to schematically indicate the relationship between the G cell and the luminal contents. As the G cell is open to the gastric lumen, chemical effectors can bind to the apical membrane or become internalized by the G cell and thus influence production of gastrin. There are a number of specific chemical components of antral contents that modulate the release of gastrin. The most effective and well studied of these is the antral luminal pH, which, at values less than 3, completely suppresses release of gastrin. This serves to terminate gastric digestion. If the antral luminal pH remains elevated in the presence of continuing stimulation, hypergastrinemia results. The presence of aromatic amino acids is responsible for luminal initiation of the release of gastrin. The presence of NH_3 produced by H. pylori *may interfere with the negative feedback of H^+ and result in increased gastrin levels. Intact protein fails to increase gastrin secretion, whereas the ingestion of peptone, a partially digested protein mix, is a powerful stimulant. In this respect, the preferential stimulation by aromatic amino acids is consistent with the preferred cleavage sites for the major gastric protease: pepsin. The effect of amino acids on gastrin release represents a direct action on the G cell, as it can be reproduced in vitro and is not blocked by atropine or other inhibitors of neural transmission.*

Food in the stomach is the primary physiologic event responsible for the release of gastrin from the antral G cells. The mechanism involved in this process comprises at least three stimulatory pathways that include central neural activation, distension of the antrum, and specific chemical components in the food. At the cellular level, these pathways regulate gastrin release through the actions of acetylcholine (ACh), gastrin-releasing peptide (GRP), somatostatin, and the direct chemical effects of H^+ and aromatic amino acids. It is likely that other cellular effectors, such as adenosine, galanin, and epinephrine, play a role, but their physiologic significance is dubious.

The presence of food in the stomach activates peripheral pathways that include mechanisms associated both with gastric distension and the chemical composition of the gastric luminal contents. Gastrin is released in response to oropharyngeal and central stimuli through the vagus nerve, and selective antral vagotomy abolishes both sham feeding and hypoglycemia-stimulated release. As selective fundic vagotomy leads to an enhanced vagal release of gastrin, it is likely that the vagus also initiates an inhibitory action mediated by the fundus. Muscarinic synapses are involved in both pathways because atropine inhibits both the antral release and the fundic inhibitory reflex. Given that bilateral truncal vagotomy leads to a sustained elevation of serum gastrin levels, it seems that peripheral mechanisms are primarily stimulatory for release of gastrin, whereas the central influence is inhibitory. Enhanced release of gastrin follows significant distension of the antral portion of the stomach, whereas distension of the fundus alone tends to inhibit gastrin secretion, suggesting that local neural reflexes mediate distension responses.

Hypergastrinemia

Elevated levels of gastrin range from modest increases with PPI therapy (threefold to fourfold) to levels that may be 200- to 300-fold above normal due to a gastrinoma. Hypergastrinemia is most commonly associated with either atrophic gastritis or the use of acid-suppressive therapy, particularly the PPI class of drugs. Less common causes include patients with renal failure or those who have undergone vagotomy, especially if the antrum has not been resected. Retained excluded

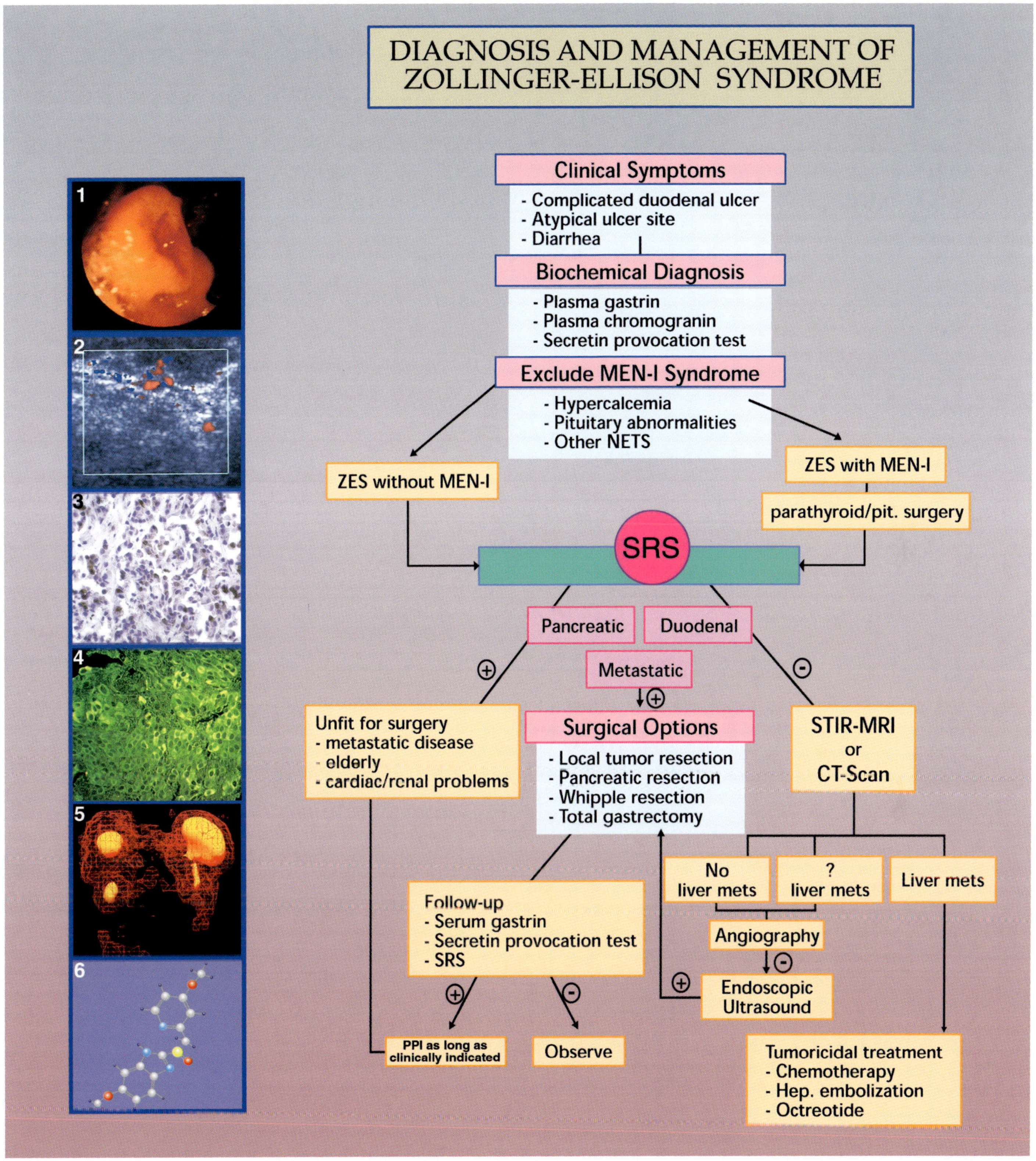

Figure 3. *— Diagnosis and management of gastrinoma. Clinical symptomatology is important in arousing suspicion of the presence of a gastrinoma. Hypergastrinemia should be confirmed to be of neoplastic origin by use of a secretin provocation test and the site of the gastrinoma then identified. Endoscopy (1) may reveal a mucosal lesion, but more often endoscopic or intraoperative ultrasound is helpful (2). It has proved particularly difficult to identify minute and often multiple duodenal gastrinomas. Endoscopic ultrasound has proved to be of use in this area, although often such lesions may only be detectable at surgery itself by transillumination of the duodenal wall, intraoperative ultrasound, or formal duodenotomy and palpation. Biopsy is useful if immunocytochemistry reveals the presence of chromogranin (3) and gastrin (4). The most effective topographic study is the somatostatin receptor scintigram (SRS) (Octreoscan) (5) that uses an isotopically labeled somatostatin receptor-2 subtype analog to detect tumors and their metastases. This study has a high sensitivity and specificity (85% to 90%) for both primary and secondary lesions and is particularly effective in the detection of lymph node and hepatic metastases. Panel 5 demonstrates a gastrinoma in the head of the pancreas (bottom left) and a metastatic lesion in the liver (top left). (The uptake on the right is splenic with some isotope also in the colon.) Computed tomography (CT) scan and magnetic resonance imaging (MRI) may be of some use but rarely provide further information than available from the SRS scan. Because 80% to 90% of gastrinomas are either metastatic at diagnosis or residual tumor is left after surgery, the treatment of choice for long-term management is a proton pump inhibitor (PPI) (6).*

antrum due to surgical technique is rare given the awareness of the need for complete antral resection and the current rarity of the need to use a Billroth II resection for peptic ulcer disease. Despite its significant biologic role in the stimulation of acid secretion and trophic regulation of the gastric mucosa, the effects of either acute or chronic hypergastrinemia appear to be minimal, especially if parietal-cell function is inhibited (acid-suppressive drugs) or absent (diminished) as in atrophic gastritis or pernicious anemia. Prolonged, albeit modest, post-vagotomy hypergastrinemia has not been associated with any adverse effects in numerous patients followed for as long as 30 to 40 years.

The prolonged elevation of gastrin levels may be associated with biologic effects that reflect the action of gastrin, particularly on gastric ECL cells. The trophic effect of gastrin on mucosal stem cells may be associated with gastric mucosal thickening and occasionally formation of polyps. No evidence has emerged to support the role of elevated gastrin levels in the genesis of colonic carcinoma, and its effects are, for the most part, only relevant to the stomach. Prolonged gastrin drive culminates in ECL cell proliferation, increased secretion of histamine, and, consequently, hypersecretion of acid. The consequences of hypergastrinemia are varying degrees of ECL cell hyperplasia but not dysplasia or carcinoids, as demonstrated in long-term clinical trials. Rarely, PPI-induced massive (10- to 20-fold) hypergastrinemia may occur, but no adverse effect has been noted, and gastrin levels have returned to pretreatment levels usually within 1 to 2 weeks after withdrawal of the PPI. The relationship between PPI-induced suppression of acid and gastrin levels is considered to be of such minimal clinical relevance that measurement of plasma gastrin levels is deemed unnecessary.

Gastrinoma

The association of an islet cell tumor of the pancreas and a peptic ulcer diathesis was previously eponymously recognized as the Zollinger-Ellison syndrome (ZES). The subsequent biologic elucidation of a gastrin-secreting neoplasm associated with acid hypersecretion facilitated the development of rational medical and surgical therapy. Pathologically, the condition consists of a neuroendocrine tumor arising in either the pancreas or the duodenum, which produces excessive amounts of gastrin, driving the parietal-cell mass to the secretion of hydrochloric acid in quantities that overcome the "mucosal barrier" of the stomach, duodenum, and upper small bowel. The duodenal or pancreatic lesions may, in rare circumstances, be part of the multiple endocrine neoplasia type 1 (MEN-1) syndrome, and, under such circumstances, consideration should be given to the previous surgical management of the associated parathyroid or pituitary problems.

In the absence of adequate suppression of acid, the condition is associated with multiple, intractable, and aggressive ulcers of the duodenum and the small bowel with dramatic episodes of bleeding or perforation. Emergency surgery resulted in anastomotic bleeding or leakage due to unrestrained secretion of acid and associated morbidity and mortality that total gastrectomy was often the only viable option. The introduction of H2-receptor antagonists led to a significant diminution in the need for gastric surgery, but the tachyphylaxis associated with competitive receptor antagonism led to a diminution of efficacy in suppressing acid secretion and an increase of complications, such as bleeding and perforation, with time. The introduction of PPI therapy has greatly diminished the occurrence of such problems. The potency at high dosage of this class of drugs has rendered them an excellent treatment in the management of gastrinomas, dramatically reducing complications and abrogating the need for total gastrectomy. In the past, diagnosis was heralded by the identification of aggressive ulceration, failure to heal, and dramatic complications. An important clinical clue is the presence of diarrhea in patients with the diagnosis of peptic ulcer disease, especially if there is no evidence of intake of antacids containing magnesium or other agents known to provoke increased gut motility or secretion.

Most patients are now identified early in the disease process either because of the presence of an ulcer in an atypical site (postbulbar) or the failure to heal on adequate therapy, particularly if *H. pylori* have been eradicated. Recurrent ulcer disease after demonstration of eradication of *H. pylori* and appropriate compliance with antisecretory therapy should lead to a high index of suspicion with early measurement of fasting gastrin levels.

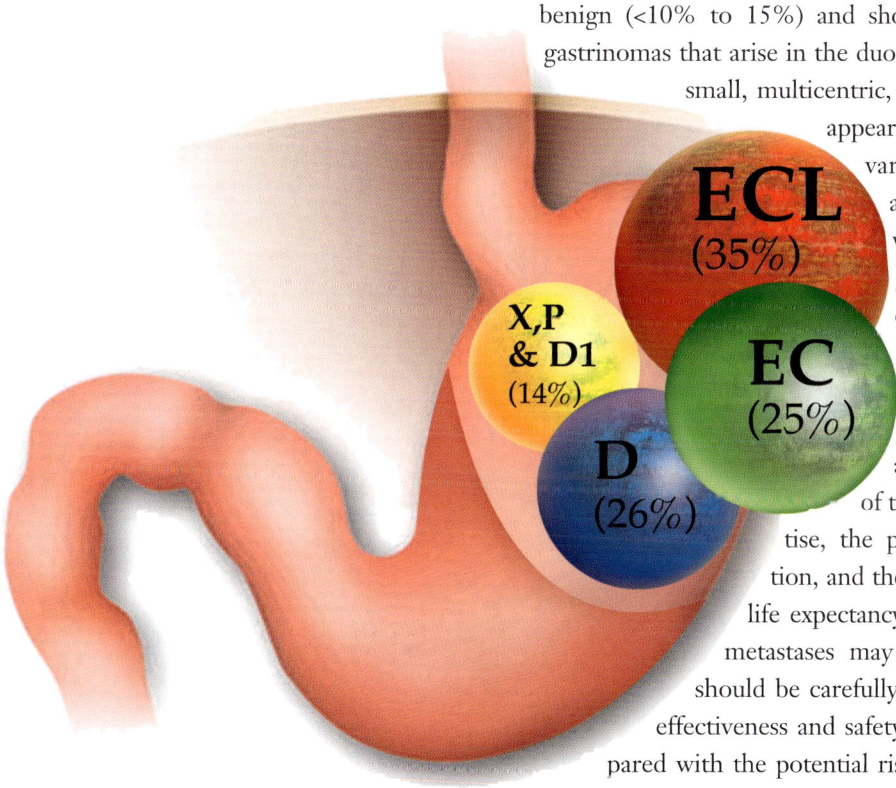

Figure 4. — The distribution of neuroendocrine cell types in the gastric fundic mucosa. The histamine secreting ECL cells are the dominant fundic neuroendocrine cell type. They function as critical regulators of parietal cell acid secretion through an H2–receptor subtype. The D cells, which secrete somatostatin, are the next most common cell type and exert an inhibitory effect on acid secretion, mostly by negative regulation of ECL cell histamine secretion by a SST_2 receptor. The precise function of the other cell types and their biologic role is as yet unclear, although it is likely that they play a role in the modulation of mucosal microcirculation and trophic regulation.

Treatment

The management of gastrinomas has evolved considerably in the last decade, particularly with the advent of PPIs. In the past, the inability to adequately suppress secretion of acid and obviate the drastic complications of aggressive peptic ulcer disease led to the widespread use of total gastrectomy to remove the target organ for gastrin. Current management strategy using maintenance PPI therapy tailored to the individual requirements of the patient has provided excellent clinical response. The incidence of acid breakthrough and complications has been insignificant if therapeutic compliance is maintained.

Nevertheless, the issue of surgery in the management of gastrinoma remains controversial. Gastrinoma tumors of the pancreas appear to be of a more malignant variety and are usually multicentric and metastatic at diagnosis. In rare instances, the lesion is solitary and/or benign (<10% to 15%) and should be resected. The gastrinomas that arise in the duodenum, although often small, multicentric, and difficult to detect, appear to be of a more benign variety and should be addressed more actively with consideration given to pancreaticoduodenectomy. The use of such operations should be carefully evaluated against the background of the local surgical expertise, the patient's overall condition, and the question of projected life expectancy. Resection of hepatic metastases may increase survival but should be carefully considered, given the effectiveness and safety of PPI therapy compared with the potential risk of major abdominal surgery and hepatic resection.

If the gastrinoma is a component of the MEN-I syndrome, gastric carcinoids may develop. This reflects the relationship between hypergastrinemia and an as yet uncharacterized genomic abnormality, as gastrinomas unassociated with the syndrome do not develop gastric carcinoids. Gastric carcinoid tumors should be identified and carefully monitored. If they are multiple, rapidly growing, or greater than 2 cm in size, consideration should be given to fundic resection to obviate the possibility of perforation, bleeding, or the development of metastases.

Gastric Carcinoid

Background

In 1988, Solcia and others delineated a system of classification for the spectrum of proliferative changes of endocrine cells of the gastric fundus. This classification defines histopathologic appearances ranging from hyperplasia to dysplasia to neoplasia of the ECL cells. The term *pseudohyperplasia* has been used to describe cell clustering unassociated with cell proliferation. The successive stages of hyperplasia are termed *simple, linear or chain-forming, micronodular, and adenomatoid.* Relatively atypical cells with features of enlarging or fusing micronodules, microinvasion, or newly formed stroma characterize dysplasia. When the nodules increase further in size to greater than 5 mm or invade into the submucosa, the lesion is classified as a neoplasm. This stage is divided into intramucosal and invasive forms. The entire spectrum of endocrine cell proliferation, from hyperplasia to dysplasia and neoplasia, has been observed in MEN-ZES and diffuse type A chronic atrophic gastritis. Both hyperplastic and pseudohyperplastic changes occurs with low frequency in the *H. pylori*-related chronic gastritis associated with ulcer disease or dyspepsia. However, because no progression to dysplastic or neoplastic lesions have thus far been documented in these latter conditions, their role in gastric endocrine tumorigenesis appears unlikely. Carcinoid tumor is thus characterized morphologically by the criteria of size and invasion. Biologically, however, the state of neoplasia is recognized by autonomy from the trophic effects of gastrin. A lesion that fails to regress once gastrin levels have been normalized should be regarded as a carcinoid tumor.

Clinical Pathology

It was apparent that a threshold value of plasma gastrin is necessary, not only for ECL-cell hyperplasia to occur but for conversion to neoplasia. This value reflects not only gastrin levels but length of exposure and other factors of which the female gender and genomic events (MEN-1) are involved. In fact, the ECL cell density does not exhibit a relation to plasma gastrin levels in normogastrinemic persons nor does it reveal any significant differences in patients with duodenal ulcer and mild hypergastrinemia. In patients on omeprazole or with sustained hypergastrinemia associated with surgical vagotomy, ECL-cell hyperplasia without progression to dysplasia or carcinoid has been noted after more than a decade of continuous treatment. Although duration of exposure appears important, it has been noted that ECL-cell hyperplasia may be stable with time, provided that gastrin levels do not increase significantly. With hypergastrinemia alone (eg, sporadic ZES) ECL-cell proliferation is usually limited to hyperplastic lesions of the simple or linear type. However, in patients with MEN-1-ZES or type A chronic atrophic gastritis, ECL cell lesions are usually dysplastic or overtly carcinoid in nature. Factors other than hypergastrinemia must therefore be involved in ECL cell transformation. In the MEN-1 syndrome, the loss of a suppressor oncogene in 11q13 may be related. The trophic sensitivity of the ECL cell is significantly influenced by female gender.

Classification of ECL Cell Proliferation

HYPERPLASIA	Simple (diffuse) Linear Micronodular Adenomatoid	
DYSPLASIA **(Pre-neoplastic stage)**	Enlarging micronodule Fusing micronodule Microinvasive lesion Nodule with newly formed strata	
CARCINOID	Intramucosal carcinoid Invasive carcinoid	

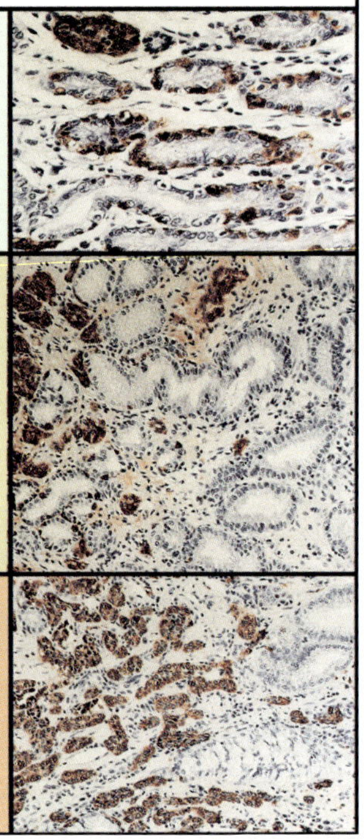

Figure 5. *— A histologic grading system for evaluation of the ECL cell proliferative changes that may occur in the fundic mucosa. The top panel (x400), demonstrates simple hyperplasia in one gland (bottom), linear hyperplasia (chains without intervening cells) (middle), and a micronodule (top). The middle panel (x200) exhibits adenomatoid hyperplasia of the ECL cells, which is defined as a cluster of five or more micronodules. In the bottom panel (x200) is an example of an intramucosal ECL cell tumor. (All micrographs immunoperoxidase for chromogranin A.)*

The hyperplastic effect of hypergastrinemia on gastric mucosal epithelial cells appears not to be restricted to the ECL cells. Foveolar cells and surface mucous cells also undergo hyperplasia in the human stomach under the influence of excessive gastrin drive, often to a considerable degree. This process may be patchy, and not infrequently results in the development of endoscopically detectable fundic gland polyps that are classified histologically as foveolar hyperplasia. Thus, in patients with these lesions, in a setting of hypergastrinemia, at least two types of mucosal polyps may occur: those due to ECL cell proliferations and foveolar hyperplasias.

Classification

Neuroendocrine tumors of the stomach account for about 0.3% of all gastric tumors and 3% to 5% of all gastrointestinal carcinoids but may be as high as 11%. This purported increase represents added awareness of the entity as well as the widespread use of diagnostic endoscopy. In reviewing the histology and pathobiology of gastric carcinoids, it is critical to distinguish among different types of gastric carcinoids. The presence of hypergastrinemia, in particular, connotes a more benign situation than lesions occurring under normogastrinemic conditions. Furthermore, patients with solitary sporadic lesions have worse prognoses than patients with multiple or diffuse microcarcinoid lesions. The latter occur relatively frequently in association with hypergastrinemic states, in contrast to the rarer sporadic gastric tumors. Gastric carcinoids can be broadly classified by behavior, histologic type, or by their relationship to associated conditions and gastrin levels.

The Munich Classification

The Munich Classification evaluated lesions on the basis of their histologic behavior and proposed four groups. (1) *Benign:* Nonfunctioning, well-differentiated tumor of small size (up to 1 cm) limited to the mucosa-submucosa and without angioinvasion; usually ECL cell tumors of the fundic mucosa associated with chronic atrophic gastritis and hypergastrinemia. (2) *Benign or low-grade malignant behavior:* Nonfunctioning, well-differentiated tumor within the mucosa-submucosa of small size (>1 up to 2 cm) without angioinvasion or of small to intermediate size (up to 2 cm) with angioinvasion; usually ECL cell tumors of the fundic mucosa associated with chronic atrophic gastritis and hypergastrinemia (rarely MEN-1 associated or sporadic ECL cell tumors). *(3) Low-grade malignant behavior* (low-grade neuroendocrine carcinoma): Nonfunctioning, well-differentiated tumor of large size (>2 cm) or extending beyond the submucosa; usually sporadic ECL cell tumors; rarely serotonin-producing tumors or others; rarely MEN-1 or chronic atrophic gastritis-associated ECL cell tumors; functioning well-differentiated tumor of any size and extension-sporadic gastrinoma, serotonin-producing tumor (EC), or others. *(4) Malignant behavior:* Functioning or nonfunctioning poorly differentiated intermediate or small-cell carcinoma.

An analysis using such a classification indicates the majority (83%) of gastric carcinoids to be well differentiated.

The Histologic Classification

Three histologic patterns of gastric carcinoid (ECL cell) tumor have been proposed: (1) *argyrophilic carcinoids* arising in type A chronic atrophic gastritis (chronic atrophic gastritis/A); (2) *argyrophilic ECL cell carcinoids* in multiple endocrine neoplasia-Zollinger-Ellison Syndrome (MEN-ZES); and (3) *sporadic argyrophil carcinoids.* This classification does not include neuroendocrine carcinomas (non-ECL cell), previously known as atypical carcinoids, which represent an unrelated aggressive neuroendocrine neoplasm.

Gastric Carcinoid Tumor Types

NOMENCLATURE	TUMOR CHARACTERISTICS	HISTOLOGY	HYPER-GASTRINEMIA	BIOLOGICAL BEHAVIOR
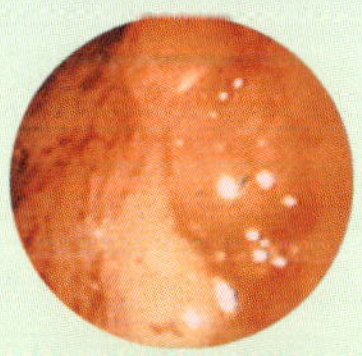 TYPE I	Generally small (<1cm) and multiple; often nodular/polypoid	ECL cell lesion. Stages of ECL cell hyperplasia, dysplasia, and neoplasia present in adjacent mucosa	Present	Slow growth, regional or distant metastases extremely rare
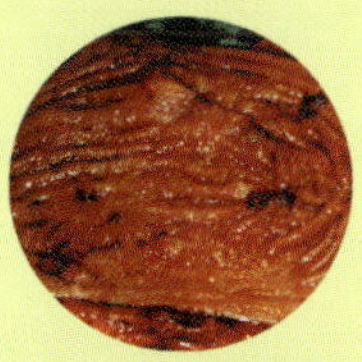 TYPE II	Generally small (<1cm) and multiple	ECL cell lesion. Stages of ECL cell hyperplasia, dysplasia, and neoplasia present in adjacent mucosa	Present	Slow growth, may metastasize more often than CAG-associated lesions
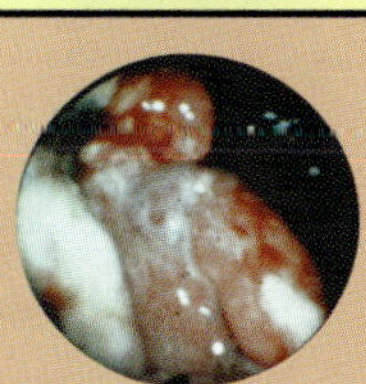 TYPE III	Solitary, often large (>1 cm)	ECL, EC, or X cells. Tumor formation w/o evidence of hyperplasia or precarcinoid dysplasia in adjacent mucosa	Absent	Relatively aggressive growth, frequent metastases to regional nodes (55%) and liver (24%)

Figure 6. *— The characteristic features of gastric carcinoid tumor types. The most common variety is Type I (80% to 85%) (top panel), which is almost always associated with chronic atrophic gastritis type A. It is rare for such lesions to exhibit anything other than benign biologic behavior. In Type II lesions associated with MEN-1 patients with gastrinoma, more aggressive growth is evident, and resection of the stomach may be necessary (middle panel). Type III lesions (bottom panel) behave much as gastric adenocarcinomas and require early and radical surgical intervention.*

Type I Carcinoids Arising in Type A Chronic Atrophic Gastritis

About 85% of gastric carcinoid tumors arise in the presence of type A chronic atrophic gastritis and constitute the most common type of gastric carcinoid. Chronic atrophic gastritis/A is characterized by chronic inflammation of the oxyntic mucosa, often associated with autoimmune diseases, such as pernicious anemia, and results in atrophy of the oxyntic glands and achlorhydria. Carcinoid tumors related to chronic atrophic gastritis/A are usually small, often multicentric, occur against a background of hypergastrinemia, and exhibit benign behavior. Patients with such carcinoids do not die of causes related to their tumors. For patients with small (<1 cm) gastric carcinoids associated with hypergastrinemia, expectant therapy with endoscopic follow-up is satisfactory. This conservative form of management reflects the benign behavior of such tumors. Antrectomy has resulted in regression of such tumors as the source of gastrin has been removed but rarely seems warranted unless the lesion is not a pure ECL cell tumor or cannot be adequately managed endoscopically.

Type II MEN-1-ZES Associated Gastric Carcinoids

About one third of patients with MEN-1-ZES develop gastric carcinoids, presumably due to a genetic predisposition (possibly loss of heterozygosity near the MEN-1 locus on chromosome 11q13) that facilitates the development of such lesions. Despite a substantial level of hypergastrinemia, patients with sporadic ZES very rarely develop such lesions. Type II tumors are composed predominantly of ECL cells, although some lesions contain a heterogeneous population of cell types. Surgical resection may be necessary, as the behavior of gastric carcinoids associated with MEN-1-ZES appears to occupy a middle ground between that of the relatively aggressive sporadic lesions and the mostly benign tumors seen in conjunction with chronic atrophic gastritis.

Type III Sporadic Argyrophil Carcinoids

Sporadic argyrophil carcinoids are isolated tumors that arise against a background of normal gastric mucosa. They tend to be larger (two to three times) than the other types of gastric carcinoids and to behave more aggressively, exhibiting deep mucosal invasion. Ultrastructurally, the lesions appear to contain a mixture of cell types. Generally, some of the cells are identifiable as ECL cells, whereas others resemble EC or X cells. Overall, lesions of this type may be regarded as bearing greater similarity to neuroendocrine carcinomas rather than carcinoids. Between 60% and 80% exhibit local or lymph node spread at diagnosis, and even minute tumors may metastasize. The biologic behavior of the Type III lesions is far more aggressive than either Type I or II, with invasive growth and metastasis predictable features in their evolution. Complete or partial gastrectomy with local lymph node resection is recommended therapy in surgical candidates with solitary, large (>1 cm) or invasive tumors. For patients with metastatic disease involving the liver, surgical resection of tumor foci may reduce symptoms and improve survival. Similarly, selective hepatic artery ligation or embolization has a beneficial effect. Chemotherapy (streptozocin, 5-fluorouracil, cyclophosphamide, and doxorubicin) alone produces a 20% to 40% tumor response rate in patients with disseminated disease. Biologic modifiers, such as leukocyte interferon or the somatostatin analog octreotide, have been of some use.

Prognosis

No reliable survival data are available, as current databases were assembled before the recognition of the different types of lesion. Overall, a survival rate of 93% for 5 years is apparent for patients with local mucosal lesions and those associated with hypergastrinemia. In Type II and especially Type III patients, regional metastases are associated with a 23% survival rate and 0% for patients with distant metastases. Overall, the outcome for the sporadic tumors may be regarded as poor compared with lesions that are purely of ECL cell origin and/or associated with hypergastrinemia that appear to be relatively benign.

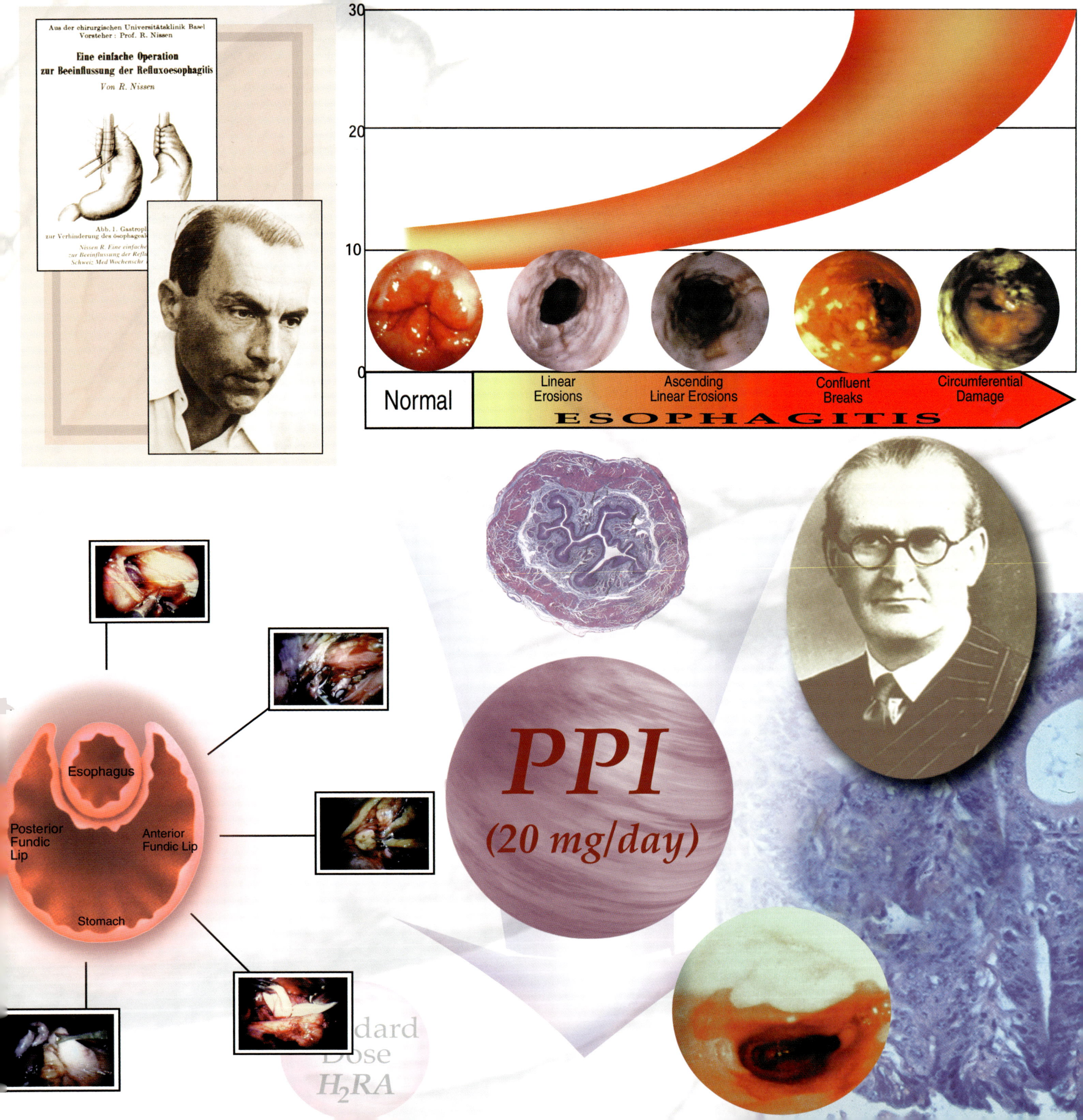

Aus der chirurgischen Universitätsklinik Basel
Vorsteher: Prof. R. Nissen
Eine einfache Operation zur Beeinflussung der Refluxoesophagitis
Von R. Nissen
30
20
10
0
Normal
Linear Erosions
Ascending Linear Erosions
Confluent Breaks
Circumferential Damage
ESOPHAGITIS
Esophagus
Posterior Fundic Lip
Anterior Fundic Lip
Stomach
PPI
(20 mg/day)
H2RA

Chapter IX

GASTROESOPHAGEAL REFLUX DISEASE

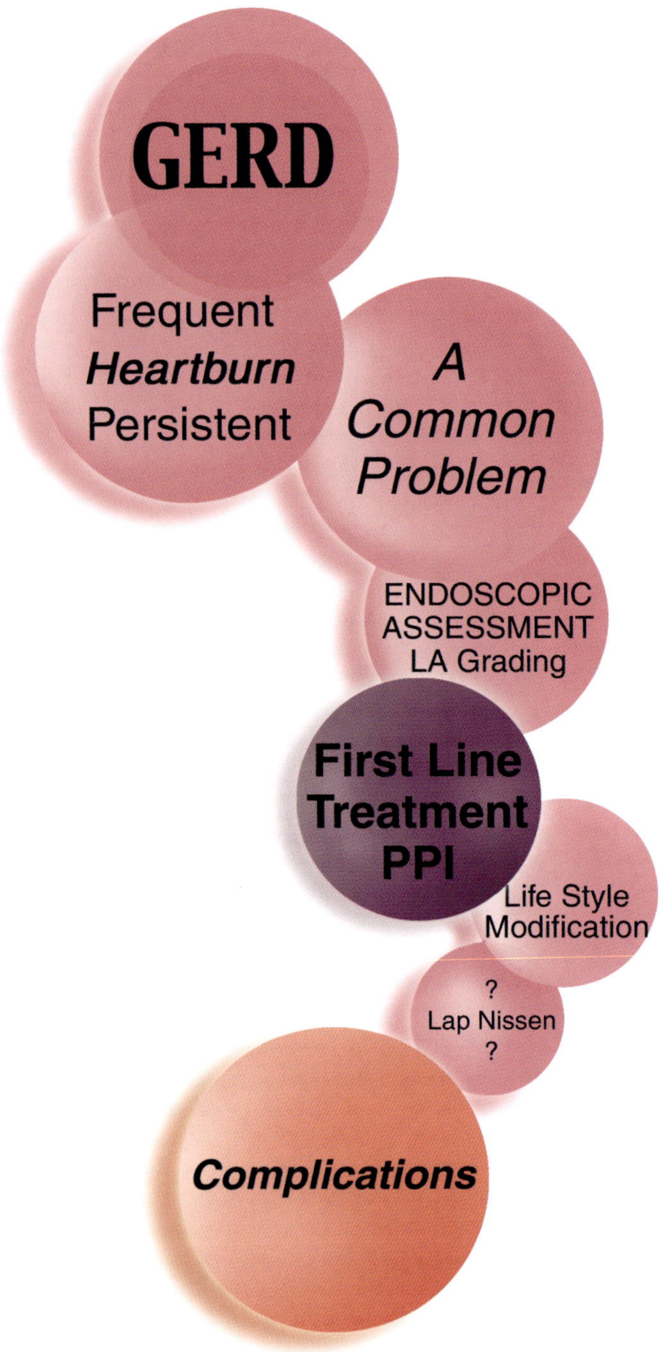
GERD
Frequent
Heartburn
Persistent
A
Common
Problem
ENDOSCOPIC
ASSESSMENT
LA Grading
First Line
Treatment
PPI
Life Style
Modification
?
Lap Nissen
?
Complications

Chapter IX

GASTROESOPHAGEAL REFLUX DISEASE

Introduction

Gastroesophageal reflux disease (GERD) refers to all symptoms, manifestations, and complications from gastroesophageal reflux. Reflux disease is often considered to be present when heartburn persistently occurs on 2 or more days a week. When heartburn is the major or sole symptom experienced by a patient, gastroesophageal reflux is the cause in at least 75% of patients, and heartburn itself is the most common symptom of reflux disease. Frequent, persistent heartburn that occurs in the absence of definitive endoscopic abnormality (esophagitis) is still most likely due to gastroesophageal reflux disease. The precise meaning of heartburn involves semiotic and semantic connotations that vary widely among patient groups depending upon ethnic and social background. In general, however, the description of the symptom of heartburn as "a burning feeling rising from the stomach or lower chest upward towards the neck" is broadly accepted as descriptive of the symptom. "True" dyspeptic symptoms, as defined by the "Rome Criteria," may be produced by gastroesophageal reflux. However, upper abdominal and lower retrosternal symptoms that are consistently relieved by antacids may be due to reflux disease even in the absence of chronic peptic ulcer and evidence of definite reflux esophagitis. The majority of reflux symptoms occur predominantly after food intake, although a subset of patients more commonly experiences nocturnal symptoms.

The diagnosis of GERD is based upon recognition of the characteristic symptom complex or confirmation by endoscopy of definite esophageal mucosal breaks (erosion or ulceration). The term *endoscopy-negative reflux* disease should be reserved for patients who satisfy the clinical definition of GERD but at endoscopy exhibit no mucosal breaks, or only minor changes such as erythema, edema, or friability. The intensity and the frequency of reflux-induced symptoms are poor predictors of the presence or severity of endoscopic mucosal breaks (erosion or ulceration).

The dominant mechanism responsible for reflux disease is the exposure of the esophageal mucosa to acid and pepsin. In the majority of patients there has been abnormally prolonged exposure of the distal esophagus to acid and pepsin. In a small number of patients, normal levels of reflux of acid and pepsin trigger reflux induced symptoms that may reflect increased esophageal sensitivity (tender esophagus).

The increasing incidence of GERD and the major focus on its medical management represent one of the most remarkable scenarios in gastroenterology in the last decade. From its being a mere curiosity, understanding, diagnosing, and treating esophagitis has become one of the great challenges of the new millennium. Although first reported by Albert in 1839, and described as peptic ulcer of the esophagus by 1906, Tilestone could identify

Figure 1. Experimental evidence has demonstrated a clear correlation between the severity of esophagitis and the amount of acid to which the esophagus is exposed.

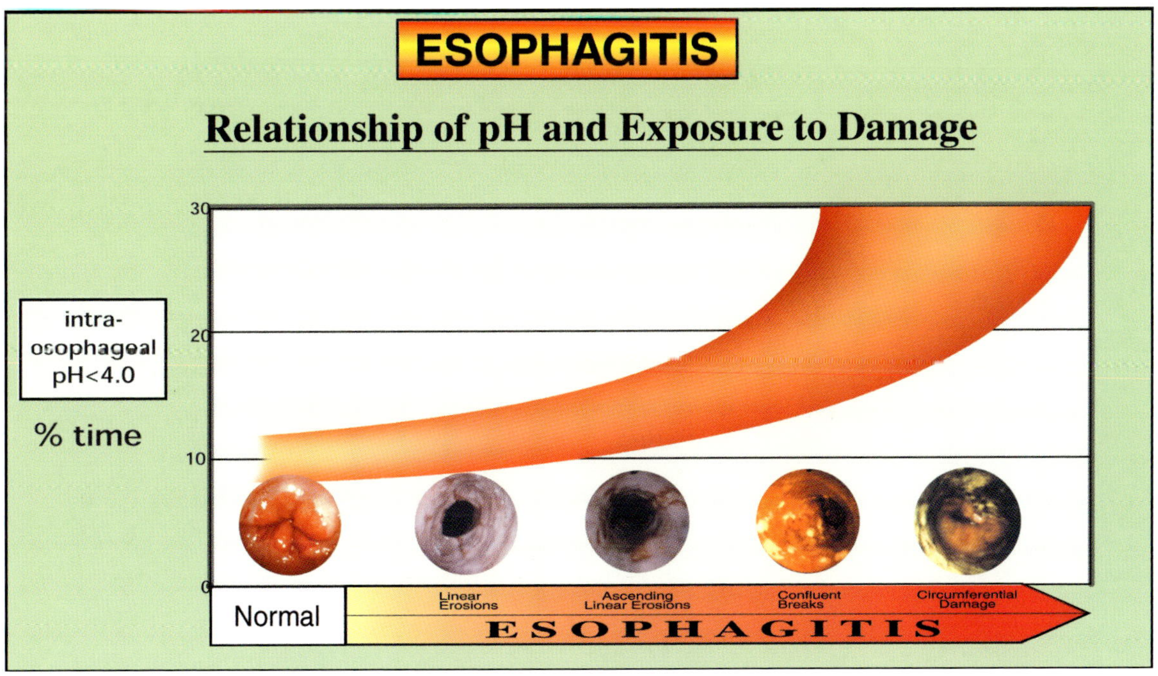

no more than eight patients with the disorder. The disease was so rare and obscure that in 1926 Von Hacker could collect only 91 cases while Stewart, 3 years later detected one esophageal ulcer in 10,000 autopsies. In Philadelphia, Chevalier Jackson reviewed 4000 consecutive esophagoscopies in 1929 and identified 88 examples (21 active and 67 healed) of esophagitis. Of particular interest was the observation in 1929 by Friedenwald that esophageal ulcers healed rapidly if hydrochloric acid was withheld from the lesion. The alteration in incidence and recognition of this disease process in the remainder of the century has been remarkable.

In recent years, there has been an increased awareness among both patients and doctors of the increasing prevalence of GERD. It has been estimated at least 10% of the US population persistently experiences at least twice weekly symptoms associated with the disease. The incidence of diagnosis appears to be increasing in a linear fashion in countries that are generally thought of as first world, whereas in less developed areas, the disease is still relatively rare. Current information suggests that the disease has increased significantly in some areas and has raised the specter of a similar increase in Barrett's esophagus and adenocarcinoma. This increase in diagnosis and awareness has been associated with recent changes in the availability of effective pharmacologic and surgical treatments and an increasing knowledge of some of the basic mechanisms underlying gastroesophageal reflux.

Symptoms

Esophageal

The spectrum of complaints in individuals with gastroesophageal reflux ranges from occasional heartburn to increasing degrees of esophageal injury with associated progressive lower sphincter dysfunction. Although up to 40% of adults complain of at least occasional heartburn, only 2% demonstrate erosive esophagitis. Complications may be more likely to develop in patients with erosive esophagitis and include ulcer, hemorrhage, or stricture. Of increasing concern is the complication of Barrett's esophagus, occurring in 5%–20% of patients with GERD who are selected for endoscopy, and the predisposition to the development of esophageal adenocardinoma. The latter disease is one of the fastest growing categories of cancer in the United States, with a threefold increase during 1983 to 1987 as compared with 1973 to 1977.

Symptomatic GERD is a chronic disease requiring long-term management in most patients. Before the introduction of the two classes of gastric acid inhibitory agents — H2-receptor antagonists and PPIs — treatment exhibited a bias toward surgical management. The safety and efficacy of antisecretory drugs resulted in more reliance on medical therapy to avoid potential complications of surgery. Relapse continues to be the significant concern in the pharmacologic management of patients with GERD; more than 80% relapse within 6 months after the cessation of therapy, and long-term drug therapy is usually necessary. The introduction of minimally invasive surgery has engendered considerable enthusiasm, although there is limited experience with laparoscopic antireflux procedures. Although it is widely believed among surgeons that a laparoscopic procedure combines the potential of excellent long-term results with low morbidity and mortality, only 6 years have elapsed since its introduction. Neither its safety nor its long-term efficacy is as yet fully determined, although it is clear that if performed by an inexperienced operator, life-threatening complications may ensue.

__Figure 2.__ — The prevalence of GERD varies considerably from country to country and reflects not only the level to which subjective symptomatology is investigated but the psyche of the population and its physicians. Overall, it may range from less than 1% in Senegal to almost 23% in the United Kingdom. Gastroesophageal reflux disease is now the most common upper gastrointestinal disorder in the Western world. Thus, 7% to 10% of the adult population may report daily heartburn, whereas 30% to 40% of patients complain of symptoms of the disease on a monthly basis.

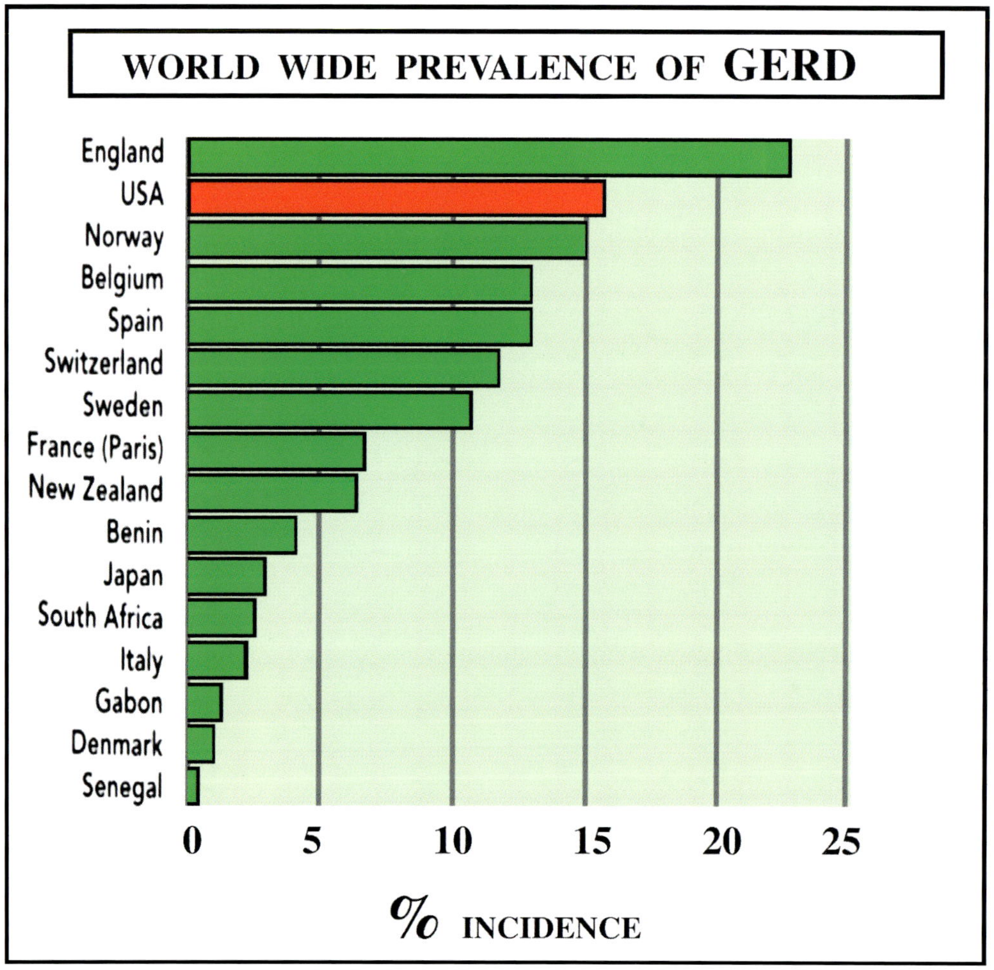

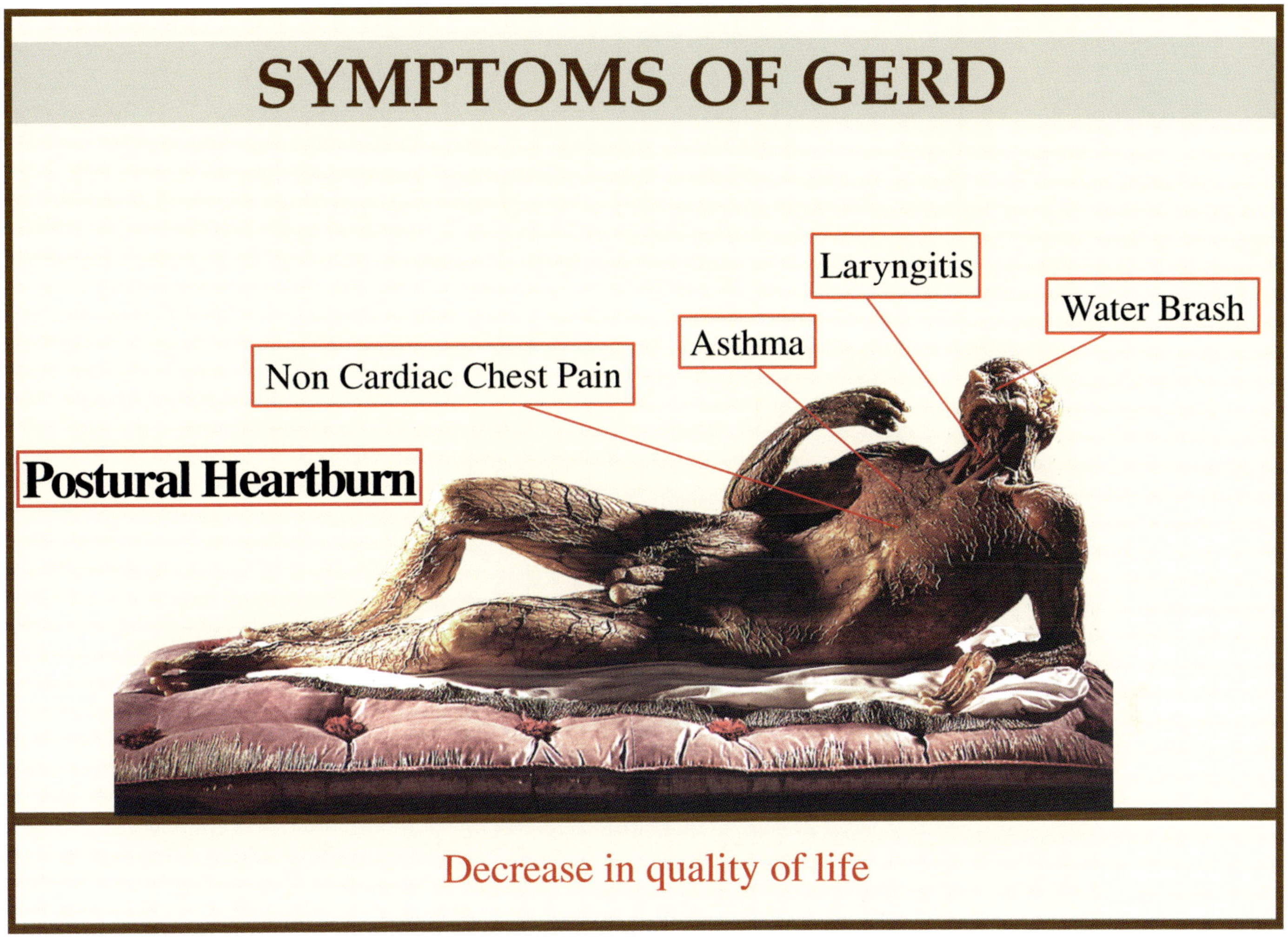

Figure 3. *— The symptoms of GERD commonly involve postural or nocturnal heartburn accentuated by certain foods such as coffee, chocolate, and alcohol. It is, however, apparent that problems, such as asthma and laryngitis—which are less well recognized as GERD-related events—can be important components of this disease spectrum. Noncardiac chest pain may also be a significant presentation in some patients.*

Nonesophageal

Although the majority of patients with GERD present with heartburn and related symptoms, an increasing percentage are now recognized to exhibit other symptoms. Atypical or noncardiac chest pain was identified as an additional presenting feature of GERD; now asthma-like symptoms, are also noted. A third group of symptoms includes ear, nose, and throat complaints, of which laryngitis may be the most common.

Noncardiac Chest Pain

Up to 20% to 30% of patients undergoing coronary angiography have been shown to have normal studies; their chest pain has been noncardiac in origin. Acid reflux has been identified in 40% to 45% of this group, and episodes of chest pain correlate with reflux episodes. In some circumstances, both coronary artery disease and reflux may occur in the same patient and require both Holter monitoring as well as pHmetry for identification. Acid infusion or the Bernstein test has proved to be relatively insensitive in establishing the diagnosis and has been replaced by esophageal pH monitoring.

Asthma

William Osler first remarked upon the association between asthma and a distended stomach a century ago, but it is only recently that the etiology has become apparent. The frequency of the association of GERD and asthma varies between 34% to 89% and it has been estimated that as many as 20% of adults have intermittent bronchospasm that may be associated with reflux. Clearly, the potential benefits of identifying a subgroup of patients with respiratory complaints whose disease is initiated by GERD is of considerable clinical relevance.

At least two mechanisms are operative in the interface between GERD and asthma. The most commonly accepted cause is microaspiration of gastric contents, but it has been proposed that a vagally mediated reflex exists whereby acid reflux into the lower esophagus initiates bronchoconstriction. The genesis of this condition represents a shared autonomic innervation between the esophagus and the bronchi based upon their common embryonic origin. Two lines of evidence support this proposal. Acid infusion of the esophagus in asthmatic children results in antacid-reversible increase in airway resistance. Also, the infusion of acid into the distal esophagus of sleeping asthmatic children induces bronchoconstriction.

Although the relationship between acid reflux and GERD can be identified by a barium esophagogram, upper gastrointestinal (GI) endoscopy, and esophageal manometry, the most useful study is pH monitoring. Increased acid reflux can be identified in more than 50% of asthmatics and may occur in 70% to 80%. Other factors are clearly involved in the genesis of asthma, as in about 50% of wheezing episodes no relationship to reflux can be established. However, many patients who have undergone fundoplication procedures were cured or significantly improved.

Laryngitis

This association is now common and particularly relevant in patients who do not respond to standard management by otolaryngologists. Patients may present with hoarseness, chronic cough, throat clearing, chronic laryngitis, and globus. Less common but well-described symptoms include vocal-cord granulomas, laryngeal or tracheal stenosis, and carcinoma of the larynx. The typical signs and symptoms of GERD may only be evident in 40% of such persons. In some circumstances, otolaryngologic complaints may be the sole manifestation of GERD. Thus, 10% of patients with persistent cough, 5% to 10% of patients with hoarseness, some patients with globus sensation, and a small number of patients with laryngeal neoplasia have GERD. At least four mechanisms have been proposed to explain this relationship: (1) a vagally mediated reflex, whereby acid in the lower esophagus mediates a response that involves chronic repetitive throat clearing and coughing that culminates in laryngeal symptoms and finally lesions; (2) aspiration of refluxate directly onto the laryngeal structures with ensuing inflammation and damage, which may be associated with decreased upper esophageal sphincter (UES) pressure and reflux into the pharynx; (3) decreased UES pressure at night with esophagopharyngeal reflux; and (4) esophageal motility disorders, which may be present in up to 60% of persons with persistent ear, nose, and throat symptoms (up to 80% may have abnormal acid clearance from the lower esophagus).

Once the otolaryngologic diagnosis has been established, the existence of GERD needs to be validated. Prolonged esophageal pH monitoring with a dual pH probe system (one in the hypopharynx or just below the UES and a second probe at the lower esophageal sphincter) is the most sensitive and specific method for diagnosing GERD-related otolaryngologic disease. Proximal pH monitoring is difficult, as the probes may dry out, or, in the large hypopharyngeal space, reflux may actually be missed.

The Genesis of Esophagitis

Esophagitis should be regarded as a mucosal inflammatory disease secondary to mechanical events that infringe upon the function (competency) of the lower esophageal sphincter. The high relapse and recurrence rate of GERD can be predicted based on the fact that the majority of current therapy is directed at dealing with the consequences (acid reflux) of sphincteric dysfunction—the pathology (inflammation/pain) and its healing rather than the actual etiology. Overall, the latter probably represents an as yet inadequately characterized mechanical or electrical phenomenon, possibly of gastric (pacemaker) origin. This is possibly analogous to a cardiac rhythm disturbance with pump failure (delayed gastric emptying) and consequent lower esophageal sphincter (LES) incompetence. The pathogenesis of GERD probably does not lend itself to reductionist thinking. Integration of both anatomic and physiologic studies of the gastroesophageal junction suggest the multifactorial nature of the anatomic disruption of the diaphragmatic hiatus, the physiologic dysfunction of the LES, and the resulting disease: esophagitis and GERD. Once reflux has occurred, the degree of mucosal damage reflects a number of variables: the ability of the esophagus to clear the reflux, the precise nature of the refluxate, and the degree of mucosal resistance. There is evidence to support a direct correlation between the exposure of the esophagus to acid and the severity of GERD. Thus, persons with severe disease exhibit longer and more frequent reflux episodes, with the consequence that their esophageal pH remains below 4 for significantly greater periods of time than those patients with milder forms of GERD.

Mechanisms

Gastric

The stomach itself is an important variable in determining GERD, and, in many patients delayed gastric emptying is not only demonstrable but the gastric emptying rate can be related to the degree of esophageal damage. Some authorities have even proposed that the entire disease process may be a consequence of disordered gastric motility. Under such circumstances, a decrease in the rate of gastric emptying, coupled with an increase in both duodenogastric reflux and the volume of gastric contents, may be critical variables in the establishment and maintenance of GERD.

Patients with GERD who are resistant to medical therapy have been demonstrated to display delayed gastric emptying of solids more often than those who respond well to treatment. In this respect, the motor function of the corpus fundus region of the stomach is little understood despite the fact that the area adjacent to the LES is primarily responsible for the regulation of intragastric pressure by modulating gastric accommodation. A loss of the regulatory interaction between the gastric fundus and the lower esophageal area that involves alteration in the function of the LES might easily therefore be a critical component of the initiating pathogenesis of this disease process. Patients with GERD exhibit a lower LES pressure response after fundic distension compared with healthy controls. Under such circumstances, delayed gastric emptying would facilitate gastroesophageal reflux.

Figure 4. — *In some patients with gastroesophageal reflux disease, there is the development of complications that are problematic for the patient and pose major management problems for the physician.*

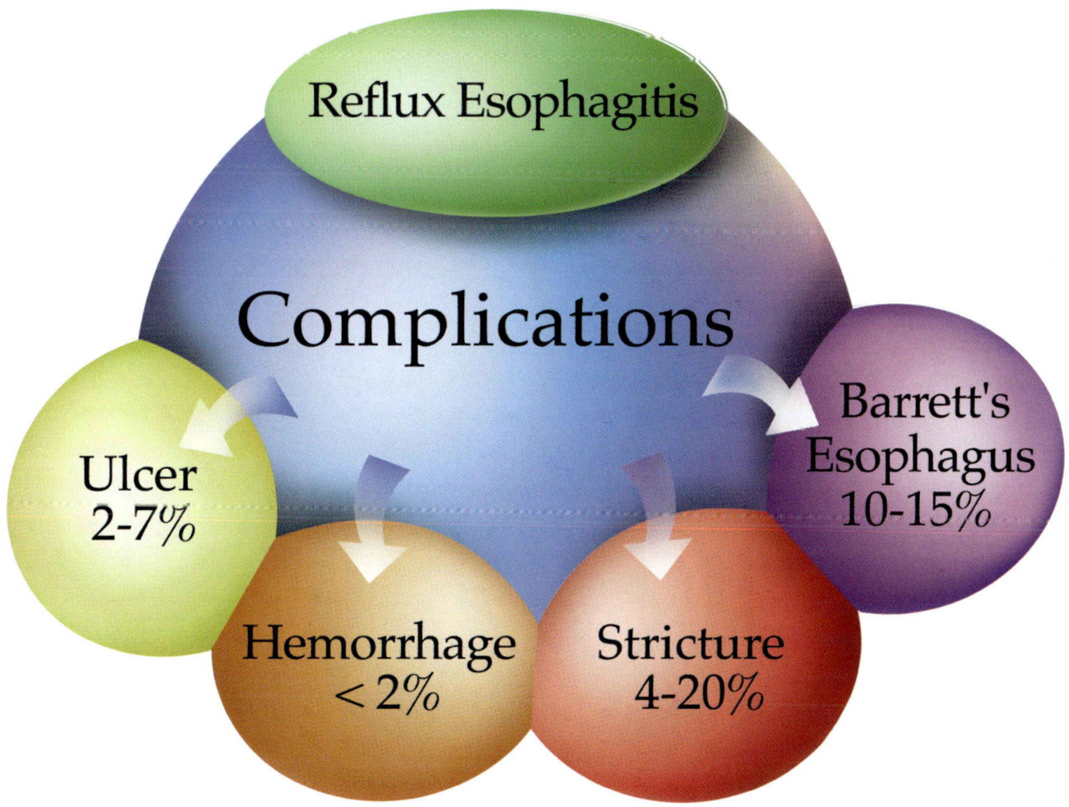

Although the stomach has a highly developed capacity (a specialized apical cell membrane and complex tight junction mechanism) to withstand low pH, a stratified squamous epithelial barrier that lacks tight junctions maintains esophageal integrity. Thus, the ability of the esophagus to withstand the presence of barrier-breaking agents — such as acid, pepsin, and, occasionally, bile — is modest. Additional protection is afforded by the secretion of glands in the lower third as well as the presence of esophageal "stripping" waves, whereby refluxate is readily and efficiently cleared from the esophagus back into the stomach. In the presence of decreased LES pressure, decreased clearance of lower esophageal contents, delayed gastric emptying, and diminution of barrier function, inflammatory sequelae are liable to occur in the lower esophagus. Because the stratified squamous epithelium of the lower esophagus does not have either the tight junctions or the apical barrier properties of the gastric mucosa, damage culminates in inflammation that is relatively resistant to healing. In fact, the pH of the lower esophagus needs to be significantly greater than that in the duodenum or stomach to ensure healing.

As a result of recurrent episodes of inflammation with incomplete healing, a loss of esophageal glands with the development of scar tissue occurs in some patients. An inexorable accentuation of the damage in these patients may result in a healing/damage cycle with alteration in the phenotype of the mucosa toward a columnar epithelium predominance and culminates in intestinal metaplasia (Barrett's esophagus). It is likely that the interface between the squamous epithelium of the esophagus and the columnar epithelium of the stomach represents a junctional zone with a degree of instability and even susceptibility to damage. The failure to generate a stabilized scar or regenerate healthy epithelium engenders a locus minoris resistentiae, which is more vulnerable and hence susceptible to further damage. Under such circumstances, the relapsing pattern and chronicity of GERD are predictable.

Lower Esophageal Sphincter

A prerequisite for the development of GERD is the passage of acid and pepsin from the stomach into the esophagus. Under normal circumstances, gastroesophageal reflux is prevented by a competent LES. Mechanically, the gastroesophageal junction is required to protect against reflux in both static and dynamic conditions, and failure to adequately prevent reflux is associated with both the initiation of GERD as well as relapse and chronicity.

The gastroesophageal junction is a complex physiologic sphincter composed of at least two anatomic elements: a diaphragmatic element and the smooth-muscle LES. Several mechanisms may engender dysfunction and render the area vulnerable. The functional integrity of this antireflux barrier has been variably attributed to intrinsic LES pressure, extrinsic compression of the LES by the crural diaphragm, intra-abdominal location of the LES, integrity of the phrenoesophageal (PE) ligament, and maintenance of the angle of entry of esophagus into the stomach (His). It is probable that competence of this barrier is attributable to more than one of these factors and that incompetence becomes increasingly severe as more mechanisms are compromised.

At this time, there are three theories that consider gastroesophageal junction incompetence or variations thereof as the critical issue in the genesis of GERD: excessive transient LES relaxation episodes, a hypotensive LES without any accompanying anatomic abnormality, or an anatomic disruption of the junction by hiatal hernia. It has been proposed that the dominant mechanism may vary as a function of severity of disease or possibly even be a determinant. Thus, transient LES relaxations may predominate in mild disease, whereas mechanisms associated with a hiatal hernia or weak sphincter may be more prevalent in patients with more severe disease.

The LES is a 3- to 4-cm segment of tonically contracted smooth muscle at the distal end of the esophagus. Resting tone varies between 10 and as much as 45 mm in normal persons and may be least in the postcibal period and greatest at night. Intra-abdominal pressure, gastric distension, peptides, hormones, various foods, and many drugs affect this pressure. LES tonic contraction itself is a property of both the surrounding muscle and the extrinsic innervation. Anatomically, the proximal margin of the LES may be effectively about 1.5 cm above the Z line, which is in close proximity to the PE. In contrast, the distal margin may be about 2 cm distal to the Z line, bounded inferiorly by the angle of His. The resultant is a segment whose distal portion herniates through the hiatus as a consequence of esophageal shortening, with the formation of the phrenic ampulla.

The crural diaphragm encircling the LES serves a sphincteric function. The diaphragm appears to augment the LES during transient periods of increased intra-abdominal pressure (eg, inspiration, coughing). Electrical and mechanical inhibition of the crural diaphragm has been demonstrated during transient LES relaxations. The concept of the intrinsic pressure zone, augmented by an extrinsic system, has enabled consideration of a dual mechanism known as the two-sphincter hypothesis of gastroesophageal junction competence.

The delineation of the mechanisms that are responsible for maintaining the LES contracted, yet allowing for transient relaxation during a swallow, are critical for the elucidation of the pathogenesis of GERD. As electrical stimulation of the LES leads to relaxation, it was initially proposed that cholinergic nerves controlled the LES. However, in humans, vagotomy does not in general alter tone. Subsequently, gastrin was considered as the modulator, but as none of the classical neurotransmitters or peptide hormones currently studied account for all LES tone, the sphincter has been regarded as possessing an inherent myogenic tone. Regulation of this "tone" has been variably attributed to nitric oxide, prostaglandins, leukotrienes, and a variety of arachidonic acid metabolites.

The clinical problem is best characterized by the loss of an efficient reflux barrier that results in the retrograde passage of gastric contents into the esophagus. Although the mean basal pressure of the LES is significantly lower in patients with GERD, especially in those with severe esophagitis, there is significant overlap between normal patients and patients with GERD. Transient inappropriate episodes of LES relaxation, not associated with swallowing, may be responsible for GERD in some patients with mild-to-moderate disease. The spectrum of

Figure 5. — The esophagus, stomach, and duodenum ideally act as a one-way system for the transit of food into the rest of the gastrointestinal tract. The stomach functions as reservoir and pump. Gastric peristalsis results in an increase in pressure, whereby the valve constituted by the pylorus opens at a lower pressure than the lower esophageal sphincter (LES). The gastric pacemaker initiates pressure waves directed toward the pyloric valve, further ensuring that food mixed with acid and pepsin exits from the gastric pump/reservoir in an aboral fashion. The reflux of gastric contents into the esophagus is an abnormal situation and generally has been accepted as reflective of failure of the esophageal valve component of the system. The failure of the pylorus to relax appropriately or the gastric peristaltic wave to be coordinated with the function of both sphincters may also play a part in the genesis of the reflux scenario. Under such circumstances, the LES, which normally opens intermittently to permit food to enter the stomach, exhibits an inability to remain closed as gastric pressure increases to force food toward the pylorus, through it, and into the duodenum. In mechanical terms (iatromathematical), reflux represents leakage of the proximal LES valve system of a one-way cycling pump (the stomach). As a result of failure of either motility coordination and/or valve competency, noxious agents (acid/pepsin) are delivered into the lower esophagus for varying periods. Under such circumstances, it may be predicted that once a certain degree of damage has been inflicted upon the lower esophageal mucosa, therapy with acid suppression is only able to suppress symptomatology and maintain or stabilize the damage and scar already present. In this respect, medical therapy, although successful in facilitating healing, can do little more than maintain a steady state, whereas the motor abnormalities of the stomach, pyloric valve, and LES persist.

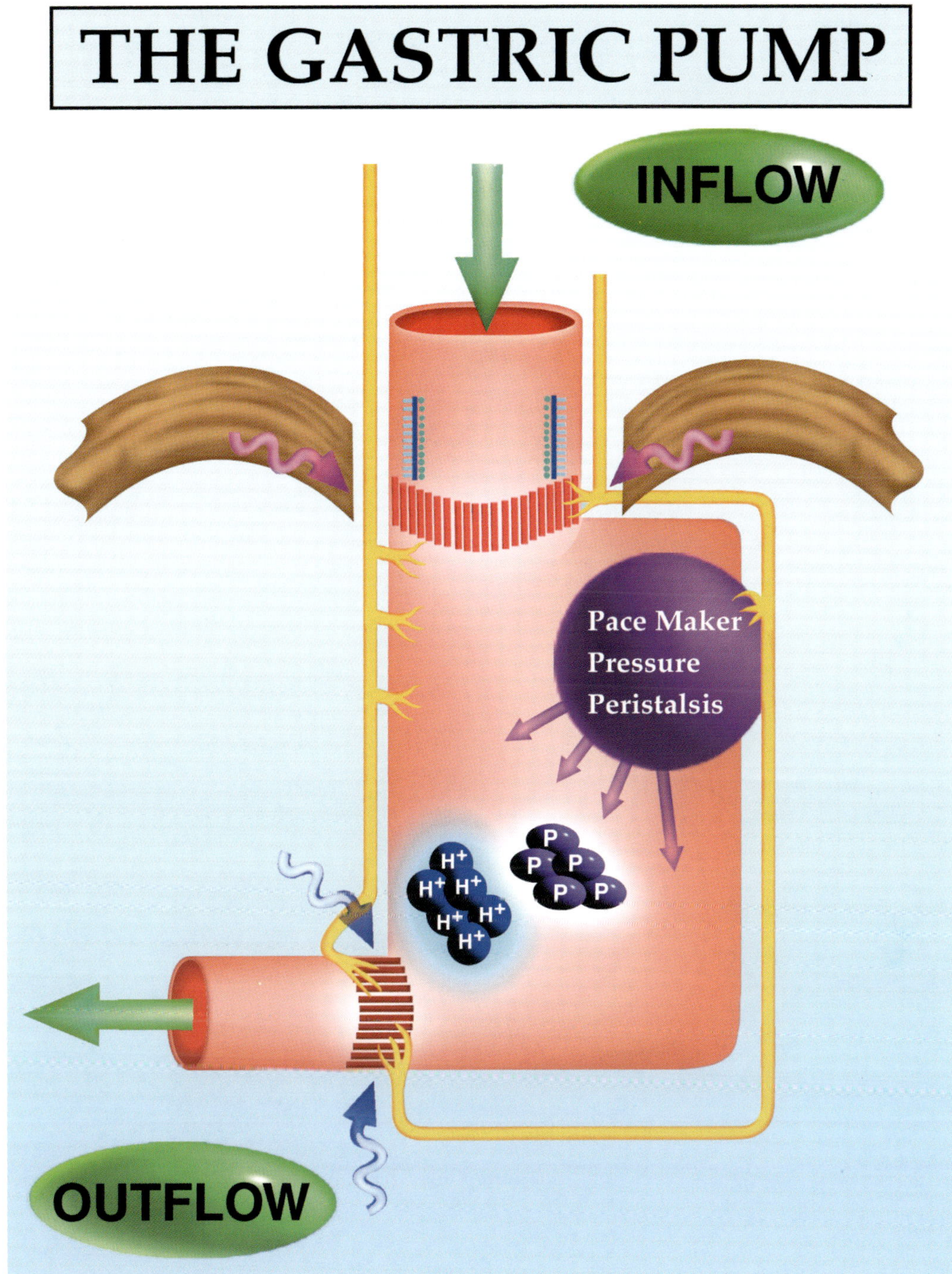

alterations in LES pressure, however, is wide. Thus, in some circumstances, basal LES pressure may be normal but the number of transient inappropriate LES relaxations abnormally high. Alternatively, in some patients, a persistent but as yet uncharacterized defect of LES control is associated with permanent low resting sphincter pressure and almost constant reflux. Indeed, in up to 80% of patients with GERD, reflux episodes are associated with transient LES relaxation. The precise regulation of transient spontaneous relaxation of the LES is unknown but includes vagal pathways, gastrin and cholecystokinin, nitric oxide, VIP, acetylcholine, and serotonin.

It seems likely that LES relaxations account for the majority of reflux events in normal persons and in patients with normal LES pressure at the time of reflux. Transient lower esophageal relaxations probably represent a physiologic response to gastric distension by food or gas and is the primary mechanism responsible for gastric gas venting. Acid reflux (at the same time) would therefore appear to be an associated phenomenon. Investigations suggest that the functional LES consists of integrated motor responses involving not only LES relaxation, but also crural diaphragmatic inhibition and contraction of the costal diaphragm. They appear to occur without an associated pharyngeal contraction, are unaccompanied by esophageal peristalsis, and persist for longer periods (>10 seconds) than do swallow-induced LES relaxations. Thus, not all LES relaxations are accompanied by reflux.

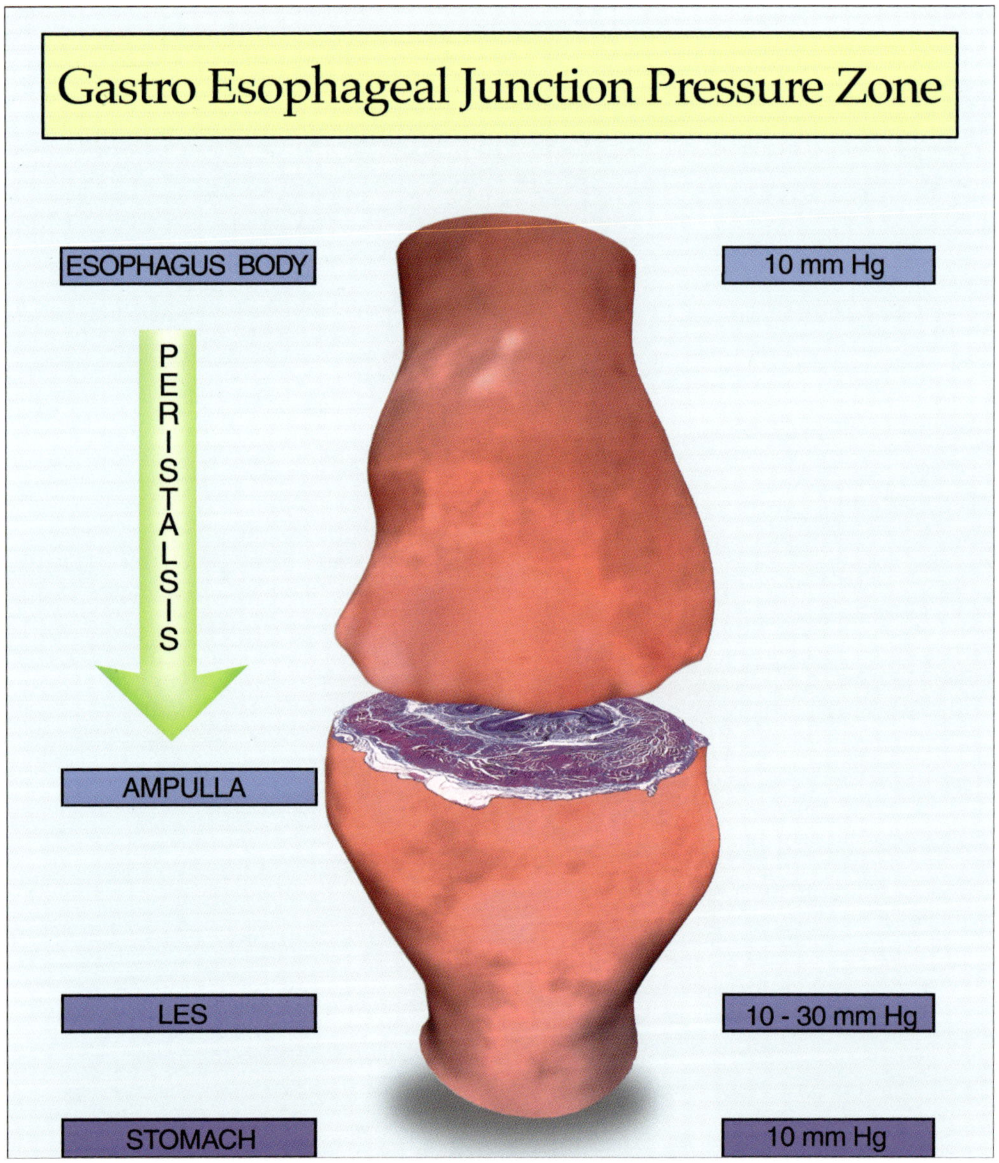

Figure 6. *— A diagram of the gastroesophageal junction pressure zone with a cross-section of the esophageal lumen illustrating the dynamic peristaltic mechanism of the ampulla. The descending esophageal peristaltic wave creates an ampullary bolus at the LES that on relaxation allows the high pressure zone of the ampulla to propel swallowed food into the stomach. The presence of a hiatal hernia and reflux creates a pressure zone disturbance that interferes with ampullary emptying. This enables the development of an "esophageal acid containing space" above the "crural sphincter" and facilitates the development of esophagitis.*

Esophageal Ampulla

The esophagus is normally a collapsed, empty tube. During swallowing, transient phrenic ampulla form as a consequence of physiologic herniation associated with longitudinal muscle contraction during peristalsis. The process of esophageal emptying slows significantly with formation of the phrenic ampulla from about 3 cm per second, characteristic of peristalsis, to about 1 cm per second. The ampulla appear to form as a result of longitudinal shortening of the esophagus, thus forming a closed chamber, bound above by the distal esophagus and below by crural diaphragm. Because the LES moves about 2 cm with each swallow, an important part of its anatomic stabilization is the elastic recoil provided by the PE ligament. Emptying of the ampulla occurs in conjunction with relengthening of the esophagus. These mechanistic descriptions have anatomic implications. There appears to be a sequential activation of esophageal longitudinal muscle with progression of the peristaltic contraction. It is possible that each longitudinal section is subsequently reelongated by contraction of the adjacent distal segment. The distal end of the esophagus is anchored to the diaphragm by the PE membrane, formed by the fused endothoracic and endoabdominal fascia. The PE membrane has elastic properties and inserts circumferentially into the esophageal musculature close to the squamocolumnar junction, normally residing within the esophageal hiatus. Thus, the PE ligament is stretched with each swallow and its elastic recoil is responsible for pulling the squamocolumnar junction back to its normal position after shortening. This repetitive stress subjects the PE ligament to substantial wear and tear, making it a plausible target of age-related degeneration.

A number of discrete observations have provided evidence to suggest that hiatal hernias may play a significant pathogenetic role in up to 50% of instances of GERD. It would appear that hiatal hernias constitute only an aberration from normal anatomy, based on the concept of the well-documented physiologic herniation observed during swallowing. It has been proposed that the PE membrane, which is stretched during each peristaltic contraction, gradually loses its elasticity with the passage of years. As the PE membrane weakens, the extent of herniation during swallowing gradually increases, with the resultant sequelae. Under such circumstances, it is plausible that large hernias may impair the normal process of esophageal emptying, thereby prolonging the clearance time of acid and increasing the mucosal acidification exposure time of the esophagus, particularly in the recumbent position. Therefore, hiatal hernias, although not an initiating factor in GERD, may be considered as providing a significant contribution to the chronicity of the disease. A critical issue, however, is the need to think in more precise terms in regard to the identification of the hiatal hernia itself. Thus axial length both at rest and during distention need to be evaluated as well as the competence of the diaphragmatic hiatus.

GERD may be due to an extremely hypotensive sphincter, but it is now understood that this abnormality is rare and that most GERD is probably due to spontaneous but excessively prolonged (30- to 60-second) relaxation of the LES. The stimulus for these prolonged relaxations may be distention of the fundus — for example, by large meals — and perhaps by signals from the pharynx. Patients with chronic reflux may have numerous episodes of these prolonged relaxations: even up to 12 per hour. It is also apparent that transient LES incompetence is more common with increased age. In this respect, hiatal hernia is again thought to have a role

The Esophageal Gland System

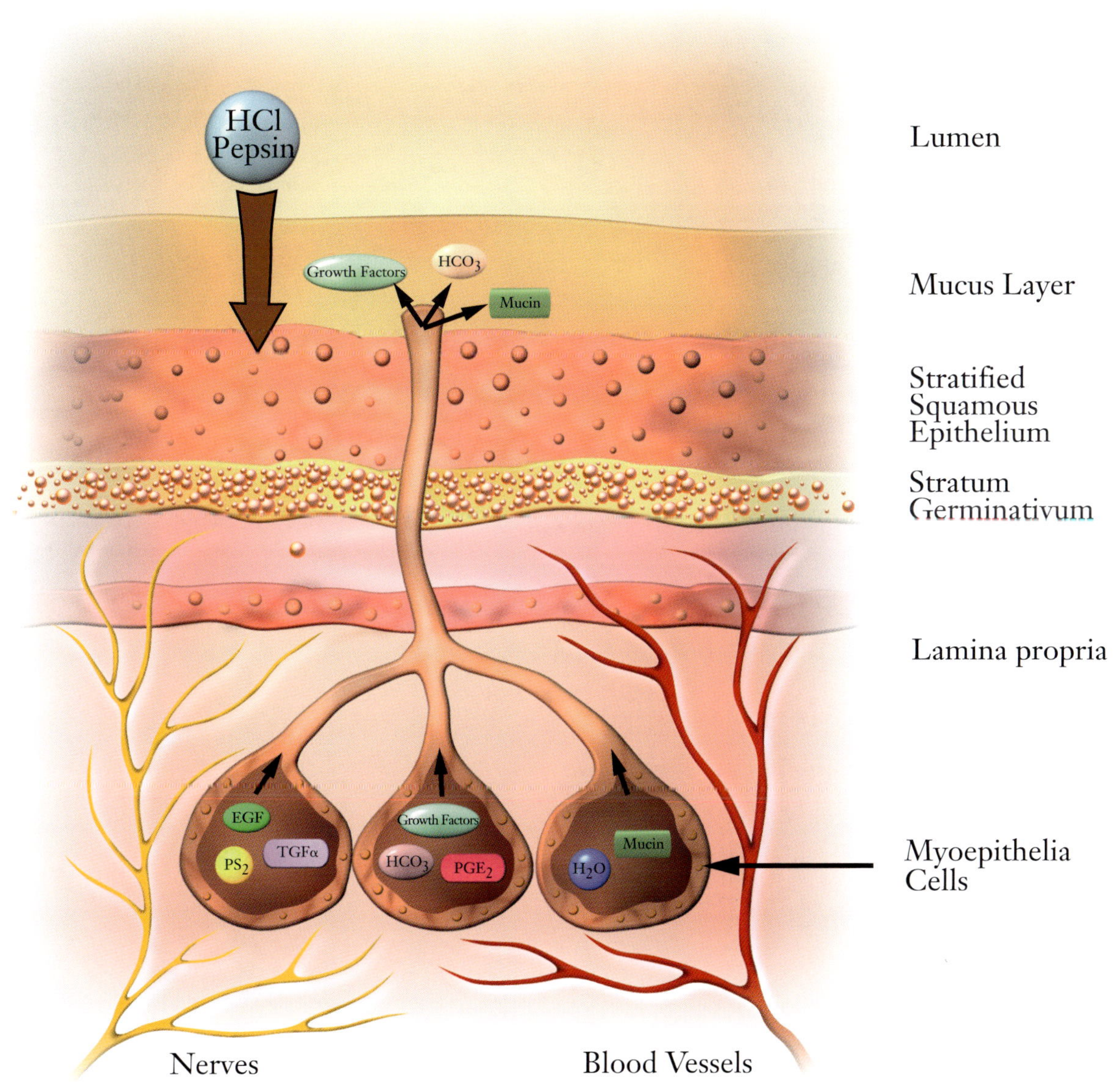

Figure 7. — Although the esophagus is lined by squamous epithelium, the presence of esophageal glands at its lower end may be of clinicopathologic relevance in determining the response to damage and the development of chronicity. It is probable that these glands function as a component of the protective and healing mechanism necessary to restore structural integrity after reflux-induced damage. Destruction of the glands after repeated episodes of esophagitis renders the epithelium even more vulnerable to damage, results in inadequate repair, and the subsequent development of fibrotic scar tissue as opposed to healthy epithelial regeneration.

in the development of GERD. Thus, the age-related increase in prevalence of hiatal hernias that are capable of interfering with normal gastric mechanoreception in the fundus may lead to delayed gastric emptying of solids and overdistention of the stomach.

When placed in the esophagus, more than 90% of acid is cleared into the stomach by a rapid peristalsis, but the other 10% is cleared more slowly by saliva and other host defenses. Most diseases of the esophagus, including GERD, do not cause a loss of peristalsis but do reduce the amplitude of the contractions of the fast peristaltic phase. A hiatal hernia may thus interfere with normal peristaltic waves, and therefore prevent complete acid clearance, because acid can become trapped in the hiatal pouch.

Esophageal Epithelium

The junctions between the squamous epithelial cells lining the esophagus differ from the junctions between epithelial cells in other regions of the gastrointestinal tract, where tight junctions link the luminal ends of columnar epithelial cells by a functional "belt" comprising specialized membrane and intracellular proteins such as occludin and Zoo 1. Such tight junctions can be classified based on the number of strands into "tight" and "leaky" tight junctions. The gastric epithelium has tight junctions with as many as 15 adhesive strands of protein. At best, the tight junctions visualized in the first layer of the esophageal epithelium contain approximately two strands and are extremely leaky. In the stratified squamous epithelium of the esophagus, adjacent epithelial cells are joined more loosely by desmosomes (gap junctions), connected by intracellular intermediate filaments. The barrier function of the cells lining the esophagus is therefore normally dependent not upon tight junctions but by the multiplicity of cell layers comprising the stratified epithelium and the intercellular spaces between these cell layers. The esophagus may be considered as analogous to "wet skin" and in this respect even behave in a similar fashion when damaged. In GERD, the spaces between squamous epithelial cells enlarge, thereby perhaps allowing luminal contents more access to the submucosa. Whether enlargement of the intercellular space is the primary event or secondary to cell shrinkage is not entirely clear and remains to be determined.

H. pylori

The increase in the reported prevalence of GERD has coincided over the last 50 years or so with a natural decline in *H. pylori* infection in the West. This has led to some speculation that the two may be causally related and that *H. pylori* may have been of some symbiotic benefit to humans. One possible mechanism by which *H. pylori* may influence GERD is through engendering an alteration in acid secretion. Although *H. pylori* increases secretion of acid in patients with duodenal ulcer disease, it may be responsible for decreasing acid secretion in those patients infected early in life who develop gastritis of the gastric corpus. Several lines of evidence support this view. Thus, in Japan the gastric cancer and *H. pylori* rates of incidence have fallen dramatically over the last 20 years, and there has been an associated increase in gastric acid secretion in the population, as well as an increasing recognition of GERD. It has been reported that the eradication of *H. pylori* in a series of subjects with duodenal ulcer disease led to some of them developing GERD for the first time, although this finding remains controversial.

Diagnosis And Management

Overview

Although most patients with GERD present to, and are managed by, general practitioners, some of their care will require referral to gastroenterologists and surgeons. The management of GERD is a continuum, with management based upon not only symptoms, but also referral patterns and, increasingly, financial constraints. The first step in the management of the patient with suspected GERD is a history and physical examination. A history of frequent and persistent retrosternal burning-type chest pain radiating from the epigastrium toward the throat is characteristic of GERD, and such symptoms have a high specificity for the diagnosis. If the patient has either atypical symptoms, or any alarm symptoms such as dysphagia, evidence of gastrointestinal bleeding, unexplained anemia, weight loss, abdominal pain, or pain that does not respond to antacids or first develops symptoms after age 50, referral for endoscopy is recommended.

The majority of patients, particularly those with infrequent symptoms, probably do not require endoscopy initially, and such patients should be counseled in regard to more simple antireflux measures, which may include elevation of the head of the bed, weight loss, and the avoidance of precipitating foods and drugs. Patients should also be advised to take antacids or over-the-counter (OTC) antisecretories at the time of symptoms and to avoid heavy meals late at night or within 3 hours of retiring. If symptoms persist after about 2 weeks of these simple measures, or if antacids or OTC antisecretories are needed often, first-line prescription therapy should be instituted with an H2-receptor antagonist or a PPI.

Endoscopy

Dyspepsia occurs in approximately half of the population, and patients who have reflux symptoms often also have ulcer-like symptoms. The endoscopic evaluation of esophagitis remains an area of both controversy and difficulty. There is no completely satisfactory classification and many schemes vie for widespread acceptance. Even within individual classifications, agreement between the classifiers is not uniform. Although agreement among observers is widespread for severe changes of esophagitis — stricture and erosions — there is often extremely poor agreement among observers for minor changes. As the prevalence of endoscopy-negative reflux disease far outweighs those who have positive endoscopic findings, the precise role of endoscopy in diagnosis needs serious consideration. Given its expense, invasiveness, and relative insensitivity as a diagnostic tool, initial enthusiasm has been replaced by skepticism. A once-in-a-lifetime endoscopy, toward the beginning of treatment rather than later, is possibly a useful maneuver, if only to rule out Barrett's esophagus or other unexpected lesions. However, repeated endoscopy in a patient with uncomplicated GERD is probably not indicated unless Barrett's esophagus has been verified. In such patients, cost-effectiveness analyses have suggested that surveillance should be performed every 5 years in the absence of epithelial dysplasia, although given the current reduction in endoscopy costs in the United States, the financial equation may change in favor of more frequent evaluation.

Figure 8. *— An easily applicable, universally acceptable, and simple grading system for esophagitis is necessary to facilitate identification of the severity of the disease and enable comparable assessment of the efficacy of therapeutic intervention. An alternative system of considerable utility is the Los Angeles classification, which although somewhat complex allows for a more detailed and precise evaluation of the extent of the disease process.*

ESOPHAGITIS

The Los Angeles Classification

GRADE	DESCRIPTION
A	One or more mucosal breaks confined to the mucosals folds, each < 5mm.
B	At least one mucosal break > 5 mm long confined to the mucosal folds, but not continous between the tops of two folds.
C	At least one mucosal break continous between the tops of two or more folds but not circumferential.
D	Circumferential mucosal break.

Health-related quality of life is impaired in patients with GERD. Also, concern about reflux-induced symptoms associated with cancer or heart disease is particularly common among patients who have not had endoscopy. In more than 50% of persons who have had heartburn two or more days per week for 6 months, endoscopic esophageal mucosal breaks are absent. Endoscopy should therefore be regarded as of relatively low sensitivity in the diagnosis of reflux disease. Minor mucosal changes noted on endoscopy — including erythema, edema, and friability — attributed to reflux disease are unreliable in the diagnosis of reflux esophagitis. Endoscopic mucosal biopsy has little if any place in the routine diagnosis of endoscopy-negative reflux disease. There is a poor correlation of biopsy findings with pH monitoring data and the amelioration of typical symptoms responsive to treatment. Nevertheless, endoscopic biopsy is useful in the diagnosis of Barrett's esophagus, as it is the only method capable of providing an acceptable sensitivity for patient management. In this respect, however, the experience and skill of the pathologist is critical.

At the time of endoscopy, particular attention should be paid to the presence of signs of esophagitis, and the relationship of the squamocolumnar epithelial junction to the gastroesophageal junction should be examined carefully. Routine biopsies should not be performed; however, if there is any suspicion of Barrett's esophagus, four-quadrant biopsies should be taken at the gastroesophageal junction and at the proximally displaced squamocolumnar junction. There is some controversy about whether or not gastric biopsies also should be obtained to explore for *H. pylori*. However, as some practitioners believe that *H. pylori* infection is common and, in most circumstances, harmless in this particular clinical context, establishing whether or not *H. pylori* is present may be irrelevant and confusing.

Evaluation of Motility

The detection of reflux and abnormal motility as well as disturbances in gastric emptying can be visualized using fluoroscopy. Although fluoroscopy displays patterns of transit secondary to motor events with excellent resolution, manometry is usually required to define the underlying patterns that may, or may not, be radiologically revealed. Imaging is useful in demonstrating obstruction and reflux but is not particularly effective in identifying "underpowered" peristalsis, which is best delineated using manometric techniques. The identification of reflux events on fluoroscopy can be misleading in the short period of such an examination and requires esophageal pH monitoring and even manometric studies to fully define and confirm the clinical relevance of such events.

Intraluminal pressures in the esophagus may be measured by either water-perfused manometric assemblies connected to external pressure transducers or recording assemblies using intraluminal transducers. The latter technique does not require water perfusion, which is an advantage. However, it is expensive, fragile, and costly to repair. The perfused manometric assemblies are most widely used because of their relative low cost, easy maintenance, and reliable function. They consist of an extrusion with multiple fine channels, each of which opens sideways at the esophageal lumen at different levels, enabling recordings of pressure simultaneously at multiple levels. The measurement of LES relaxation is of particular importance not only in the early diagnosis of achalasia and the assessment of dysphagia following antireflux surgery but to determine the appropriateness of LES contraction and relaxation. Although conditions, such as achalasia or diffuse esophageal spasm, can be easily defined, in some instances a nonspecific motor defect is evident and includes "underpowered" peristalsis, which results in the failure of development of an adequate propulsive force to clear the esophagus.

The identification of a manometric abnormality is important in defining the precise characteristics of GERD in specific patients or when acid suppressive medication fails to provide adequate relief and healing. For those patients who meet the criteria of abnormal LES for elective surgery, manometric evaluation may be useful as a quantitative tool to evaluate potential benefits of the surgery or define causes for its failure. Under circumstances in which a defined motor abnormality is evident, the use of surgery should be carefully considered, as wrap procedures performed may not function adequately.

pH Monitoring

Esophageal pH monitoring is not essential for all patients with suspected GERD. Endoscopy and biopsy are the investigations of first choice because they are the most sensitive means of diagnosing erosive esophagitis and Barrett's esophagus. Esophageal pH monitoring is most useful for patients with troublesome symptoms but without endoscopic signs of esophagitis for whom a trial of medicinal therapy has failed, patients with atypical symptoms that cannot be clearly related to reflux, and patients who are being considered for antireflux surgery. Normal acid exposures are recorded in up to 25% of patients with otherwise typical reflux esophagitis and in about one third of patients with endoscopy-negative reflux disease. In addition, the repetition of the study in such patients indicates that a minority of patients may even change from a normal to abnormal acid exposure measurement. Overall, the evaluation of the association of symptoms with actual documented reflux episodes provides a valuable clinical advantage in pH monitoring. Nevertheless, the practical difficulties associated with the evaluation of symptoms are such that it alone can not be used effectively as a gold standard for the diagnosis of reflux disease in all patients.

Esophageal pH monitoring is also useful in assessing the adequacy of acid suppression in patients who fail to respond to what would appear to be adequate levels of acid suppressant therapy. Esophageal pH monitoring is an important adjunct to clinical assessment and endoscopy in the diagnosis of reflux disease. Although it is the gold standard for the measurement of esophageal exposure to acid and assessment of relationships of symptoms to reflux, the weaknesses in both these functions should be understood when applying this test for the diagnosis of reflux disease. Methods of esophageal pH monitoring have advanced substantially in the last decade. Better and more versatile recording equipment has been developed and is now widely marketed. Computers and purpose-designed software have extended the scope of interpretation of the recordings and made this process more time dependent.

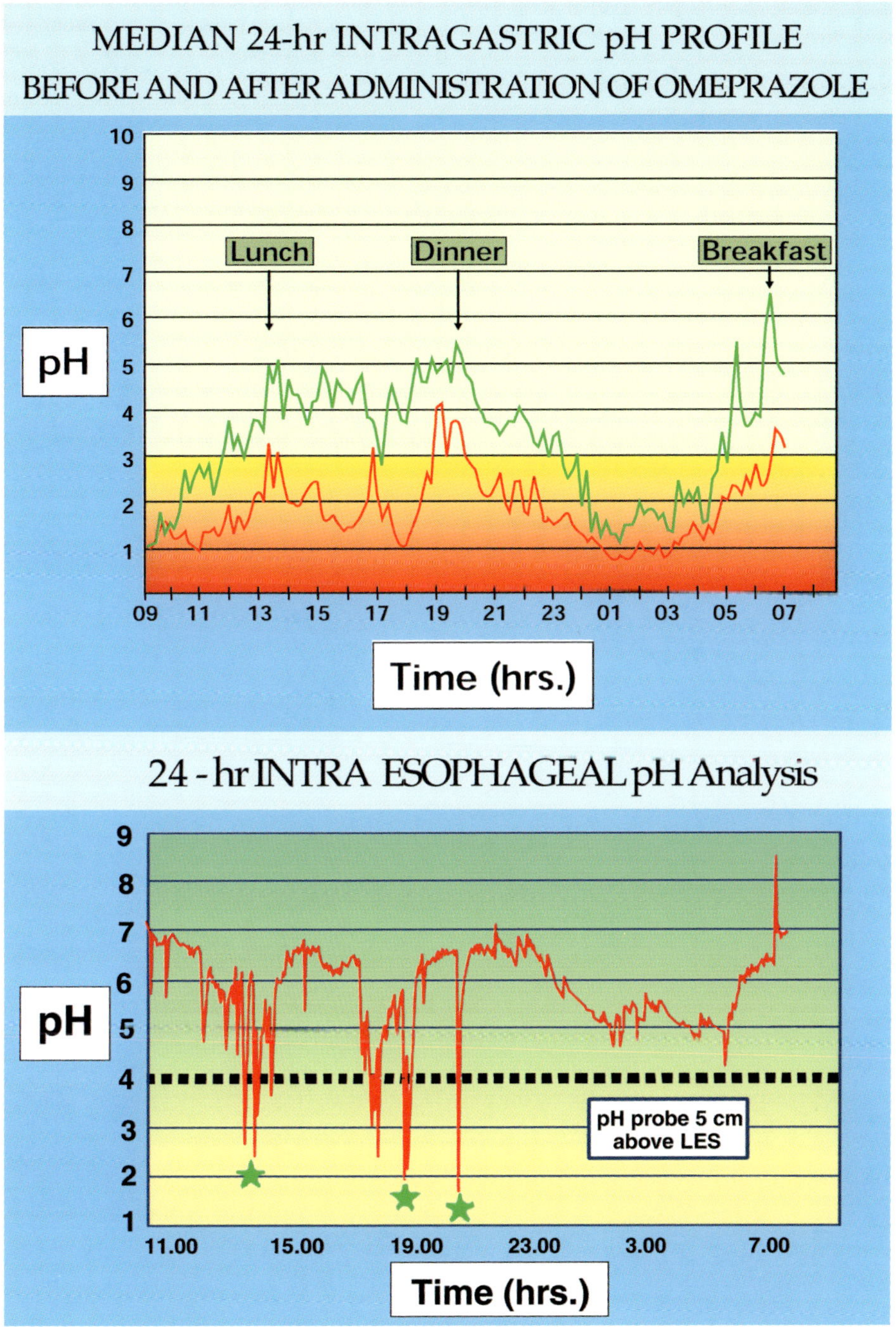

Figure 9. — *The ability of a PPI such as omeprazole to increase the intragastric pH to levels to >3 for a substantial percentage of a 24-hour period (top panel) is of critical relevance in promoting the healing of duodenal or gastric ulceration. In patients with GERD (bottom panel), the use of a PPI does not decrease the number of reflux episodes themselves (documented by asterisks) but the significant increase in the gastric pH lessens the esophageal acid load during a reflux event. This results in an increased percentage of the 24-hour period during which the esophageal lumen is exposed to a pH of >4 and consequently facilitates healing.*

In contrast to endoscopy or the Bernstein test, ambulatory esophageal pH monitoring records spontaneous reflux events and directly measures the degree of esophageal acid exposure—fundamental factors in the pathogenesis of this disease. It is not surprising that it is widely regarded as the gold standard for the diagnosis of reflux disease. However, there are methodologic limitations and inappropriate approaches to analysis and interpretations of results.

There are two major considerations in the analysis of pH recordings: measurement of the amount of reflux, and the relationship between the patient's symptoms and reflux. These two issues are not necessarily related and rather appear often to be complementary aspects of the analysis and interpretation of pH recordings.

Traditionally, GERD is diagnosed when esophageal pH falls below 4 for a specified portion of a 24-hour period. This threshold is clinically relevant because heartburn occurs at pH lower than 4, and peptic activity diminishes rapidly above this level. It is common for buffering of gastric contents early in the postprandial period to lead to reflux of gastric contents with a pH greater than 4. In addition, decreases in pH that do not reach pH 4 can also be symptomatic, and in some circumstances (eg, gastric resection), it may be appropriate to set the threshold above pH 4 or 5. The end of the reflux period is defined as the point at which esophageal pH rises above 4 (or 5); it is recommended that a minimum time (18 seconds) should elapse before a new reflux period is scored. Reflux events occurring at pH above 4 are not currently identifiable but do not have an adverse impact on the clinical importance of pH monitoring. Shifts in esophageal pH greater than 7 (alkaline pH events) have been interpreted as reflux of alkaline duodenal contents. However, more recent analysis has suggested that these may be as a result of swallowed saliva. Inclusion of such events in the final analysis is therefore potentially inappropriate.

The duration of pH under 4, usually expressed as a percentage of the recording time, is the variable most often used in the analysis of esophageal pH recordings. It is a measure of the degree of esophageal exposure to acid and correlates with the severity of esophagitis. The overall 24-hour esophageal acid exposure appears to be the best single determinant to discriminate between normal subjects and patients with esophagitis. The upper level for normal for total duration of esophageal acid exposure ranges between 5% and 7%. Reasonable intrasubject reproducibility (75% to 86%) has been recorded in patients with esophagitis. However, actual values may differ as much as threefold. Unfortunately, reproducibility is lowest in endoscopy-negative patients or those with atypical symptoms as well as in studies of less than 24 hours.

Although much emphasis has been placed on the measurement of esophageal acid exposure to classify patients as either normal or having reflux disease, this approach has its limitations. Levels of exposure to acid do not indicate whether the symptoms are related to reflux. This suggests the necessity of a symptom analysis. Minor increases in the level of exposure above normal should be interpreted with caution.

Assessment of the relationship between reflux and the patient's symptoms has proven to be a significantly greater challenge than quantification of acid exposure. The problem lies in the potentially independent relationship of these two variables. Despite the many attempts to express the relationship objectively (symptom specificity index, symptom sensitivity index, symptom-associated probability, and binomial symptom index), an ideal approach has yet to be devised.

Barrett's Esophagus

There has been considerable controversy in the past decade regarding the diagnosis and management of Barrett's esophagus, particularly as it relates to the possible evolution of malignant disease. To a large extent, the issue has been fueled by the extraordinary rise in incidence of adenocarcinoma of the esophagus and the esophagogastric junction and gastric cardia in particular.

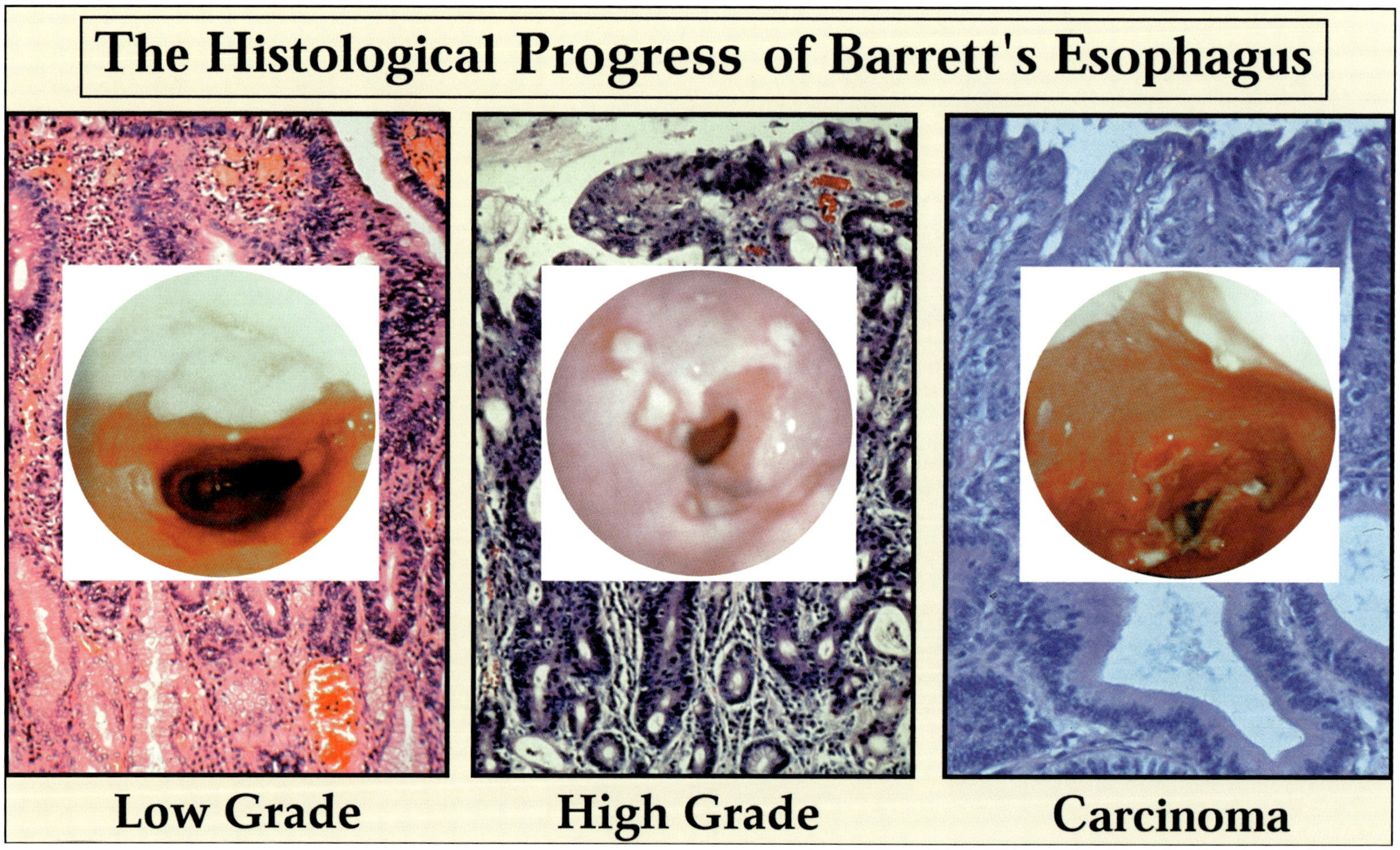

Figure 10. *— The histologic evolution of Barrett's esophagus is represented as a background to three endoscopic views of the complications of Barrett's esophagus. Sustained damage to the esophagus over time culminates in cell lineage and phenotype transformation, resulting in a histologic spectrum that may vary from various grades of dysplasia to carcinoma. Although histologic alterations are often associated with topographic alterations, the endoscopically evident appearance may not be related to the histology, and biopsy is necessary to confirm the precise nature of the lesion.*

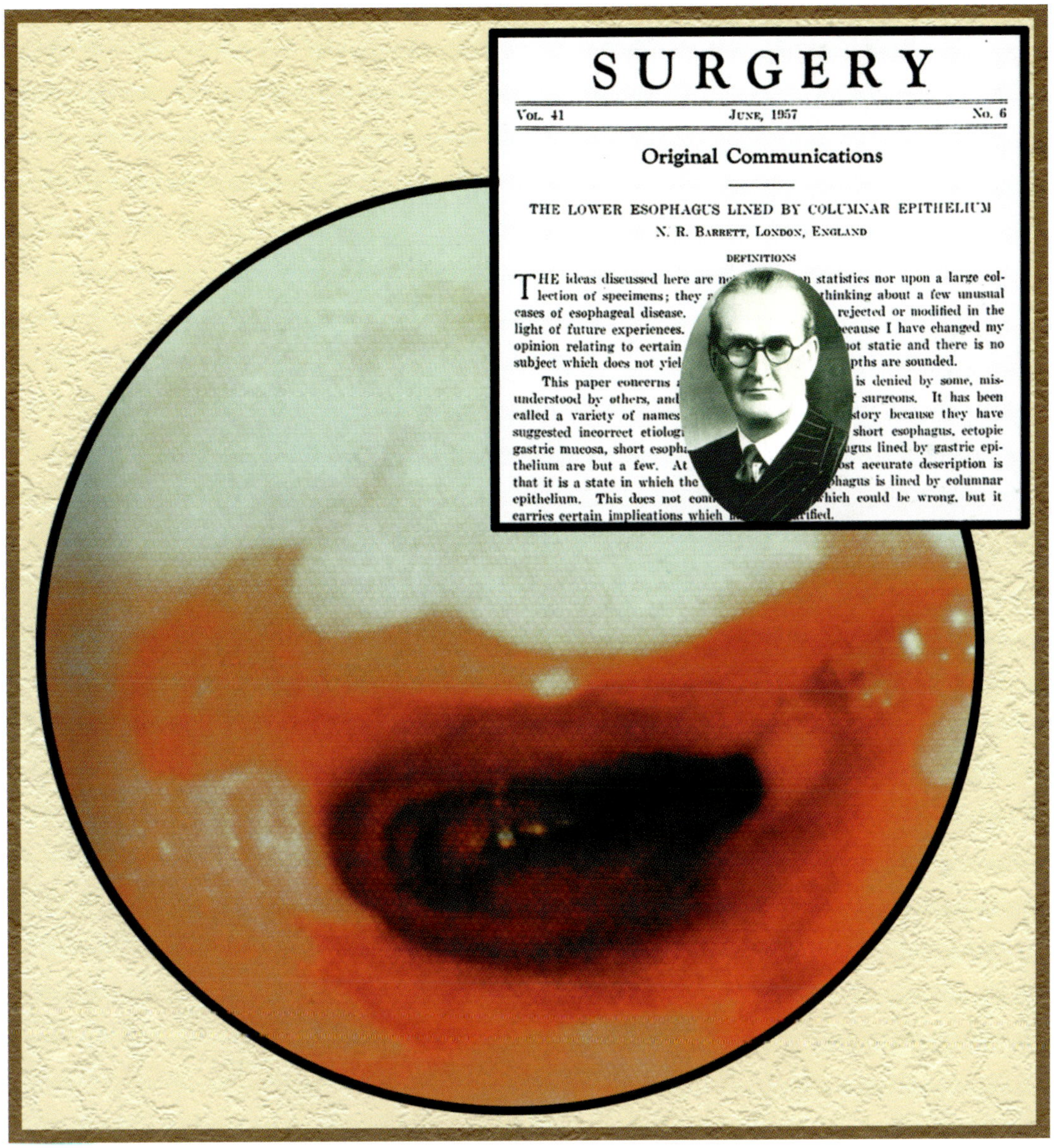

Figure 11. — Norman "Pasty" Barrett, in 1950, published a report in the British Journal of Surgery, in which he defined the esophagus as "that part of the foregut, distal to the cricopharyngeal sphincter, which is lined by squamous epithelium." He described a number of patients who had ulcerations in a tubular interthoracic organ that appeared to be to the esophagus, except that its distal portion was lined extensively by a gastric type of columnar epithelium. Because the esophagus was, by definition, a squamous-lined structure, Barrett believed that the columnar lined organ was a tubular segment of stomach generated by traction induced by a congenitally short (squamous-lined) esophagus and tethered within the chest. In this report, Barrett did not identify intestinal features (goblet cells) in the columnar lining of the tubular organ nor did he raise the question of intestinal metaplasia. Based on criticism of the conclusions of his work, Barrett, 7 years after his original report, reversed himself and concurred that the columnar lined organ that he had previously believed to be the stomach was, in fact, the esophagus. He suggested that the condition now be called "lower esophagus lined by columnar epithelium." Despite this about-face, the condition is still known as Barrett's esophagus and continues to evoke as much confusion as when initially described.

The precise definition of Barrett's esophagus by the identification of the extent of esophageal columnar lining has not been confirmed. Furthermore, problems in defining Barrett's esophagus by the presence of intestinal metaplasia require certainty regarding biopsy-sampling sites and histologic identification. Also, there is considerable confusion in regard to the relationship between the extent of the esophageal columnar lining, specialized intestinal metaplasia, and gastroesophageal reflux disease. The greater the length or extent of the esophageal columnar lining of the esophagus, the greater the frequency of the finding of intestinal metaplasia.

Barrett's esophagus had been identified primarily in patients with the signs and symptoms of GERD and in whom endoscopic examination revealed a long segment of columnar epithelium extending well up into the esophagus. Biopsy specimens taken from the columnar lining usually reveal an unusual form of intestinal metaplasia called specialized intestinal metaplasia, and the intestinal lining is invariably evident in the columnar epithelium surrounding Barrett's adenocarcinomas. As a result of such observations, Barrett's esophagus with specialized intestinal metaplasia became recognized as a major risk factor for adenocarcinoma of the esophagus and the gastroesophageal junction. The similar recognition that the incidence of these cancers was increasing at a dramatic rate in the United States and western Europe led to the development of a high level of interest in pathology and early identification. Patients who undergo esophagectomy for adenocarcinoma at the gastroesophageal junction often do not exhibit endoscopically apparent Barrett's esophagus; more often, they have short, inconspicuous segments of specialized intestinal metaplasia only evident at histologic examination. This observation accords with reports that in 18% of elective endoscopy patients with no evidence of Barrett's esophagus (columnar lined epithelium less than 3 cm of the distal esophagus), biopsies of the Z line (squamocolumnar junction) revealed specialized intestinal metaplasia. It is evident from this and similar studies that short, inconspicuous segments of specialized intestinal metaplasia can be frequently found at the Z line in predominantly white populations.

The precise relevance of the metaplasia is not certain. In particular, the question as to whether columnar metaplasia develops as a sequela of GERD is not proved. Thus, different studies have variously reported an association with GERD symptoms, no association with GERD, no association with endoscopic esophagitis, and an occasional association with histologic esophagitis. Given these inconsistent observations, the traditional concept that intestinal metaplasia develops as a consequence of GERD requires further scrutiny. Similarly, the risk of cancer for patients with short segments of intestinal metaplasia is unknown. Given the relatively high prevalence rates reported for intestinal metaplasia at the Z line and the infrequency of cancers at this location (irrespective of the rise in incidence), it seems likely that the risk associated with the short segments of specialized intestinal metaplasia may be quite small.

As with neoplasia elsewhere, the transformation from normal to a malignant mucosa occurs through a series of morphologic changes accompanied by specific molecular genetic events. The histologic changes in the squamous mucosa exposed to gastroesophageal reflux include an increase in the height of the rete pegs and an increase in the number of cycling epithelial cells. Whether the latter phenomenon is a direct effect of exposure of the gastric contents to the esophageal squamous epithelium or whether it is indirect is not known. Similarly, whether direct damage including erosions are necessarily the stimulus for transformation from squamous to columnar epithelium, as in Barrett's esophagus, is not clear. At present, it is thought that the development of a Barrett's-type mucosa containing gastric and/or small intestinal and/or colonic-type cells, often together in the same metaplastic esophageal gland, is due to an altered process of differentiation from the pluripotent epithelial stem cell. The presence of abundant growth factors in the esophageal gland system suggests that a process analogous to that described for the ulcer-associated cell lineage sytem may be implicated in the local repair process.

Because of the confusion regarding the term Barrett's esophagus, an alternative classification, which does not rely on arbitrary and imprecise endoscopic measurements, has been proposed by Spechler. When columnar epithelium is detected in the esophagus, regardless of its extent, the condition should be called *columnar-lined esophagus*, as originally proposed by Barrett. Once biopsy samples have been obtained from this esophageal columnar lining, the use of histologic criteria can be used to classify the condition as either columnar-lined esophagus with specialized intestinal metaplasia or columnar-lined esophagus without specialized intestinal metaplasia. This proposal provides considerable improvement in clarity for both physicians and pathologists in regard to the entity under consideration in a particular patient. Although both conditions may be associated with GERD, the association is variable and appears to be related to the extent of the columnar lining. Patients with long segments of esophageal columnar lining often exhibit both severe GERD and specialized intestinal metaplasia. Signs and symptoms of GERD, however, may be absent in patients with short segments of columnar lining in the distal esophagus, even when biopsy specimens reveal specialized intestinal metaplasia.

Endoscopic surveillance for adenocarcinoma may be recommended in patients who have columnar-lined esophagus with intestinal metaplasia irrespective of the extent, whereas columnar-lined esophagus without specialized intestinal metaplasia does not require endoscopic surveillance. When a distal esophagus appears to be normal and specialized intestinal metaplasia is identified at the squamocolumnar junction, which does not extend appreciably above the anatomic junction of the esophagus and the stomach, the condition should be called *specialized intestinal metaplasia* at the esophagogastric junction. It has not been established whether this condition is related to GERD nor is it evident that the risk of cancer applies to patients with this condition.

The issues in regard to neoplasia in relation to GERD and Barrett's esophagus remain a source of concern. In 1990, Cameron and colleagues showed that for every case of Barrett's esophagus in patients with esophageal cancer, many more are unrecognized. Similarly, in at least five separate studies, it has been demonstrated that of all patients undergoing endoscopy, up to one in five will have specialized intestinal metaplasia at the gastroesophageal junction, whether or not abnormalities are evident at the time of endoscopy. Despite the screening recommendations for the management of Barrett's esophagus, it has been suggested that the yield of a Barrett's surveillance program may be too low to justify economically. Interesting issues have been raised in regard to the relationship between *H. pylori* and GERD and in particular between these two disease entities and the possible relationship to adenocarcinoma at the gastroesophageal junction. At this time, any such pathogenic linkage is speculative, and rigorous studies are required before such relationships can be substantiated.

At present, because of advances in endoscopic detection and a better understanding of metaplasia, the definition and pathogenesis of Barrett's esophagus seem less clear than previously envisaged. The definition of Barrett's esophagus solely by the presence of specialized intestinal metaplasia, regardless of its extent, may serve to significantly overestimate the disease process. It is probably more realistic to restate the observation in terms of the identification of a condition known as "columnar epithelium-lined esophagus with specialized intestinal metaplasia." Upon identification of such an entity, a specific focus can be developed to identify cellular or molecular markers consistent with the development of dysplastic and neoplastic transformation.

If the principal issue is to have impact upon the incidence of adenocarcinoma of the esophagus, which is currently the most rapidly increasing cancer in the United States, and amplify therapeutic gain, a different strategy is required. Better tests are needed to identify at-risk patients than endoscopy in patients with known Barrett's esophagus. In particular, the identification of molecular markers of cell transformation in the esophagus are mandatory to facilitate the identification of patients whose metaplasia is of pathologic significance.

Patients found to have Barrett's esophagus at biopsy, but with no dysplasia, should be placed in a surveillance program with approximately 5-year intervals between surveillance endoscopies. This opinion is, to a large extent, based upon cost-effectiveness analysis data and may need to be modified with the significant alterations in endoscopic charges. If a pathologic diagnosis of Barrett's esophagus also identifies the presence of dysplasia, the material should be reviewed by two expert independent pathologists to confirm the diagnosis and to establish whether the changes conform to a pattern consistent with low- or high-grade dysplasia. The identification of low-grade dysplasia mandates repeat biopsy at 3 to 6 months to determine whether there is progression to high-grade dysplasia. If, at this point, multiple biopsies fail to identify evidence of dysplasia, the patient should return to the normal surveillance program; if low-grade dysplasia persists, endoscopy and biopsy should again be repeated in 3 to 6 months. If there is a diagnosis of high-grade dysplasia at the initial or any follow-up biopsy, an attempt to confirm this diagnosis should be made within 1 to 3 months. If the repeat biopsy confirms high-grade dysplasia, the patient should be referred for consideration of surgery. Some experts have noted that careful, repeated endoscopic surveillance of high-grade dysplasia can be performed to monitor for and biopsy for any visible mucosal abnormality. Under such circumstances, surgery might be obviated until a carcinoma is discovered. However, most physicians are uncomfortable with this approach and express a preference for prophylactic surgery once the presence of a high-grade lesion had been reliably identified. Ablation therapy by laser, bicap, heater probe, or photodynamic therapy for Barrett's esophagus and/or dysplasia should be regarded as experimental, but encouraging results have been reported.

Acid and Esophagitis

pH and Symptoms

It is well recognized that whereas GERD is due to impaired function of the LES, the pathologic effects of this are mostly or entirely mediated by acid and pepsin reflux. The esophageal epithelium appears more susceptible to acid damage than either the gastric or duodenal epithelium, and the explanation for this is found in the structural and secretory properties of the squamous lining of the esophagus adjacent to the stomach.

Malfunction of the LES results in acid reflux into the esophagus. Reflux is mostly episodic, so that the esophagus is not often presented with a continuous acid load. Prediction of esophageal disease related to reflux takes into account the pH of the refluxate and the duration of reflux. Expulsion of the refluxate back into the stomach shortens the time of exposure. The volume of reflux is also an important parameter for estimation of the acid load on the esophageal epithelium. It is the magnitude of this acid load that determines the presence or absence of pathology or symptoms. Intraesophageal pH monitoring provides an approximate measure of the acid load to the lower esophagus.

The human esophageal epithelium is a multilayered, stratified, squamous epithelium. Afferent nerves are present reaching into the superficial layers of the mucosa. With incompetence of the LES, acid reflux results in pain and damage to the epithelium, depending on the pH of the refluxate. Rather than being protected by a continuous tight junction, this epithelium has largely regional cell-to-cell contact through desmosomes, but being multilayered provides a winding path for proton diffusion into the epithelium. It is nevertheless significantly more acid sensitive than the gastric epithelium that is provided with "tight" tight junctions.

The threshold of acidity for damage and pain may be different. A higher acidity is likely needed for damage to the epithelial cells compared with the acidity required for stimulation of the pain fibers. This is probably because the epithelial cells have acid recovery mechanisms (such as Na/H or anion exchange) mostly absent in the pain fibers. Dependent on the location of the pain fibers and access thereto of H^+, patients will have different sensitivities to luminal acidity.

The central hypothesis regarding the pathogenesis of esophagitis is dependent upon the extent of esophageal injury that itself is a reflection of the mucosal acidification time. Overall motility disorder as a basis for esophagitis can therefore be considered as either due to a markedly increased propensity to incur reflux events (LES abnormality) or a markedly impaired acid clearance (peristaltic dysfunction). The dominant abnormality leading to the development of esophagitis and GERD can vary from patient to patient and may even evolve with time as scarring and damage progresses.

pH and Reflux

There is a clear predictive relationship between intragastric pH and intraesophageal pH, as both correlate with the severity of esophagitis. The conventional pH threshold for aggressive versus nonaggressive reflux is regarded as pH 4, and this has been supported by pH measurements in patients with defined severities of GERD. Overall, it is apparent that the severity of mucosal injury in GERD is dependent on the pH of the reflux material and its dwell time in the esophagus. In this respect, 24-hour esophageal pH monitoring has proved to be the most effective measurement of gastroesophageal reflux, as it records both the pH of the reflux and the duration of the exposure. It is evident that the daily duration of time for which the intragastric pH is elevated to 4 or higher correlates closely with the healing of erosive reflux esophagitis. Nevertheless, esophageal pH monitoring studies reveal the presence of GERD in some patients despite normal or near-normal acidic exposure values.

This paradox probably reflects alterations in reflux patterns that vary from day to day as well as variations in pH among different regions of the esophagus. Esophageal pH generally rises as the distance from the LES increases, and pH appears to be lower at the peaks of the esophageal folds that are exposed to acid as opposed to the tufts, where there is a greater degree of protection afforded by bicarbonate and mucus. This variation in esophageal pH is presumably responsible for the linear distribution of erosive esophagitis evident at endoscopy in some patients. Overall, it does not appear that patients with GERD are acid hypersecretors. Nevertheless, repeated measurements of 24-hour intragastric acidity in individual patients reveal considerable variations.

In some patients, abnormal duodenogastric reflux may make gastric juice especially aggressive to esophageal mucosa. In this respect, delayed gastric emptying may contribute significantly to pathologic gastroesophageal reflux. Similarly, abnormally frequent transient LES relaxation, as well as inappropriate esophageal clearing and the presence of a hiatal hernia, may contribute to the development of GERD. Twenty-four hour esophageal pH monitoring in endoscopically negative or mild reflux disease has shown that most acid exposure occurs during the day postprandially. Furthermore, several esophageal pH monitoring studies have demonstrated that patients with Barrett's esophagus exhibit high levels of esophageal exposure to gastric reflux. Rigorous data supporting that Barrett's esophagus is linearly related to the level of acid reflux are not available.

The key role of acid in the development of GERD is best exemplified in patients with gastrinoma disease in which peptic esophagitis is related to the level of acid exposure. Other pH-related factors involved in the development of GERD include the ability of the esophagus to clear acid and to deal with activated pepsinogen. In up to 50% of patients with GERD, it has been demonstrated that the higher the acid concentration in the refluxate, the longer the required clearance. The reasons for the diminished rate of clearance is unclear but may represent either abnormally low swallowing rates and ineffective primary or secondary peristalsis. Although salivary bicarbonate is of importance in determining esophageal acid clearance, little information is available on salivary gland function in patients with GERD. The pH necessary to activate pepsinogen is an important variable in the sensitivity of the esophageal epithelium through acid peptic insult. The higher the pH, the further outside the optimal pH profile for activation of pepsinogen and the lower the likelihood of damage. A similar pathogenesis is probably involved in damage caused by bile acids, but this usually reflects a smaller subgroup of patients who have had previous gastric surgery or exhibit major motility disorders.

pH and Healing

As the degree of exposure to esophageal acid correlates almost linearly with the severity of esophagitis, the primary aim of acid-suppression therapy is to raise the pH of the refluxate. A number of meta-analytic studies have indicated that a threshold of pH 4 appears to be the critical determinate for ensuring esophageal healing. Thus, the longer the esophageal acid exposure to a pH greater than 4, the more likely it is that healing will occur. The rapid relapse of esophagitis upon withdrawal of acid-suppressive therapy indicates that the duration of therapy is of critical relevance in determining complete healing. In this respect, agents such as the PPI class of drugs are effective given their ability to not only provide a higher degree of acid suppression but maintain pH levels elevated both during the day and the night regardless of stimulation by meals. At this time, the suppression of gastric acid secretion will remain the primary goal of GERD therapy.

Figure 12. *— The recurrence rate of erosive esophagitis is substantial following initial healing with, and then withdrawal of, omeprazole therapy.*

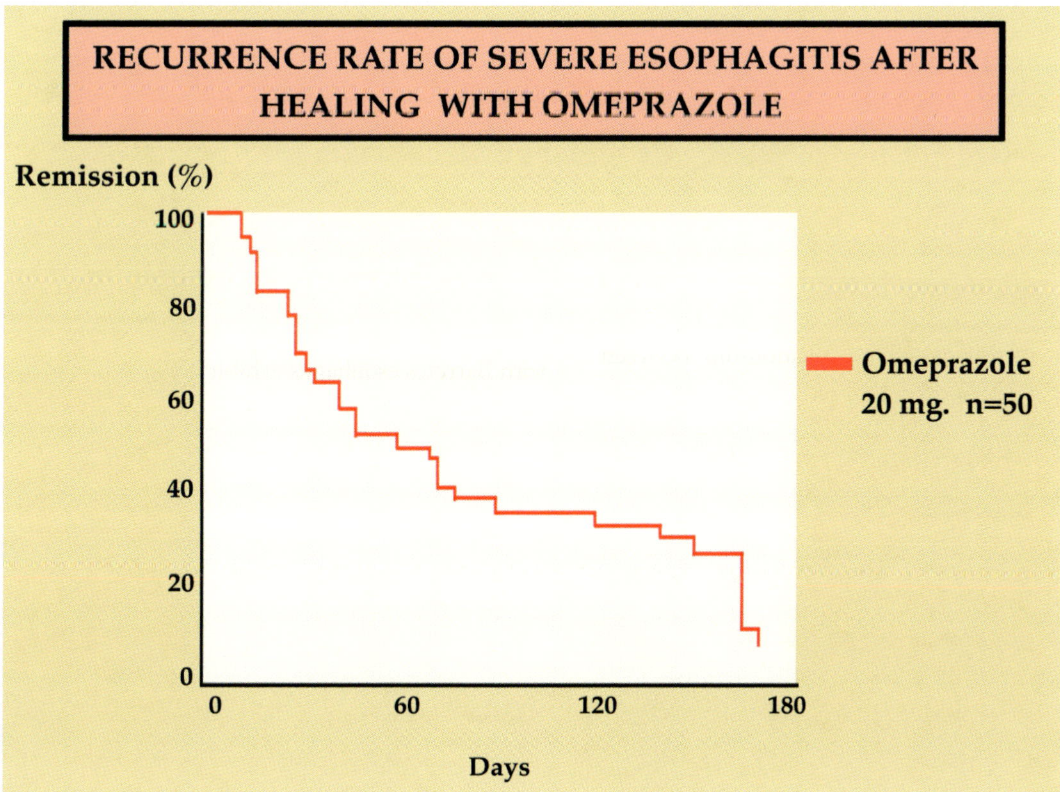

Treatment

The recognition in the first part of this century that mucosal damage was caused by acid and that this acid could be decreased by luminal neutralization resulted in application of antacid preparations, bland diets, and milk infusion as therapeutic options. The subsequent categorizing of the H2-receptor and the development of agents specifically capable of blocking this receptor improved the management of acid-related diseases and virtually abrogated surgery as a therapeutic option for peptic ulcer except in cases of emergency. However, the relapse rate for GERD in patients on H2-receptor antagonists therapy still engendered considerable enthusiasm for surgical intervention in the management of reflux disease. The more recent identification of the specific molecular mechanism of acid secretion — the proton pump (H^+, K^+ATPase) — resulted in the development of a new class of therapeutic agents, the PPI class of drugs, of which omeprazole was the first. Within a relatively short period it was apparent that PPIs were more effective in the treatment of GERD symptoms and maintaining healing of erosive esophagitis than the H2-receptor antagonists, and were more potent inhibitors of acid secretion.

Antisecretory drugs clearly are the best therapeutic agents for the treatment of GERD. Similarly, the development of agents that might be used to increase the LES tone, thus further diminishing the ability of gastric contents to regularly enter the lower esophageal area, would confer obvious advantage. The current failure to identify a specific agent capable of targeting the LES has to date hindered the widespread clinical use of this strategy.

Treatment Targets In GERD

The theoretical goals of GERD management are to abolish symptoms, heal erosive esophagitis, maintain healing, and prevent reflux and pathologic sequelae. Current options available include neutralization or inhibition of acid secretion. This requires the introduction of a therapeutic strategy that targets the defective mechanisms that facilitate reflux is a goal for the future. Although drugs can be delivered by existing anatomic routes, the surgical option includes all the sequelae of general anesthesia and invasion of the peritoneal cavity. The introduction of laparoscopic surgery engendered initial enthusiasm because of its relative noninvasiveness; however, early results are no better than noted with open surgery. Surgery restores a barrier between the esophagus and the stomach, thus ameliorating reflux. Laparoscopic fundoplication appears to have some advantage in decreasing hospital stay.

The wide variety of modifications of the surgical options available to increase the pressure zone of the incompetent sphincter suggest that no option is perfect. The recent advent of laparoscopic surgery has not altered the principles of the procedure but simply facilitated access to the gastroesophageal junction. Indeed, individual surgeons performing what they believe to be the same operation often disagree on the precise details, and it has been difficult to compare surgical results among centers and among patients. Complications may include bleeding, perforation of the esophagus, splenic injury, sepsis, dysphagia, and a disabling inability to belch. The rate of complications varies between 10% and 15% and the mortality rate is 0.5% to 1%. Generally, the more procedures the surgeon undertakes, the more likely is the patient to be cured of reflux, as the learning curve for this operation is somewhat lengthy.

An experienced surgeon and selection of the appropriate patient are the most important determinants of surgical success. Given the potential problems of surgery, a careful preoperative assessment of the patient is mandatory as is a joint discussion with a gastroenterologist to determine that an appropriate management strategy is in place. It is necessary to make a positive diagnosis of GERD before surgery, either by endoscopy or 24-hour pH measurement. Similarly, delineation of peristaltic function and LES pressure by manometry is important. The identification of patients with poor motor function who will not benefit from surgery is critical to avoid iatrogenically induced exacerbation of GERD. Treatment response to antisecretory drugs may be a useful predictor of likely surgical success; if the patient's symptoms are markedly improved by such therapy, the symptoms will probably also be helped by surgery.

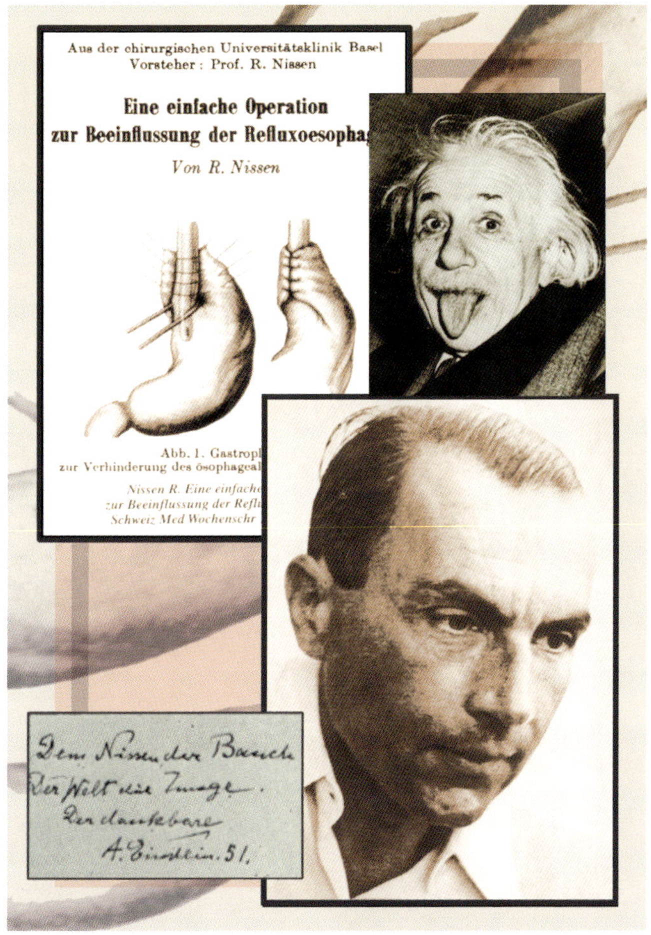

Figure 13. — *In 1956, Rudolf Nissen (bottom) published from Zurich his description of the operation that he had initially called "gastroplication." Its efficacy in treating the hitherto unresolvable problem of reflux esophagitis led to initial widespread enthusiasm for the procedure. Although trained in Berlin, Nissen had fled to the United States during the Nazi regime. In New York, on December 31, 1948, he operated on Albert Einstein, who had developed untreatable dyspepsia and an abdominal mass. At operation, the causation of symptoms was identified as an aortic aneurysm. In gratitude, Einstein sent him a card (bottom left) inscribed "To Nissen my gratitude, for the world-my tongue!" On April 18, 1949, Einstein died of a leaking aortic aneurysm, having adamantly declined to accept any further surgical intervention.*

The Lower Esophageal Sphincter

Study of the LES and esophageal peristalsis is usually reserved for patients who fail acid suppressive therapy, exhibit obvious symptoms consistent with motility problems, or for whom surgery is contemplated. The determination of the function of the LES and the motility status of the esophagus are important in the management of these patients. Current knowledge of sphincter physiology is limited, and, in the case of the lower esophagus, this is particularly apparent. The LES in GERD appears to malfunction either by exerting a pressure zone that is too low to prevent reflux from the stomach or to produce transient episodes of relaxation that are either prolonged or occur with excessive frequency. Initial surgical strategies for dealing with the problem focused on reduction of the hiatal hernia with its subsequent fixation in the abdomen and repair of the crural defect. In the 1950s, novel surgical techniques were developed that added a wrap of a mobilized portion of gastric fundus around the LES (Nissen, Belsey) in an attempt to increase LES pressure and obviate reflux. Numerous permutations of this procedure failed to provide a reliable or predictable high-pressure barrier zone to reflux, and the morbidity of the open procedure was substantial (12% to 18% rate of complications). A particular difficulty continues to be the inability to precisely calibrate the increase in lower esophageal pressure generated by the wrap. An arbitrary determination based upon the size of an intraesophageal bougie has led to failures either due to excessive wrapping or inadequate increase of pressure. It is, however, apparent that in certain patients, a mechanical defect associated with decreased LES pressure may merit consideration for surgical repair.

Fundoplication

When a patient is young, requires maintenance acid-suppression therapy, is fit for surgery, and desires an operation, manometric testing should be undertaken to exclude esophageal peristalic abnormalities and confirm the presence of decreased LES pressure. If all the criteria for surgery are met, the most appropriate operation at this time appears to be a Nissen fundoplication undertaken by laparoscopic technique. This consists of the introduction of a number of ports into the upper abdomen whereby dissection and mobilization of the fundus and esophagus of the stomach can be undertaken. It is essential to avoid damage to the stomach and esophagus as well as the vagal nerves. The diameter of the esophagus embraced by the wrap is determined by insertion of a large bougie through the gastroesophageal junction from the mouth. Results using this technique have been reported as initially successful in up to 85% to 90% of patients with a morbidity level less than between 10% and 15%. Under some circumstances, however, both physicians and patients would prefer to avoid surgery.

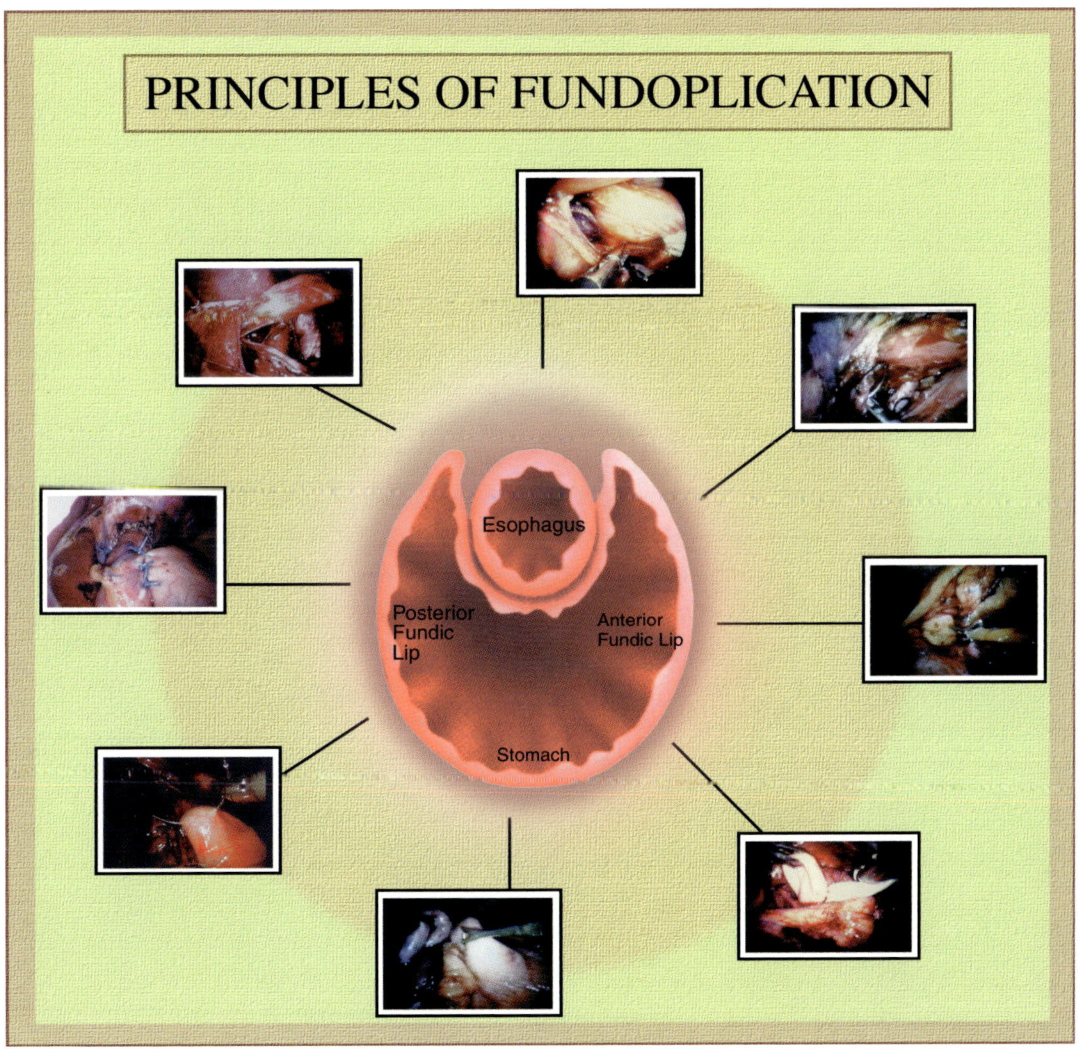

Figure 14. *— The most commonly performed antireflux procedure is the laparoscopic Nissen fundoplication. The essential elements of the procedure are illustrated in a clockwise fashion, starting at 11 o'clock.*

1. *Crural dissection with identification and preservation of the vagal nerves.*
2. *Circumferential dissection of the esophagus.*
3. *Suture closure of the crura*
4. *Division of the short gastric vessels and fundic mobilization.*
5. *Traction of the greater curve of the fundus behind the esophagus.*
6. *Creation of a short, loose fundoplication over the esophagus containing a 60F bougie.*
7. *Suture of the two fundic lips to each other and to the anterior gastric wall.*
8. *Completed procedure with wrap sutured over the lower esophagus*

Gastric Acidity

It is evident that gastric juice is harmful to esophageal squamous mucosa and that hypersecretion is not the cause of the disease, as the amount of acid, pepsin and bile is no different in persons with or without GERD. Most experimental models suggest that it is not acid alone that is injurious, and other "barrier-breaking agents" of the refluxate — including pepsin, bile, ingested material, and lysolecithin — may be implicated. Although acid may have a direct effect on the esophageal mucosa its main function may be to facilitate the damage initiated by pepsin and bile and as well as activating pepsinogen to pepsin.

Therapeutic Strategy

Medical

Within broad parameters, GERD may be diagnosed on the basis of a history and physical examination. The general algorithm employed under some circumstances for the diagnosis of GERD in other patients includes initial evaluation by endoscopic examination with biopsy and possibly followed by 24-hour pH monitoring and measurement of LES pressure.

A number of different proposals have been considered for treatment of GERD. Once this diagnosis has been established, an attempt at life-style modification — including weight loss, cessation of smoking, dimunition of alcohol intake, and eating at least 3 hours before sleeping head elevation of the bed — is recommended. Such treatment may be undertaken with or without antacids, mucosal-protectant agents, or alginic acid. The failure to gain relief with this regimen culminates in the introduction of first-line prescriptive acid-inhibitory agents such as an H2-receptor antagonist or a PPI. PPIs, such as omeprazole, may be prescribed for 4 to 8 weeks, and additional 4 to 8 week courses may be prescribed for recurrences of GERD symptoms. The most common adverse events associated with the use of omeprazole are headache, nausea, diarrhea, and abdominal pain.

In a substantial number of patients, especially those with erosive esophagitis, relapse is common, and therefore the issue of maintenance therapy is of considerable relevance. In this respect, a number of studies, using either omeprazole or other PPIs have demonstrated that

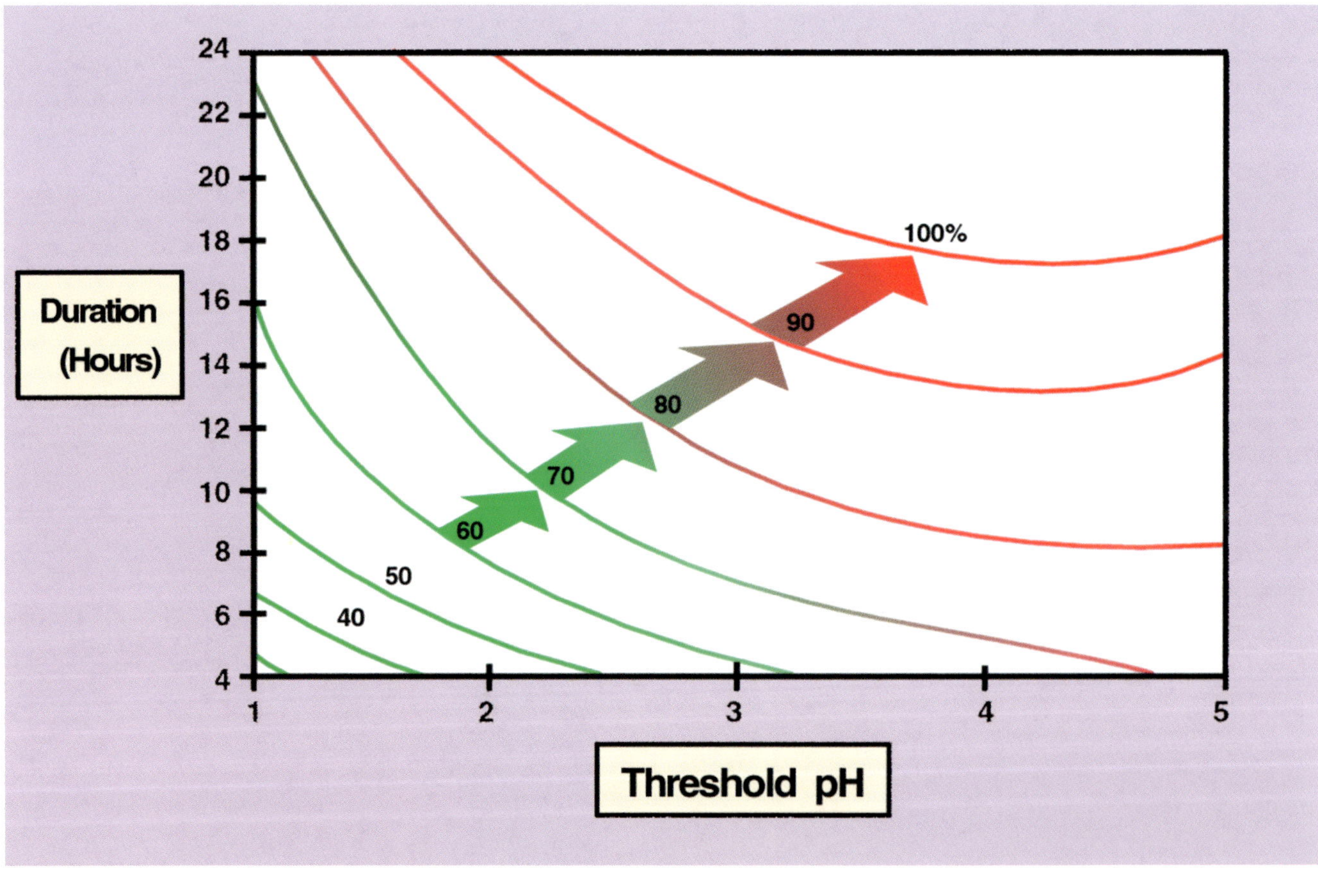

Figure 15. — The predictive value for healing of esophagitis can be calculated based upon the duration of time that esophageal pH is elevated by antisecretory therapy.

the perpetuation of esophageal healing is superior when compared with H2-receptor antagonists. Numerous clinical studies have defined the relative efficacy of the various treatment choices by comparison of healing of rates. In these studies, the results of healing represent a proportion of those healed compared with those treated at any given point. As the duration of therapy becomes prolonged, the larger proportion of patients with esophagitis are healed, and the speed of healing decreases, as there are fewer patients left to be healed.

When considered from the vantage point of the patient, the issue of symptom relief may, in the short term, be more critical than the issue of healing. In head-to-head clinical trials, PPIs are more effective than H2-receptor antagonists in producing complete relief of heartburn in patients with GERD.

Depending upon the severity of symptoms, level of therapeutic compliance, number of relapses, age of the patient, and the physician's level of concern, modification of management may be considered. This may lead to the discussion of surgery. For the most part, the latter option now entails laparoscopic surgery. At initial diagnosis of GERD, the use of short-term (4- to 8-week) PPI therapy before consideration of surgical intervention is prudent. Using this general strategy, it appears that between 85% and 95% of all patients can be medically managed. The remainder who either exhibit complications or are nonamenable to long-term PPI therapy may require surgery. This may reflect the fact that such patients present for treatment at a point well into the evolution of the disease. Under such circumstances, the gastroesophageal area is so damaged that the healing process cannot achieve or maintain mucosal integrity in the presence of anything other than the presence of the most limited amounts of acid or pepsin.

Figure 16. — Apart from the predictable nonspecific complications of any surgery, specific complications related to this procedure are of significant morbidity and even mortality in some instances

SURGICAL	Range (%)	Mean (%)
Esophageal or gastric perforation	0 - 5.1	1.5
Hepatic lesion	0 - 10	0.6
Splenic lesion	0 - 6.9	2.5
Splenectomy	0 - 1.7	0.7
Inadvertent vagotomy	0 - 6.3	0.6
Wound infection	0 - 4.4	2.2
Incisional hernia	0 - 1.9	0.3
Intraperitoneal, mediastinal abscess	0 - 1.9	0.6
Herniation into chest	0 - 1.0	0.2
Severe stricture	0 - 1.0	0.2
Postoperative bleeding	0 - 3.4	0.6
NON SURGICAL	**1.2 - 11.4**	**4.3**

n= 3123 patients (23 studies)

Surgical

It is critical that clearly defined requirements for an antireflux procedure be fulfilled before consideration of fundoplication. These include (1) pathologic esophageal acid exposure on 24-hour pH monitoring, (2) significantly decreased LES pressure, (3) normal parameters of esophageal contractility, and (4) normal esophageal length. Information that symptoms are ameliorated by acid suppression therapy (PPI) may also provide support. Surgical intervention is for the most part regarded as a laparoscopic Nissen fundoplication, although a variety of modifications, including the Toupet, have been used with some success. The rigorous evaluation of surgical techniques has been difficult, as few studies have been performed in a prospective randomized fashion and even fewer evaluated by blinded observers.

The current surgical data available for laparoscopic fundoplication has a limited long-term evaluation (the procedure was introduced in 1991) and the initial series published are those of experts in the field. Over the last 5 years, antireflux surgery has substantially shifted to the use of laparoscopic procedures. Although follow-up is limited, it is apparent that between 85% and 95% of all patients can be predicted to improve after surgery, regardless of the technique used.

Surgery is an attractive option for patients under 40 years of age and for patients who do not want to take long-term medication. Patients who require PPI therapy continually for a year are unlikely to be able to manage without these medications. Before surgery, both the gastroenterologist and the surgeon should meet with the patient and engage in a full and frank discussion regarding all the risks and benefits of long-term medical versus surgical therapy. Preoperative motility studies are essential both to precisely delineate the state of the sphincter as well as to facilitate follow-up if there is post-surgical relapse. Although there are as yet no major studies with long-term data available, laparoscopic fundoplication appears to be safe and preferable to open surgery. The critical determinant is the choice of surgeon. The "wrap" type procedure appears satisfactory, and no data exist to suggest that the addition of any form of vagotomy is required. Above the age of 60, and in the presence of comorbid conditions, the risks of surgery, general anesthesia, and violation of the peritoneal cavity probably outweigh the benefits. If Barrett's esophagus is a component of intractable GERD symptoms, it is essential to continue the surveillance program even if the patient is asymptomatic after surgery, as Barrett's esophagus may progress even after successful surgery. A failed fundic wrap increases the costs of the surgical procedure, significantly complicates further treatment, and considerably increases the risk if reoperation is undertaken.

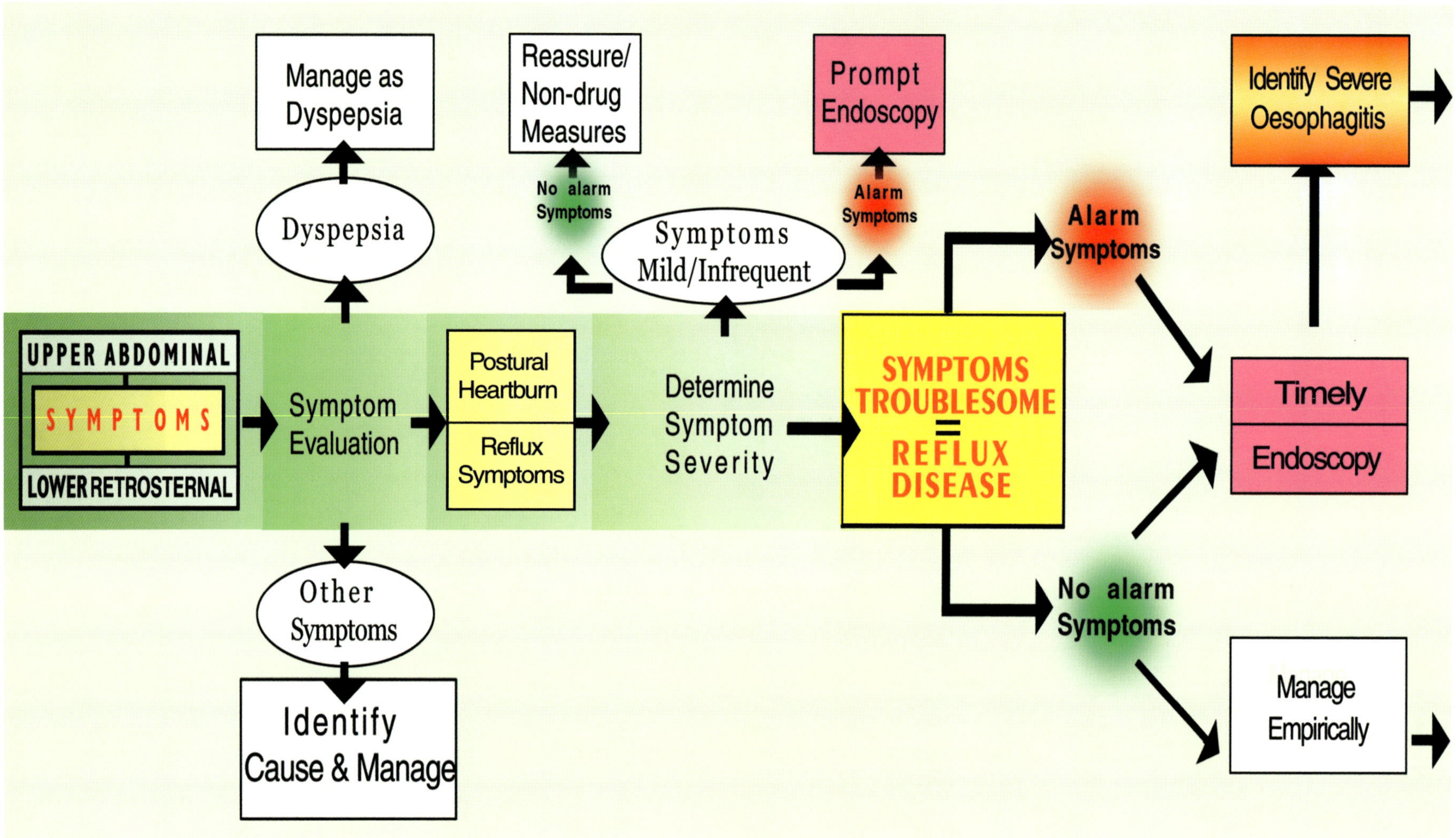

Figure 17. — Patients with reflux disease should be distinguished from those with mild, infrequent symptoms as a result of gastroesophageal reflux. In the absence of alarm symptoms, there is controversy as to whether endoscopy or empiric therapy should be the initial management of choice. This decision is influenced by individual patient issues as well as access and cost factors in a particular area.

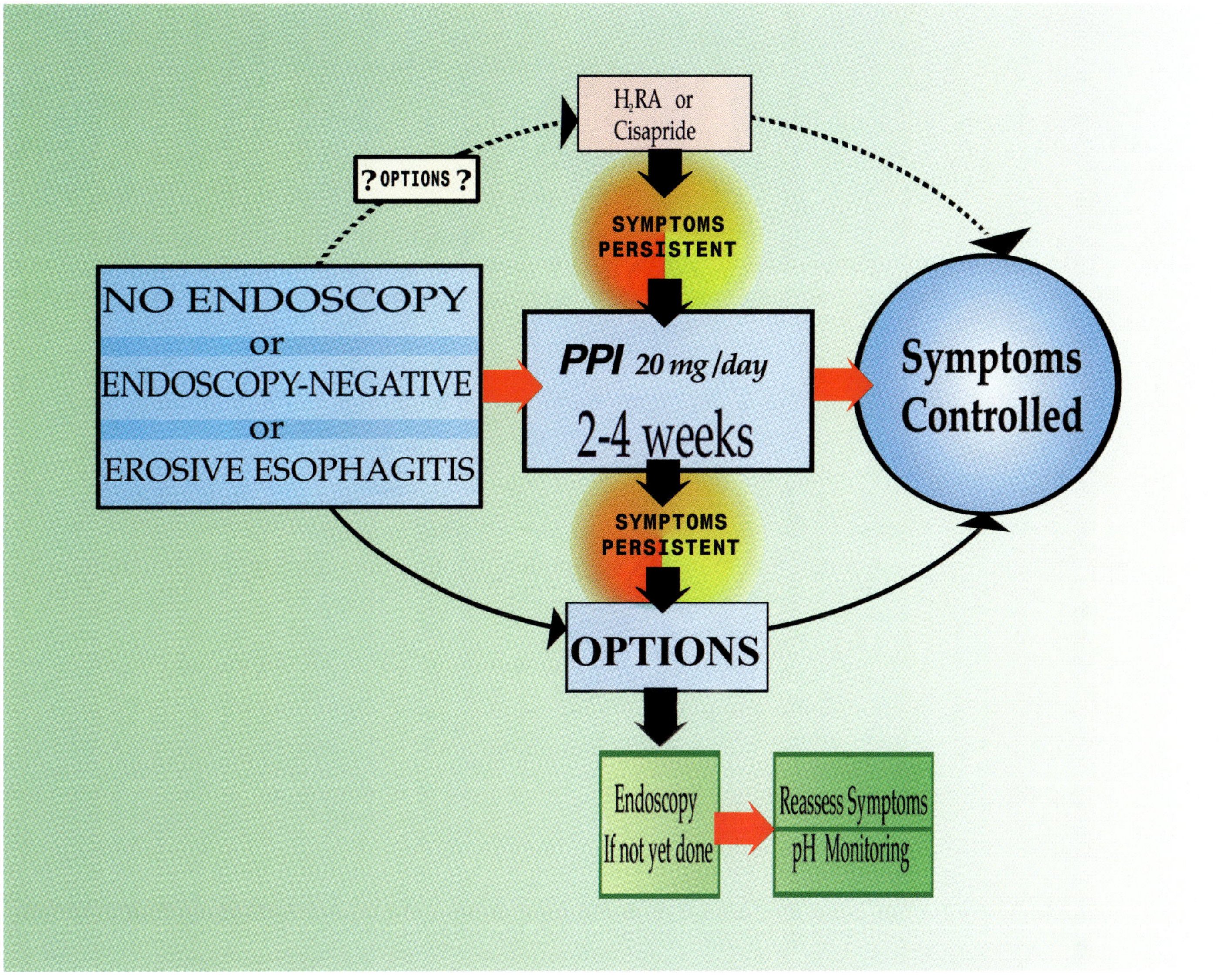

Figure 18. *— PPI therapy is effective as the initial treatment option for patients with GERD. The goals of treatment are healing erosive esophagitis and complete relief of GERD-related symptoms. In the event of failure of therapy to control symptoms, endoscopy should be undertaken, particularly if this was not previously performed.*

The data for open wrap indicate that a defective fundic wrap occurs in 7% after 7 months, 23% after 77 months, and 29% after 20 years. Thus, the potential rate of reoperation may be predicted to be as high as 5% to 10% for patients who have undergone a laparoscopic fundoplication. Because concerns have been raised regarding adverse effects of long-term medical therapy, viability of fundic wrap requires serious consideration.

Treatment Overview

Patients who have reflux disease are frequently led to believe that they should be able to cure themselves by correction of an inappropriate life style. This is probably unrealistic. However, the avoidance of particular foods and alcoholic drinks that provoke reflux-induced symptoms can produce a therapeutically useful amelioration of symptoms. It is controversial as to whether cessation of smoking or bed head elevation is of any lasting benefit. As most reflux is postprandial, only a small subgroup (identifiable by either nocturnal symptoms, major nocturnal acid exposure, or severe esophagitis) may benefit from bed head elevation. The demonstrated impact of bed head elevation on the nocturnal acid exposure of the esophagus is small compared with the effect of PPI therapy.

Clinical Strategy

Patients with dyspepsia should be separated from those with heartburn at the initial assessment, as the primary decision pathway differs for the management of these two symptom patterns. Alarm symptoms that include dysphagia, weight loss, or hematemesis warrant early endoscopic evaluation to exclude esophageal stricture, peptic ulcer, or malignancy. The risk of the development of esophageal adenocarcinoma in association with Barrett's esophagus is so small that in

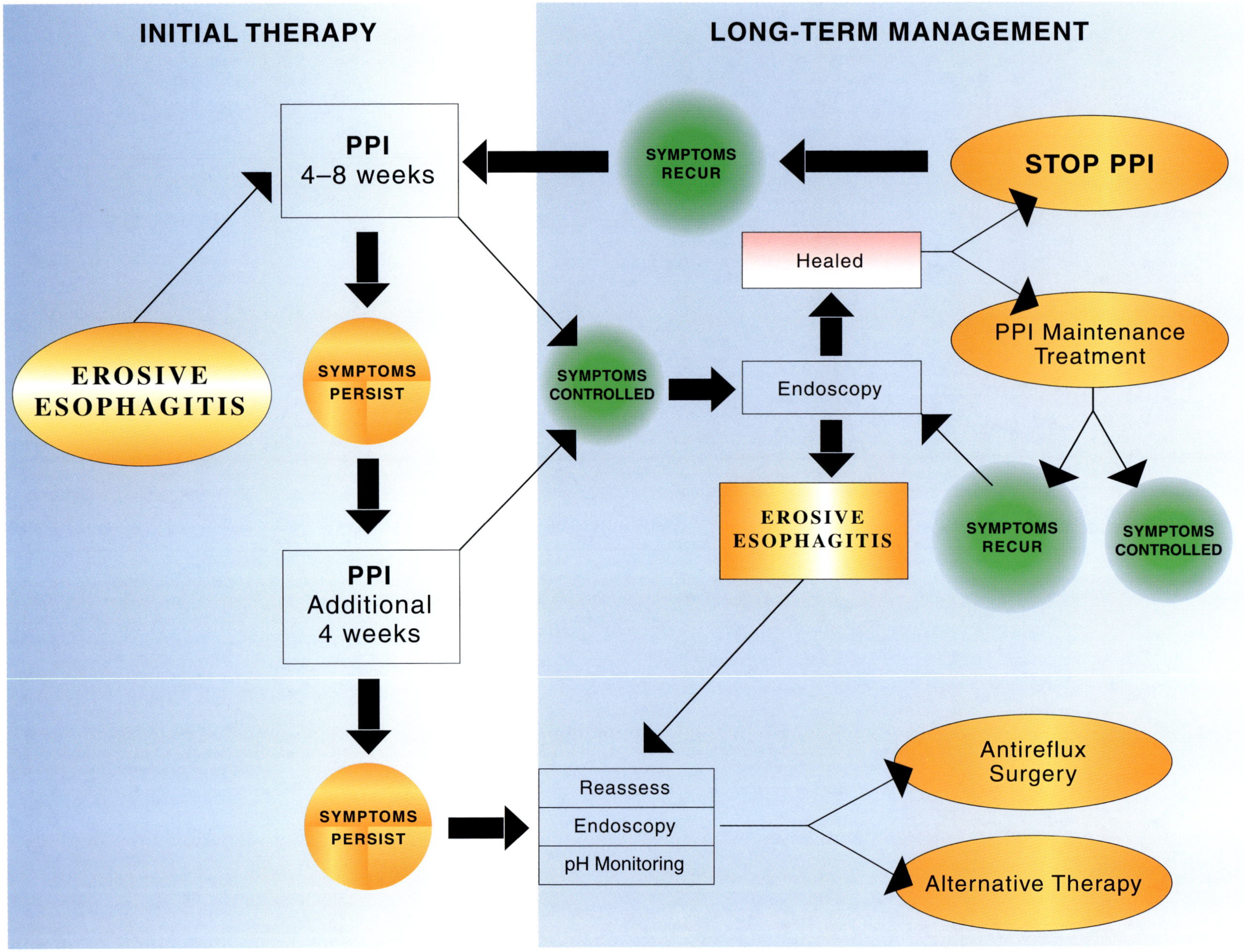

Figure 19. *— PPI therapy is the treatment recommended for patients with erosive esophagitis. Although consideration may be given to the use of antireflux surgery at any point in the algorithm, this is best reviewed after the efficacy of initial management strategies have been evaluated and with consideration to patient preference, fitness for surgery, and the level of laparoscopic expertise available. This management strategy does not factor in adjustments necessary to deal with patients noted to have Barrett's esophagus.*

unselected patients presenting with typical symptoms of reflux disease without previous therapy, the risk should not be considered as a primary determinant of whether to undertake endoscopy. Nevertheless, prompt endoscopy is probably the best clinical strategy in those who have experienced reflux symptoms at least twice a week for at least some years and who have not had previous endoscopy.

For the diagnosis of erosive reflux esophagitis, the greatest diagnostic value is obtained from an endoscopy that is undertaken before antisecretory therapy. Although treatment effect may confound an important baseline assessment of esophagitis, treatment-induced healing of esophagitis may facilitate endoscopic recognition of Barrett's esophagus. Nevertheless, endoscopy should also detect abnormalities unrelated to reflux disease that respond to acid suppression.

Principles of Initial and Long-Term Medical Therapy

Overall contemporary management decision pathways should be directed toward minimizing the use of endoscopy in the interest of both cost effectiveness and patient comfort and convenience. As the majority of people with reflux disease are *H. pylori* negative, the eradication of *H. pylori* infection does not heal or prevent reflux or relapse of reflux disease. However, when a

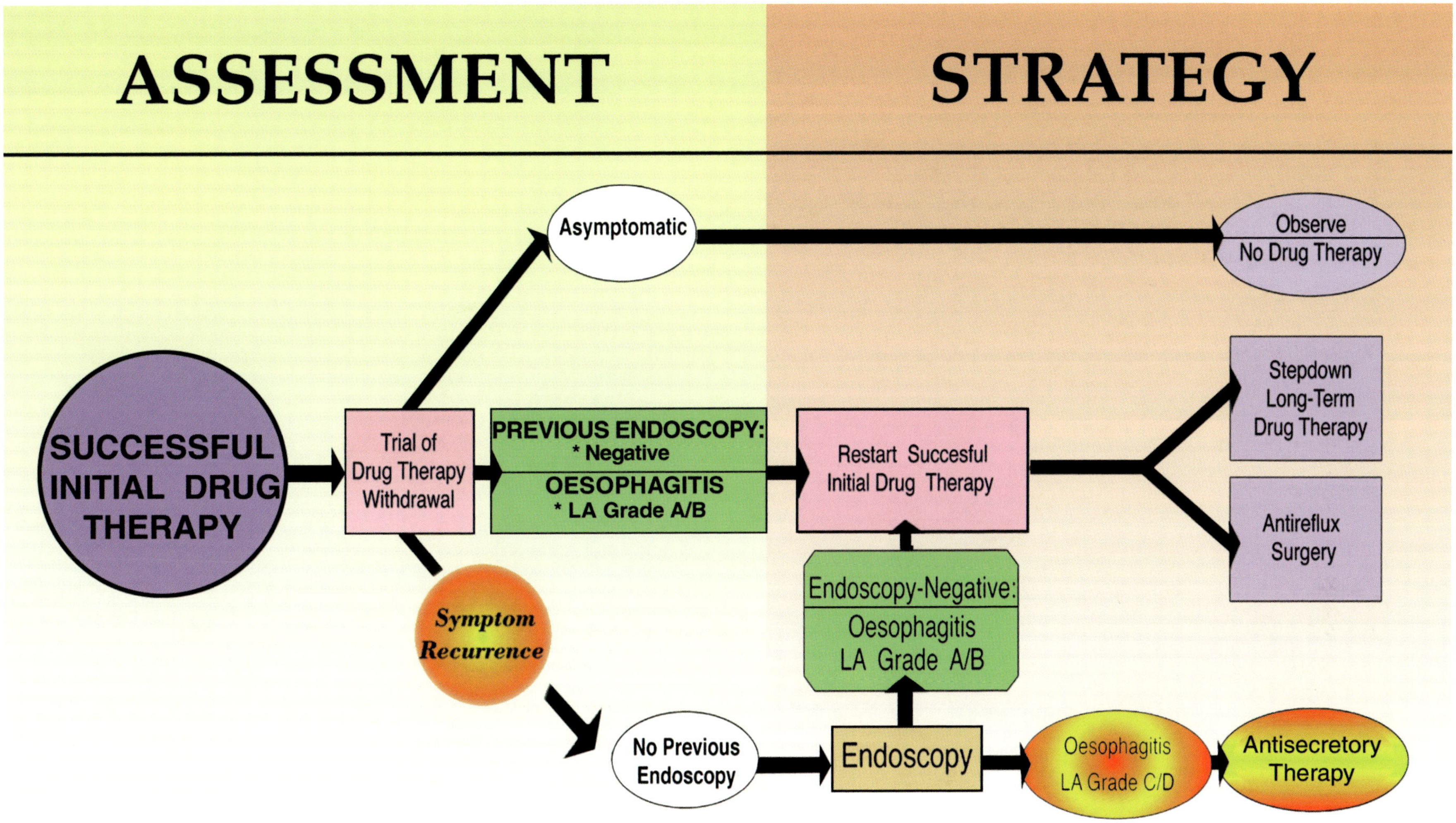

Figure 20. *— A major difficulty is the management of patients who have undergone successful initial drug therapy and thereafter develop recurrence of their symptoms. It is necessary that the recurrent nature of GERD be established before long-term therapy or antireflux surgery is considered. Although it is evident that the avoidance of certain types of food and alcoholic beverages may provide a therapeutically useful reduction in symptomatology, such patients are best managed with long-term PPI therapy. A select group may be considered as candidates for laparoscopic fundoplication surgery.*

patient with reflux disease has *H. pylori* infection, it appears that there may be a clinically relevant interaction between the two with the possibility that reflux disease is exacerbated by *H. pylori* eradication. The data on this subject are limited and contradictory.

Goals of treatment include complete healing of esophagitis and complete relief of symptoms. By and large, symptom response to PPI treatment can guide the physician in longer-term management decisions including either step-down treatment or maintenance treatment with a PPI, and considerations of diagnostic testing or of surgical intervention in selected patients.

Envoi

If medical advances made in the management of acid inhibition and the control of gastric mucosal inflammatory disease in the last 5 years are reviewed, it could be predicted that there will be significant pharmacologic advances in the medical management of GERD. With the rate of scientific and medical advance, it is probable to propose that more specific pharmacotherapeutic probes targeting the LES will become available. Mucosal healing is a subject under extensive investigation, and the development of agents capable of amplifying the healing process or altering the quality of the healed mucosa is on the horizon.

At the turn of the 20th century, Ismar Boas had just founded gastroenterology as a discipline, and Elsner had for the first time viewed the interior of the stomach with a rigid endoscope, while x-rays were regarded as novel in the study of a patient. Dyspepsia was a diagnosis of futility, as few could discern a cause, and therapy had little to offer other than chalk, herbs, and bland diets. Such was the intellectual destitution of the times that the quixotic notion of surgery as a cure for ulcer was even offered by Billroth, Moynihan, and their sanguine colleagues. One wonders what the thinkers of the time dreamt of for the future resolution of the suffering faced by their patients with "stomach problems." Certainly, there was the desire to see the pathology and define it, the need to understand the causation and address the pathogens therapeutically, and the means to intervene in the face of dramatic clinical events such as bleeding or perforation. All have come to pass as endoscopes, acid secretory regulation, and omeprazole were introduced and *H. pylori* was discovered.

Now, as we stand at the doors of the 21st century, we face an entirely different series of challenges. It is foolish to imagine that we can predict either the logical or serendipitous progress of science. Imagine the turn of the last century. Certainly, Darwin and Mendel had made their epochal discoveries, but physics was Newtonian, subatomic structure had yet to be dreamed of, the periodic table of elements was unspecified, biochemistry was nonexistent, radio and television were a dream, although the telephone and electricity and the automobile were spreading throughout civilization. We could not have predicted the advances of the first 20 years of the 20th century, or even the advances in the last 20 years, although this would appear a lesser challenge.

What might we contemplate for the dawn of the new century? The elucidation of cell growth and the pharmacologic regulation of healing? The identification of the pathogenesis of the erosive disease of the lower esophagus and the development of therapeutic probes able to reverse the damage or restore smooth muscle contractility? Endoscopes capable of optical biopsies and the application of optical coherence tomography and spectroscopy to the mucosa rather than to organs so that disease can be identified in a timely fashion?

The major revolution in the understanding and treatment of ulcer disease in the last quarter of this century was fueled by a number of events. The drivers of this late-breaking revolution were several: understanding of the regulation of acid secretion and its mechanism, improved visualization of the lesions using flexible endoscopes, advanced surgical approaches, more sophisticated pharmaceutical research, and the discovery of *H. pylori* and its implication in duodenal ulcer disease, to name but a few. Although we are still arguing about the personality of *H. pylori*, the revelations afforded by its identification have been substantial. Is it always a pathogen? Is it merely a commensal on occasion, hindering rather than helping to initiate disease?

The early part of the century should provide an answer to many current conundrums and enable the resolution of some issues presently unresolved. Although the treatment of acid-related disease has been successful, treatment of gastric or esophageal malignancies has for the most part been a failure. The development of robotic surgery with its nanometer precision coupled with imaging technology may bring a level of exactitude enabling levels of curative extirpation impossible today. Nevertheless, excision is an invasive modality, and strategic targeting of specific cellular regulatory domains will probably be more fruitful.

We await the complete human genome, with its more than 100,000 genes. From this, we will learn about — perhaps more rapidly than we can understand — the changes in gene expression in different cell types that orchestrate growth and differentiation and that diagnose the presence or predict one or more of life's many ills. A host of new therapeutic targets will be recognized, and strategies for appropriate delivery systems, as well as agents, will be developed. The number and variety of oncogenes that have been described, the various cell growth and multiplication cascades still confuse as much as they illuminate. The emergence of novel disciplines, such as proteomics and their offshoots, will amplify the possibilities in solving the puzzle of tumor generation. Once this is resolved, rational and targeted therapy of malignancies will emerge much as the understanding of bacterial growth spawned the development of entire classes of antibiotics.

Seed the mucosa with growth factors, implant stem cells, transplant the gut, infect it with organisms that prey upon pathogens, patrol it with remote controlled self-propelling video pills capable of optical biopsy: Who knows? For a new idea to be correct it must be both a dream and utterly absurd. An immortalized gastrointestinal tract, dying old while young, eternal life? Dare we anticipate these? One is reminded of the excruciatingly enantiodromic answer: "Nes. Yo."

Whose names, whose pictures will illustrate the historical part of this book 100 years from now as our descendants ponder the extraordinary vision of the long past dreams of the physicians of yesterday?

NOTE TO PRESCRIBER

PRESCRIBING CONSIDERATIONS

BIAXIN® (clarithromycin) PRESCRIBING CONSIDERATIONS: Because of the risk of potentially serious drug interactions, concomitant use of Biaxin with Propulsid® (cisapride), Orap (pimozide), or Seldane® (terfenadine) is contraindicated, and concomitant administration of Biaxin with Hismanal® (astemizole) is not recommended. Biaxin is also contraindicated in patients with a known hypersensitivity to any macrolide antibiotic.

WARNING: CLARITHROMYCIN SHOULD NOT BE USED IN PREGNANT WOMEN EXCEPT IN CLINICAL CIRCUMSTANCES WHERE NO ALTERNATIVE THERAPY IS APPROPRIATE. IF PREGNANCY OCCURS WHILE TAKING CLARITHROMYCIN, THE PATIENT SHOULD BE APPRISED OF THE POTENTIAL HAZARD TO THE FETUS. (See WARNINGS in prescribing information for Biaxin.)

Clarithromycin may elevate digoxin serum concentrations. Serum digoxin levels should be carefully monitored while digoxin and clarithromycin are taken concomitantly.

AMOXICILLIN IS CONTRAINDICATED IN PATIENTS WITH A HISTORY OF ALLERGIC REACTION TO ANY OF THE PENICILLINS.

Consult complete prescribing information for Biaxin and amoxicillin.

The most frequently reported adverse events with PRILOSEC® (omeprazole) are headache, diarrhea, and abdominal pain. The most frequently reported adverse events with combination PRILOSEC and Biaxin therapy are taste perversion, nausea, and headache. The most frequently reported adverse events using combination therapy with PRILOSEC, Biaxin, and amoxicillin are diarrhea, taste perversion, and headache.

A minority of patients may have DU recurrence after successful eradication of *H. pylori.* In patients who fail therapy, susceptibility testing should be done. If resistance to clarithromycin is demonstrated or susceptibility testing is not possible, alternative antimicrobial therapy should be instituted. Atrophic gastritis has been noted occasionally in gastric corpus biopsies from patients treated long term with omeprazole. PRILOSEC is contraindicated in patients with known hypersensitivity to any component of the formulation.

For patients on PRILOSEC receiving concomitant warfarin, phenytoin, or a benzodiazepine, please see *Drug Interactions* section of full Prescribing Information.

Before prescribing PRILOSEC, please see accompanying full Prescribing Information.